OXFORD MEDICAL PUBLICATIONS

Oxford Handbook of
Midwifery

Published and forthcoming Oxford Handbooks in Nursing

Oxford Handbook of Midwifery 2e
Janet Medforth, Susan Battersby, Maggie Evans, Beverley Marsh, and Angela Walker

Oxford Handbook of Mental Health Nursing
Edited by Patrick Callaghan and Helen Waldock

Oxford Handbook of Children's and Young People's Nursing
Edited by Edward Alan Glasper, Gillian McEwing, and Jim Richardson

Oxford Handbook of Prescribing for Nurses and Allied Health Professionals
Sue Beckwith and Penny Franklin

Oxford Handbook of Cancer Nursing
Edited by Mike Tadman and Dave Roberts

Oxford Handbook of Cardiac Nursing
Edited by Kate Johnson and Karen Rawlings-Anderson

Oxford Handbook of Primary Care Nursing
Edited by Vari Drennan and Claire Goodman

Oxford Handbook of Gastrointestinal Nursing
Edited by Christine Norton, Julia Williams, Claire Taylor, Annmarie Nunwa, and Kathy Whayman

Oxford Handbook of Respiratory Nursing
Terry Robinson and Jane Scullion

Oxford Handbook of Nursing Older People
Beverley Tabernacle, Marie Barnes, and Annette Jinks

Oxford Handbook of Clinical Skills in Adult Nursing
Jacqueline Randle, Frank Coffey, and Martyn Bradbury

Oxford Handbook of Emergency Nursing
Edited by Robert Crouch, Alan Charters, Mary Dawood, and Paula Bennett

Oxford Handbook of Dental Nursing
Kevin Seymour, Dayananda Samarawickrama, Elizabeth Boon and Rebecca Parr

Oxford Handbook of Diabetes Nursing
Lorraine Avery and Sue Beckwith

Oxford Handbook of Musculoskeletal Nursing
Edited by Susan Oliver

Oxford Handbook of Women's Health Nursing
Edited by Sunanda Gupta, Debra Holloway, and Ali Kubba

Oxford Handbook of Perioperative Practice
Suzanne Hughes and Andy Mardell

Oxford Handbook of Critical Care Nursing
Sheila Adam and Sue Osborne

Oxford Handbook of Neuroscience Nursing
Edited by Sue Woodward and Catheryne Waterhouse

Oxford Handbook of General and Adult Nursing
Ann Close and George Castledine

Oxford Handbook of Learning & Intellectual Disability Nursing
Edited by Bob Gates and Owen Barr

Oxford Handbook of
Midwifery

SECOND EDITION

Edited by

Janet Medforth

Senior Midwifery Lecturer and Lead Midwife Educator
Faculty of Health and Well Being
Sheffield Hallam University, UK

Susan Battersby

Independent Lecturer/Researcher Infant Feeding, UK

Maggie Evans

Freelance Lecturer and Consultant in Midwifery
and Complementary Therapies, UK

Beverley Marsh

Senior Midwifery Lecturer, Faculty of Health and Well
Being, Sheffield Hall University, UK

Angela Walker

Lecturer in Midwifery, Contraception and Sexual
Health and Independent/Supplementary Nurse/Midwife
Prescribing; Clinic Nurse Co-ordinator, Contraception
and Sexual Health Service, Derbyshire Community Health
Services NHS Trust, Chesterfield, UK
Previously Senior Midwifery Lecturer, The University of
Sheffield (retired)

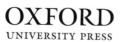

OXFORD
UNIVERSITY PRESS

OXFORD
UNIVERSITY PRESS

Great Clarendon Street, Oxford OX2 6DP.

Oxford University Press is a department of the University of Oxford.
It furthers the University's objective of excellence in research, scholarship,
and education by publishing worldwide in

Oxford New York

Auckland Cape Town Dar es Salaam Hong Kong Karachi
Kuala Lumpur Madrid Melbourne Mexico City Nairobi
New Delhi Shanghai Taipei Toronto

With offices in

Argentina Austria Brazil Chile Czech Republic France Greece
Guatemala Hungary Italy Japan Poland Portugal Singapore
South Korea Switzerland Thailand Turkey Ukraine Vietnam

Oxford is a registered trade mark of Oxford University Press
in the UK and in certain other countries

Published in the United States
by Oxford University Press Inc., New York

British Library Cataloguing in Publication Data
Data available

Library of Congress Cataloging-in-Publication-Data
Data available

Typeset by Glyph International, Bangalore, India
Printed in China
on acid-free paper through
Asia Pacific Offset

ISBN 978–0–19–958467–3

10 9 8 7 6 5 4 3 2 1

Foreword from the first edition

Midwifery is the art of the possibility. It requires insight, understanding and empathy. Above all it is about delivering the information and services, which women and their families need. In the rapidly changing field of health and social care this is no mean feat and in spite of the advances of technology and information retrieval, access to a handbook is as invaluable as ever.

I have been privileged to be involved in the development of the first *Oxford Handbook of Midwifery* and am aware of the enthusiasm, commitment and attention to detail that the authors have strived for in bringing this publication from 'conception to birth'. Throughout they have sought to provide an important, informative and evidence based tool for midwives and others working in maternity and family health services. In its construction, the handbook reflects the woman's journey through childbirth as well as the context in which maternity and midwifery care is delivered.

It is my view that the *Oxford Handbook of Midwifery* will provide an important foundation upon which current and future student midwives might begin to plan and develop their professional knowledge and practice skills. For qualified midwives, junior doctors and other healthcare professionals the handbook provides a framework and ready reference upon which they can advance their knowledge and understanding. It enables easy access to essential elements of midwifery care and will certainly help midwives more effectively structure the information and advice they give to women.

This is a welcomed addition to the midwifery literature and a resource which is likely to become part and parcel of the midwife's 'bag of tools'. I commend this work to the profession and trust that it will aid midwives and other healthcare professionals in meeting the demands and challenges of health service provision in the 21st century.

Professor Paul Lewis
Academic Head of Midwifery & Child Health
Bournemouth University

Preface

Since the first edition of the *Oxford Handbook of Midwifery* was published in 2006, maternity services and midwifery education face further challenges and developments. The structure of the health service is to undergo radical change and midwifery education is now offered at degree level in all UK universities. Influential Department of Health initiatives focus on the wider public health role of the midwife and strengthen the place of the midwife as the key organiser of care for all pregnant women, regardless of the risk factors women may face[1].

This book continues to be a handy reference guide for both Midwives and Student Midwives. It has been updated to reflect current guidelines and protocols in both obstetric and midwifery practice. New chapters are included on the impact of obesity during pregnancy and diabetes. Many chapters have been substantially revised or rewritten to reflect the changing nature of midwifery practice. There is a brand new section on sexual health with many aspects included for the first time and the contraception section provides the latest advice on new contraceptive methods.

This edition provides concise, practical and accessible content about the essential elements of midwifery practice in a pocket sized format. Chapters provide information on assessment, diagnosis, management and advice to give to the mother and family. The chapters are arranged so that the journey from pregnancy to birth and beyond can be followed easily. The page-to-a-topic format, followed through the majority of the book, means that information is easily available without the need to scan large volumes of text to find relevant principles. In the centre of the book there is a useful section on emergencies, marked by full-length blue page borders, so that it can be found quickly.

Although the book is intended for use by midwives and students it will also prove useful to others who work with women and families such as health visitors, community nurses, general practitioner trainees, childbirth educators and medical students. The book is illustrated throughout by diagrams, checklists and algorithms for key interventions.

1 Department of Health (2010). *Midwifery 2020: Delivering expectations*. London: Department of Health.

Acknowledgements

In producing a second edition of the book we are indebted to a number of people who have assisted us along the way. As authors we could not have produced the book without the excellent support of the editorial team at Oxford University Press. Anna Winstanley and Beth Womack have very patiently guided us through the process once again. Many thanks for your patience and support. Thanks also to Michael Hawkes for last minute advice and guidance.

Grateful thanks also to the Jessop Wing Maternity Unit, Sheffield Teaching Hospitals NHS Trust; for access to guidelines, evidence based protocols and care pathways.

Angela Thurlby contributed chapters on neonatal care in our first edition and has kindly reviewed and updated these; thank you Angela.

Finally, our search for illustrations and the process of gaining permission to use the work of others has proved more arduous than expected. We are therefore particularly indebted to Stella Medforth for producing such beautifully clear drawings at very short notice to illustrate the care in labour chapters.

Contents

Detailed contents

Contributor

Angela Thurlby
School of Nursing and Midwifery,
The University of Sheffield

Symbols and abbreviations

►	important
►►	very important
❶	warning
☛	note
📖	cross reference
♨	online resource/web address
ACTH	adrenocorticotropic hormone
AEDs	antiepileptic drugs
AFP	A-fetoprotein
AIDS	acquired immune deficiency syndrome
ALT	alanine transaminase
APH	antepartum haemorrhage
APT	alkaline phosphatase
ARM	artificial rupture of the membranes
AST	aspartate transaminase
B-hCG	B-human chorionic gonadotrophin
BFI	Baby Friendly Initiative
BFR	Bach flower remedy
BHIVA	British HIV Association
BMI	body mass index
BPD	biparietal diameter
bpm	beats per minute
BV	bacterial vaginosis
CAF	Common Assessment Framework
CCT	controlled cord traction
CESDI	Confidential Enquiry into Stillbirths and Deaths in Infancy
CNS	central nervous system
CPAP	continuous positive airway pressure
CPR	cardiopulmonary resuscitation
CRP	C-reactive protein
CSF	cerebrospinal fluid
CT	complementary therapy
CTG	cardiotocograph
CVP	central venous pressure
DIC	disseminated intravascular coagulation
EBM	expressed breast milk

ECG	electrocardiogram
ECV	external cephalic version
EDD	expected date of delivery
EFM	electronic fetal monitoring
eGFR	estimated glomerular filtration rate
EPAU	early pregnancy assessment unit
FBC	full blood count
FBS	fetal blood sampling
FDP	fibrin degradation product
FFP	fresh frozen plasma
FGM	female genital mutilation
FHR	fetal heart rate
FSH	follicle-stimulating hormone
G&S	group and save
G6PD	glucose 6-phosphate dehydrogenase
GBS	group B haemolytic streptococcus
GDM	gestational diabetes
GP	general practitioner
GUM	genitourinary medicine
Hb	haemoglobin
HBV	hepatitis B virus
HDN	haemolytic disease of the newborn
HDU	high-dependency unit
HFOV	high-frequency oscillation ventilation
HIV	human immunodeficiency virus
HPV	human papillomavirus
HSV	herpes simplex virus
IAP	intrapartum antibiotic prophylaxis
ICM	International Confederation of Midwives
IUD	intrauterine device
IUGR	intrauterine growth restriction
IUS	intrauterine system
IV	intravenous(ly)
IVF	*in vitro* fertilization
LAM	lactational amenorrhoea method
LCP	long-chain fatty acid
LFT	liver function test
LH	luteinizing hormone
LMP	last menstrual period
LMWH	low-molecular-weight heparin

LSA	local supervising authority
LSCS	lower segment caesarean section
MAS	meconium aspiration syndrome
MCADD	medium-chain acyl CoA dehydrogenase deficiency
mcg	micrograms
MEWS	maternity early warning scoring
MMR	measles, mumps, rubella
MRSA	meticillin-resistant *Staphylococcus aureus*
MSH	melanocyte stimulating hormone
MSU	mid-stream urine sample
NEC	necrotizing enterocolitis
NHS	National Health Service
NICU	neonatal intensive care unit
NMC	Nursing and Midwifery Council
NRT	nicotine replacement therapy
NST	non-shivering thermogenesis
NTD	neural tube defect
pCO_2	partial pressure of CO_2
PGD	patient group direction
PID	pelvic inflammatory disease
PIH	pregnancy-induced hypertension
PKU	phenylketonuria
POCT	point of care test
POP	progesterone-only pill
PPH	postpartum haemorrhage
PPROM	preterm, prelabour rupture of the membranes
PTV	patient-triggered ventilation
PV	per vagina
RBC	red blood cell
RCM	Royal College of Midwives
RCOG	Royal College of Obstetrics and Gynaecology
RDS	respiratory distress syndrome
RNI	reference nutrient intake
SCBU	special care baby unit
SIDS	sudden infant death syndrome
SIMV	synchronous intermittent ventilation
SOM	supervisor of midwives
SROM	spontaneous rupture of the membranes
STI	sexually transmitted infection
TBM	transcutaneous bilirubinometer

TEDS	thrombo-embolic deterrent stockings
TENS	transcutaneous nerve stimulation
U/E	urea and electrolytes
VBAC	vaginal birth following previous caesarean
VTE	venous thromboembolism
WHO	World Health Organization

Part 1

Introduction

Introduction

Definition of a midwife

The official definition of a midwife comes from the International Confederation of Midwives (ICM):[1]

'A midwife is a person who, having been regularly admitted to a midwifery educational programme, duly recognised in the country in which it is located, has successfully completed the prescribed course of studies in midwifery and has acquired the requisite qualifications to be registered and/or legally licensed to practise midwifery.

The midwife is recognised as a responsible and accountable professional who works in partnership with women to give the necessary support, care and advice during pregnancy, labour and the postpartum period, to conduct births on the midwife's own responsibility and to provide care for the newborn and the infant. This care includes preventative measures, the promotion of normal birth, the detection of complications in mother and child, the accessing of medical care or other appropriate assistance and the carrying out of emergency measures.

The midwife has an important task in health counselling and education, not only for the woman, but also within the family and the community. This work should involve antenatal education and preparation for parenthood and may extend to women's health, sexual or reproductive health and child care.

A midwife may practise in any setting including the home, community, hospitals, clinics or health units.'

(Adopted by the International Confederation of Midwives Council meeting, 19 July, 2005, Brisbane, Australia. It supersedes the ICM 'Definition of the Midwife' (1972) and its amendments of 1990).

This definition tells us that midwives have a very diverse role and it is one that is expanding to meet the needs of modern society.

There are a number of little known facts about what midwives do and these are just a few examples from the Association of Radical Midwives:

- The midwife is the senior professional attendant at over 75% of births in the UK.
- Midwives can give total care to mother and baby from early pregnancy onwards, throughout childbirth, and until the baby is 28 days old.
- Midwives may legally set up in practice and advertise their midwifery services, either alone or in partnerships.
- It is not necessary to be a nurse in order to become a midwife, although many practising midwives also hold nurse qualifications in addition to their midwifery registration.
- Midwives are the only professionals concerned solely with maternity care. The only other people legally allowed to deliver babies are doctors (who need not have had specialist training in this field).

---

1 International Confederation of Midwives. Core documents. Available at: ℅ www. internationalmidwives.org/Documentation/Coredocuments/tabid/322/Default.aspx (accessed 10.3.10).

Role of the midwife

The role of the midwife can be summed up in just two words: 'delivering babies'! This is the common view of the public and other professionals of what midwives do.

The Royal College of Midwives (RCM)—our professional organization—dedicated to promoting midwifery, and supporting mothers and babies by helping midwives in their professional sphere, says the following about the role of the midwife:

'A midwife does more than just deliver babies. Because she is present at every birth, she is in a position to touch everyone's life. A midwife is usually the first and main contact for the expectant mother during her pregnancy, and throughout labour and the postnatal period. She helps mothers to make informed choices about the services and options available to them by providing as much information as possible.

The role of the midwife is very diverse. She is a highly trained expert and carries out clinical examinations, provides health and parent education and supports the mother and her family throughout the childbearing process to help them adjust to their parental role.

The midwife also works in partnership with other health and social care services to meet individual mothers' needs, for example, teenage mothers, mothers who are socially excluded, disabled mothers, and mothers from diverse ethnic backgrounds.

Midwives work in all health care settings; they work in the maternity unit of a large general hospital, in smaller stand-alone maternity units, in private maternity hospitals, in group practices, at birth centres, with general practitioners, and in the community.

The majority of midwives practice within the NHS, working with other midwives in a team and other health care professional and support staff. Midwives can also practice independently and there is a small group of midwives who do so.

In any one week, a midwife could find herself teaching antenatal classes, visiting women at home, attending a birth, providing parenting education to new mothers or speaking at a conference on her specialist area. So there is more to the role than delivering babies, even though this is a very important aspect of the work of the midwife.'

In 2008 in England there were 672 807 livebirths. This is an increase of 2.7% from the previous year. In the same year there were 19 639 full-time equivalent midwives working in the National Health Service (NHS). This represents that for each of these working midwives there were 34 births, however not all working midwives offer the full range of services to women. This is because midwives fulfil many varied roles such as managerial or other specialist roles.

Principles for record keeping

Record keeping is an integral part of midwifery practice, designed to assist the care process and enhance good communication between professionals and clients. The Nursing and Midwifery Council (NMC)[1] has published guidelines for record keeping, the main recommendations of which are given below.

The principles of good record keeping apply to all types of record, regardless of how they are held. These can include:

- Handwritten clinical notes
- Emails
- Letters to and from other health professionals
- Laboratory reports
- X-rays
- Printouts from monitoring equipment
- Incident reports and statements
- Photographs
- Videos
- Tape-recordings of telephone conversations
- Text messages.
  Patient and client records should:
- Be factual, consistent, and accurate
- Be written as soon as possible after an event has occurred
- Be written clearly and so that the text cannot be erased
- Be dated accurately, timed, and signed, with the signature printed alongside the first entry
- Not include jargon, abbreviations, meaningless phrases, or offensive subjective statements
- Identify problems that have arisen and the steps taken to rectify them
- Be written with the involvement of the mother
- Provide clear evidence of the care planned, decisions made, care delivered, and information shared with the mother.
  Alterations or additions should be dated, timed, and signed so that the original entry is still clear.

Record keeping is part of the midwife's legal duty of care and should demonstrate:

- A full account of the assessment, and any care planned and provided for mother and baby
- Relevant information about the condition of the mother/baby and any measures taken in response to needs
- Evidence that all reasonable steps have been taken to care for the mother/baby and that their safety has not been compromised
- Any arrangements made for continuing care of the mother/baby.
  You need to assume that any entries you make will be scrutinized at some point. It is normal practice for mothers to carry their own records in the antenatal period and have access to their postnatal notes while under the care of the midwife.

Other members of the team involved in the care of the mother and baby will also make entries into the care record, and information about the mother and baby is shared on a need-to-know basis. The ability to obtain information while respecting the mother's confidentiality is essential.

Midwives should at all times give due regard to the way in which information systems are used, issues of access to records, and keeping their personal and professional knowledge and skills for record keeping responsibilities up to date.

It is a requirement of the NMC Midwives Rules and Standards (2004) that records are kept for at least 25 years.[2]

---

1 Nursing and Midwifery Council (2009). *Record Keeping: Guidance for Nurses and Midwives.* London: Nursing and Midwifery Council.

2 Nursing and Midwifery Council (2004). *Midwives Rules and Standards.* London: Nursing and Midwifery Council.

Statutory midwifery supervision

Statutory supervision of midwives provides a system of support and guidance for every midwife practising in the UK and is a legal requirement.[1] The purpose of supervision of midwives is to protect women and babies by:
• Promoting best practice and excellence in care
• Preventing poor practice
• Intervening in unacceptable practice.
   The practising midwife's responsibilities are to:
• Ensure the safe and effective care of mothers and babies
• Maintain fitness to practise
• Maintain registration with the NMC.
   Your responsibility in maintaining current registration with the NMC is to:
• Identify and meet the NMC requirements for PREP
• Meet at least annually with your named supervisor of midwives
• Notify your intention to practise annually to the local supervising authority (LSA) via your named supervisor of midwives (SOM)
• Have a working knowledge of how NMC publications affect your practice.[2]

1 The Nursing and Midwifery Order (2001). *Statutory Instrument 2002/253.*

2 Nursing and Midwifery Council (2008). *Modern Supervision in Action.* London: Nursing and Midwifery Council.

Role of supervisor of midwives

The potential SOM is nominated by peers and supervisors in their place of work and must undergo a selection process led by the LSA midwifery officer and university programme leader and which must include a user representative. The midwife must:

- Have credibility with the midwives she/he will potentially supervise and with senior midwifery management
- Be practising, having at least 3 years' experience, at least one of which shall have been in the 2-year period immediately preceding the appointment
- Be academically able
- Have demonstrated ongoing professional development.[1,2]

Having successfully completed the preparation programme, the midwife must then be appointed by the LSA midwifery officer as a supervisor to the LSA and to whom the SOM is responsible in that role.[2] Good communication skills and an approachable manner are essential to the role. Each supervisor is responsible for supervising a maximum of 15 midwives.

SOMs:

- Receive and process notification of intention to practise forms
- Provide guidance on maintenance of registration
- Work in partnership with mothers and midwives
- Create an environment that supports the midwife's role and empowers practice through evidence-based decision making
- Monitor standards of midwifery practice through audit of records and assessment of clinical outcomes
- Are available for midwives to discuss issues relating to their practice and provide appropriate support
- Are available to mothers to discuss any aspects of their care
- Arrange regular meetings with individual midwives at least once a year, to help them evaluate their practice and identify areas of development
- Investigate critical incidents and identify any action required
- Report to the LSA midwifery officer serious cases involving professional conduct, and when it is considered that local action has failed to achieve safe practice
- Contribute to confidential enquiries, risk management strategies, clinical audit, and clinical governance.

1 Nursing and Midwifery Council (2006). *Standards for the Preparation and Practice of Supervisors of Midwives.* London: NMC

2 Nursing and Midwifery Council (2004). *Midwives Rules and Standards: Rules 9–16.* London: NMC.

Role of the LSA and LSA midwifery officer

The LSA is a body responsible in law for ensuring that statutory supervision of midwives and midwifery practice is employed, within its boundaries, to a satisfactory standard, in order to secure appropriate care for every mother.[1]

Each LSA appoints an LSA midwifery officer to undertake the statutory function on its behalf. This must be a suitably experienced SOM,[1] who has the skills, experience, and knowledge to provide expert advice on issues such as structures for local maternity services, human resources planning, student midwife numbers, and post-registration education opportunities.

The functions of the LSA are to:
• Appoint supervisors of midwives and publish a list of current supervisors
• Ensure that every practising midwife has a named SOM
• Determine the appropriate number of supervisors to reflect local circumstances
• Receive the annual notification of intention to practise from all midwives within the LSA boundary and forward the completed forms to the NMC
• Operate a system to ensure that each midwife meets the statutory requirements for practice
• Provide continuing professional development and updating for all SOMs for a minimum of 15h in each registration period
• Ensure that systems are in place to investigate alleged suboptimal care or possible misconduct, in an impartial and sensitive manner
• Determine whether to suspend a midwife from practice
• Where appropriate, proceed to suspend a midwife from practice whom it has reported to the NMC
• Investigate and initiate legal action in cases of midwifery practice by unqualified persons.

---

1 Nursing and Midwifery Council (2004). *Midwives Rules and Standards: Rules 9–16*. London: NMC.

Drug administration in midwifery

Under the Medicines Act (1968), medicines can only be supplied and administered under the directions of a doctor. Midwives are exempt from this requirement in relation to certain specified medicines, provided they have notified their intention to practise, and the drugs are for use only within their sphere of practice. This allows midwives to supply and administer these drugs without the direction of a doctor.

Changes to the midwives exemptions list came into force on 1 June 2010; these changes will ensure appropriate and responsive care can be given to women safely as part of a midwife's normal sphere of practice, and especially during emergencies.

The medicines to which this exemption applies are as follows:
• Diclofenac
• Ergometrine maleate
• Hydrocortisone acetate
• Miconazole
• Nystatin
• Phytomenadione
• Adrenaline
• Anti-D immunoglobulin
• Cyclizine hydrochloride
• Diamorphine
• Ergometrine maleate
• Hepatitis B vaccine
• Hepatitis B immunoglobulin
• Lidocaine
• Lidocaine hydrochloride
• Morphine
• Naloxone hydrochloride
• Oxytocins, natural and synthetic
• Pethidine hydrochloride
• Phytomenadione
• Prochloperazine
• Carboprost
• Sodium chloride 0.9%
• Gelofusine®
• Haemaccel®
• Hartmann's solution.

Midwives can also supply and administer all non-prescription medicines, including all pharmacy and general sales list medicines, without a prescription. These medicines do not have to be in a patient group direction (PGD) for a midwife to be able to supply them.

Patient group directions

PGDs are detailed documents compiled by a multidisciplinary group of a local trust or hospital. They allow certain drugs to be given to particular groups of clients without a prescription to a named individual.

This arrangement is very useful as it allows the midwife to give a drug listed in the PGD to a woman without having to wait for a doctor to come and prescribe it individually. The midwife is responsible for following the instructions related to dosage and contraindications provided in the PGD.

Examples of drugs included in a PGD are:

- Dinoprostone (Prostin E2® gel) for induction of labour. 1mg or 2mg gel can be repeated after 6h. Give a lower dose if cervix is favourable
- Ranitidine 150mg tablets.

It is recommended that if a drug is on the midwives exemption list it does not need to appear in a PGD. Under medicines legislation there is no provision for 'standing orders', therefore these have no legal basis.

The NMC has published *Standards on Medicines Management* (2008)[1] which includes, dispensing, storage and transportation, administration, delegation, disposal, and management of adverse events and controlled drugs. Registered midwives must only supply and administer medicines for which they have received appropriate training.

There is clear instruction on the role of the midwife in *directly supervising student midwives during drug administration* and that only a registered midwife may administer a drug which is part of PGD arrangements. Student midwives may administer any medicines that have been prescribed by a doctor (including controlled drugs), or those on the midwives exemptions list (with the exception of controlled drugs).

Further reading

Medicines for Human Use (Miscellaneous amendments) Order 2010. Available at: ℘ www.opsi. gov.uk/si/si2010/uksi_20101136_en_1 (accessed 17.6.10).

Department of Health (2010). CNO letter to SHA Directors of Nursing implementation of Medicines for Human Use (Miscellaneous Amendments) Order 2010 Midwives Exemption List. Available at: ℘ www.dh.gov.uk/prod_consum_dh/groups/dh_digitalassets/documents/ digitalasset/dh_116516.pdf (accessed 17.6.10).

Nursing and Midwifery Council (2009). Supply and/or Administration of Medicine By Student Nurses and Student Midwives in Relation to Patient Group Directions (PGDs). Circular 5/2009. London: NMC.

1 Nursing and Midwifery Council (2008). *Standards for Medicines Management.* London: NMC.

Pre-conception care

Taking a menstrual history

Important points to remember
- A menstrual history is usually undertaken as part of the initial booking interview, ensuring privacy for the discussion.
- Allow sufficient time for discussion.
- Find out whether the woman has been keeping a recent diary record of her menstrual pattern or knows her normal menstrual cycle—the number of days between the first day of one menstrual period and the next.
- Find out what form of contraception, if any, she has been using—most hormonal methods will influence the menstrual pattern and may take several months to return to normal after discontinuation.
- An accurate menstrual history is essential to calculate the expected birth date, or expected date of delivery (EDD), as accurately as possible. This is a particularly important consideration where ultrasound examination to determine dates is not available or the woman makes an informed choice to decline this procedure.
- An accurate calculation of the expected birth date, as near to the beginning of pregnancy as possible, will subsequently allow you to calculate gestational age accurately at any point in the pregnancy and assess fetal growth.
- Abdominal assessment of uterine growth at each antenatal visit takes into account the estimated gestational age calculated from the expected birth date.
- It is important that the woman understands that her baby may be born anywhere between the beginning of the 38th week and the end of the 42nd week and be at term. The calculated expected birth date is only 1 day within that time frame.

Calculation of expected birth date
- Conventionally undertaken using Naegele's rule, which calculates the duration of pregnancy as 280 days.
- Nine calendar months and 7 days are added to the first day of the last menstrual period (LMP).
- Research by Nguyen et al.[1] into the accuracy of this method of calculation, compared with that of ultrasound measurement of fetal biparietal diameter (BPD), recommended that dating is more accurate by adding 282 days to the LMP.

Naegele's rule
- To the first day of the LMP add 9 months and 7 days.
- Or subtract 3 months and add 7 days (not forgetting to add a year!).
- To be more accurate, as discussed above, add 9 days instead of 7.
- If available, use an obstetric calendar, but add an additional 2 days.
- Naegele's rule assumes a 28-day menstrual cycle.

- Ovulation occurs 14 days before menstruation; in a 28-day cycle that is day 14.
- If the woman's normal menstrual cycle is shorter or longer than this, you will need to add or subtract days accordingly. Calculate according to Naegele's rule above, then add or subtract the required days.

Examples

- For a regular 25-day cycle, subtract 3 days from the calculated expected birth date.
- For a regular 35-day cycle add 7 days to the calculated expected birth date.
- For an irregular cycle that has no definite pattern it is advisable to send a woman for an early dating scan, before 12 weeks of pregnancy, if this service is available; or do your best to calculate and use other clinical signs and symptoms of early pregnancy to help you.
- Remember that a woman may be quite clear that she knows exactly when she conceived. Use this information as part of your judgement.

When calculation is difficult

- The woman does not know the date of her LMP.
- Cycles are irregular.
- A normal cycle has not resumed since she stopped using hormonal contraception:
    - Combined oral contraception, 'the pill', may confuse withdrawal bleeding with a normal period; anovular cycles may lead to inaccuracy in calculation of expected birth date.
    - Cerazette® progesterone-only pill may have the same effect—it is designed to inhibit ovulation, unlike other progesterone-only pills.
    - After Depo-Provera® injections it may take several months before menstrual bleeding and ovulation return; anovular cycles may lead to inaccuracy in calculating the expected birth date.
    - After the removal of the Mirena® intrauterine system or an Implanon® or Nexplanon® implant, the woman's hormonal levels return to normal with 72h of removal and will not inhibit early conception.
    - A copper intrauterine device does not affect the woman's hormonal levels.

1 Nguyen T, Larsen T, Enghollm G, et al. (1999). Evaluation of ultrasound-estimated date of delivery in 17,450 spontaneous singleton births: do we need to modify Naegele's rule? *Ultrasound in Obstetrics and Gynaecology* **14**(1), 223–8.

Nutrition

For women of childbearing age, the estimated average requirement (EAR) for energy is approximately 2000kcal/day. A healthy diet contains a variety of foods including protein and starchy carbohydrates such as bread, breakfast cereals, potatoes, pasta, rice, and a daily helping of at least five fruits or vegetables. Foods containing excess fat should be used sparingly and foods containing sugar should be eaten infrequently, in small amounts. (📖 See also Chapter 4.)

Good nutrition is an essential requirement to a successful outcome of pregnancy. In the ideal situation, the woman will have good body stores of the vitamins and minerals the embryo requires in order to develop into a healthy fetus. Poor nutritional status can cause problems with fertility and conception, and the extremes of body weight, e.g. being underweight or very overweight, are associated with adverse pregnancy outcomes, such as low birthweight, or developing complications of pregnancy such as high blood pressure, gestational diabetes, and preterm labour. Women in these categories are advised take steps to modify their body weight towards the normal range in preparation for pregnancy.

Other categories of women who may be in need of nutritional counselling include:

- Those with **closely spaced pregnancies**. If the gap between births is only about 1 year, there is an increased risk of the next baby being born prematurely and/or of low birthweight. Two or three years between births allows the repletion of body stores. Until then, vitamin and/or mineral supplements may be appropriate.

- **Vegans/vegetarians**. These diets can be extremely healthy; however, if meat or fish or dairy foods are avoided, essential nutrients must be replaced from other food sources, such as cereals and pulses, nuts, and seeds. Yeast extracts, such as Marmite®, are fortified with vitamin B_{12}.

- **Adolescents**. A main influence on pregnancy outcome is the number of years between the menarche and pregnancy: the shorter this interval, the greater the potential for nutritional deficiencies. Nutritional deficiencies are also more likely during pregnancy as adolescents need enough nutrients to complete their own growth as well as to fulfil the demands of a growing baby.

- Those with **a low income**. Several surveys have shown that women tend to 'go without' food themselves in order to ensure that other members of their family get enough to eat.[1]

- Those with **a pre-existing disease**, e.g. diabetes and epilepsy. Food allergies should always be diagnosed medically, and malabsorption syndromes, such as Crohn's disease, ulcerative colitis, or cystic fibrosis, require dietetic consultation.

- Those with *eating disorders*—anorexia nervosa, bulimia nervosa, or binge eating.
- *Immigrants/ethnic minorities.* Vegetarianism and fasting are common practices in those of Asian origin. Their diets are often low in calcium, with a low intake of dairy foods and a higher intake of wholewheat cereals, which are high in phytate, an inhibitor of calcium absorption. Because many Asian women cover their head and body, they do not manufacture much vitamin D in their skin, so may require a supplement of 10micrograms/day.

1 Northwest Community Hospital (1995). *Going Hungry: The Struggle to Eat on a Low Income.* Available at: ℘ www.nch.org/uploads/documents/going-hungry.pdf (accessed 20.3.10).

Lifestyle

Changes in lifestyle

A person's lifestyle can impact on their health and well-being and a healthy lifestyle is the ideal for everyone. It is even more appropriate during pregnancy to consider the impact of lifestyle choices. Couples who are planning a pregnancy may seek advice prior to conception.

The aim of pre-conception care is to prepare the body for a successful pregnancy. This preparation should take place at least 3–4 months prior to conception. The following lifestyle changes may be suggested:

- Advise the woman and her partner to give up smoking, as women who smoke reduce their chance of a successful pregnancy by 40% compared with non-smokers. Smoking reduces sperm motility and can lead to higher numbers of abnormal sperm. Offer referral to a smoking cessation programme (NHS smoking helpline is 0800 169 0169).
- Advise a reduction or elimination of alcohol from the diet. Women who drink more than 10 units per week have a reduced chance of successful pregnancy and increased risk of miscarriage compared with women who drink fewer than 5 units per week. Excess alcohol consumption by the mother is associated with fetal alcohol syndrome.
- Advise the woman to avoid using illegal drugs and if she is taking prescribed medications to ask for her general practitioner's (GP's) advice.
- Some occupations may reduce male and female fertility. Exposure to heat, X-rays, chemical pesticides, or solvents may contribute to reduced fertility. Advise avoiding such exposure as far a possible.
- If the man or woman is obese, advise weight reduction prior to pregnancy as excessive weight reduces fertility in both men and women, and the woman is at a greater risk of pregnancy and delivery complications.

Medical considerations

- The woman can be offered a blood test to determine her rubella immune status and offered vaccination 3 months prior to pregnancy if she is not immune. The vaccination can also be offered after the birth although there is no indication that the vaccine is teratogenic.
- Perform a full blood count to screen for anaemia, which can be corrected prior to pregnancy.
- Measure blood pressure to screen for hypertension.
- Perform a cervical smear test if more than 5 years have elapsed since her last test.
- Test a urine sample for the presence of protein (indicator of renal disease or infection) and glucose (indicator of diabetes).
- Offer the couple screening for genital infection as many of these are asymptomatic.

Medical conditions

Certain medical conditions may complicate pregnancy, and women who have these should be referred to their GP before embarking on a pregnancy so that any concerns can be addressed, medications reviewed, and treatment adjusted to enable a successful pregnancy to be achieved.

Type 1 diabetes

- Diabetes can have serious consequences for the mother and fetus, and the severity of the problems is linked directly to the degree of the disease and the mother's blood glucose control.
- High blood glucose levels prior to and around the time of conception increase the risk of fetal abnormality and intrauterine death in macrosomic babies.
- Advise the mother to aim to keep her blood glucose within the range of 6–8mmol/L before she conceives and during the pregnancy.
- Fetal macrosomia results from high blood glucose in the mother and increased insulin levels in the fetus. This promotes excessive growth of the fetus and can lead to delivery problems (shoulder dystocia) and early problems for the newborn, such as respiratory difficulties and hyperglycaemia.

Hypertension

- Pre-existing hypertension can cause problems in the mother and fetus during pregnancy.
- Hypertension can lead to placental complications, slow growth of the fetus, and renal complications in the mother.
- Pregnancy-induced hypertension can occur alongside existing hypertension, requiring earlier intervention or antenatal admission.
- Women with hypertension need to continue taking antihypertensive medication and may need to switch to a safer drug during pregnancy.

Epilepsy

- Advise women with epilepsy to seek advice prior to becoming pregnant so that their anti-epileptic drugs can be adjusted, if necessary. This is because there is a threefold increase of congenital malformations in babies of women with epilepsy.
- Anti-epileptic drugs are known to cause folic acid deficiency. Therefore, women with epilepsy should take folic acid supplements pre-conceptually and during the first 12 weeks of pregnancy. They will require a higher dose than normal, 5mg/day.

Infections

- Pre-conception screening for rubella antibodies gives those women who are unprotected the opportunity to be vaccinated prior to pregnancy. After the rubella vaccine is given, pregnancy should be avoided for 3 months.
- Hepatitis B vaccine and a tetanus booster should also be available.
- Sexually transmitted diseases such as herpes, genital warts, and chlamydiosis can be screened for, and treated, prior to pregnancy.

Sexual health

Bacterial vaginosis

- Bacterial vaginosis (BV) is the most common cause of vaginal discharge in women of childbearing age.
- It is caused when the normal lactobacilli of the vaginal flora are replaced with anaerobic flora such as *Gardnerella vaginalis*.
- It often co-exists with other sexually transmitted infections (STIs), but may occur spontaneously, often repeatedly, in both sexually active and non-sexually active women.
- It is often diagnosed in an asymptomatic form, by the detection of 'clue cells' when analysing a high vaginal swab taken for an STI screen.
- Commonly, women report it to be more of a problem in the perimenstrual period.
- It is more common in black women than white, those with an intrauterine device (IUD) and women with pelvic inflammatory disease (PID).
- In those who have undergone termination of pregnancy it may cause post-termination endometritis.
- On examination the vaginal mucosa is not inflamed.
- The main symptom is a malodorous, greyish watery discharge, although 50% of women are asymptomatic. In practice, it is not usually treated unless there are symptoms.
- The 'fishy' odour is characteristic and more pronounced following sexual intercourse, due to the alkaline semen.
- About one-third of women with active BV may also have vulval irritation.
- Treatment is usually metronidazole 2g stat or alternatively a course of clindamycin may be given.
- All these treatments have been shown to be 70–80% effective in controlled trials, however, recurrence of infection is common.
- While undergoing treatment the woman should avoid drinking alcohol for the duration of the treatment and for the next 48h, as it may cause nausea and vomiting.
- She should also abstain from sexual intercourse for the duration of the treatment and the next 7 days.
- In order to preserve vaginal acidity the woman should be advised to avoid use of shower gel in the vulval area or of bath foam, antiseptic agents, or shampoo in the bath. Similarly, she should avoid vaginal douching.

BV in pregnancy

- About 20% of pregnant women have BV in pregnancy, with the majority being asymptomatic.
- There is substantial evidence that BV is associated with preterm rupture of the membranes, preterm labour, and birth.
- Other evidence suggests an association with late spontaneous abortion, intra-amniotic infection, and postnatal endometritis.

- It is recommended that women with a history of repeat second trimester miscarriage or preterm birth be screened for BV.
- The manufacturers of the treatment recommend caution in pregnancy, but only against high doses and there is no evidence of teratogenic effects.

Fetal and neonatal infection
- There is no evidence of direct fetal or neonatal infection.
- Care should be taken when prescribing treatment while breastfeeding.

Candidiasis

- The causative organism is usually *Candida albicans*, normally a commensal organism found in the flora of the mouth, gastrointestinal tract, and vagina, which under certain circumstances become pathogenic and can cause symptoms.
- It may be sexually transmitted, but most cases occur spontaneously. Colonization from the lower intestinal tract is common.
- Culture from a high vaginal swab is currently the best method of diagnosis for vulval vaginal infection. Similarly, a mouth/throat swab should be taken for oral infection.
- The condition is not usually treated unless the woman is symptomatic, which is indicated by a thick, white, discharge and vaginal and vulval irritation.
- There is no need to treat the partner unless he is symptomatic.
- Common in diabetes mellitus, due to increased glycogen levels in uncontrolled diabetes.
- Found more commonly in the luteal phase of the menstrual cycle.
- There is no evidence that women using the combined oral contraceptive have an increased incidence of colonization. Other contraceptives, such as diaphragms and caps, may carry the infection and cause reinfection, if not cleaned and stored properly.
- Impaired immunity, such as that found with human immunodeficiency virus (HIV) infection, will increase the incidence.
- Broad spectrum antibiotics increase yeast carriage by 10–30%.
- Vaginal deodorants, disinfectants, perfumed shower, and bath gels may exacerbate the problem by increasing irritation and vulval excoriation and dermatitis.
- Washing and wiping the vulval area should always be from front to back.
- The wearing of tight, synthetic clothing should be avoided.
- Application of plain yoghurt may soothe the irritation in the short term, but has not been shown to be effective as treatment. Daily oral ingestion of 8oz of active yoghurt has been shown to decrease incidence of candidal colonization and infection, but this has not been replicated in other studies.

Candidiasis in pregnancy

- Vaginal candidiasis is the most common cause of troublesome vaginal discharge and vulval irritation in pregnancy.
- It occurs 2–10 times more frequently in pregnant than in non-pregnant women and is more difficult to eradicate.
- The problems are worst in the third trimester, with over 50% having a significant colonization due to increasing vaginal glycogen and the changing pH of the vagina in pregnancy.
- A Cochrane review of topical treatments for vaginal candidiasis[1] concluded that topical imidazole drugs are more effective than clotrimazole and that treatment over 7 days is more effective than single dose or 3–4-day treatment.

Fetal and neonatal infection

- The baby may become colonized from an infected birth canal, but is more likely to become infected from poor hand washing hygiene by those caring for or handling the baby, including visitors, or inadequately sterilized or contaminated feeding bottles.
- A breastfeeding baby may become infected from a sore nipple that becomes infected.

1 Young GL, Jewell D (2001). Topical treatment for vaginal candidiasis in pregnancy. (Cochrane review). In: *Cochrane Library*, Issue 3. Oxford: Update Software.

Chlamydia

- *Chlamydia trachomatis* is the most common cause of bacterial STI in the UK, affecting both men and women, and a leading cause of PID.
- Prevalence is highest, but not exclusive, in young sexually active adults, especially those under 25, hence the introduction of the current National Chlamydia Screening Programme in England for the 16–25-year age group.
- 80% of women and 50% of men have no symptoms and, left untreated, chlamydia can, in women, lead to infertility, ectopic pregnancy, and chronic pelvic pain. In men it may cause urethritis and epididymitis. In both sexes it can cause arthritis—Reiter's syndrome.
- In the symptomatic woman it may cause mucopurulent cervicitis, postcoital and/or intermenstrual bleeding.
- Because of the prevalence of chlamydia in the sexually active population and lack of symptoms, **it is good midwifery practice to routinely offer a chlamydia screening test**, using a 'first catch' urine sample, both at the beginning of pregnancy and again by 36 weeks, to detect and treat affected women. The newer nucleic acid amplification test (NAAT) is 95% sensitive.
- Alternatively, an endocervical swab can be taken.
- It is also good practice to screen the male partner(s) and to refer both partners to the local sexual health service for further STI screening, contact tracing, and follow-up.
- Antibiotic treatment in pregnancy is usually with a course of erythromycin 500mg twice daily for 14 days, but exact treatment will be decided by the doctor or nurse with prescribing rights. Azithromycin should be used with caution in pregnancy and breastfeeding.[1]

Chlamydia in pregnancy

- In the pregnant woman the increased vascularity of the cervix may lead to postcoital or irregular spotting or bleeding per vaginam and any woman with such bleeding should be screened for chlamydia.
- Chlamydia in pregnancy can cause amnionitis and postnatal endometritis.
- The evidence on its role in spontaneous abortion, preterm rupture of the membranes, preterm birth and neonatal death is unclear from studies to date.

Fetal and neonatal infection

- Although there is some evidence that intrauterine infection can occur, the major risk to the baby is during vaginal birth through an infected cervix.
- Up to 70% of babies born to mothers with untreated chlamydia will become infected: 30–40% will develop chlamydial conjunctivitis and 10–20% a characteristic pneumonia.
- Chlamydial ophthalmia neonatorum is a notifiable infection.
- Chlamydial ophthalmia neonatorum is now much more common than gonococcal ophthalmia, although in practice the two may occur together; 50% of those with gonococcal ophthalmia also have chlamydia.

- Chlamydial ophthalmia has an incubation period of 10–14 days, much longer than gonococcal ophthalmia, which is evident in about 48h.
- **It can permanently affect vision and can even cause blindness.**
- The orbit of the eye is swollen and there is a mucoid discharge, often known as a 'sticky eye'.
- The midwife must take swabs from both eyes, for chlamydia, gonococcal infection and general culture and sensitivity, and ensure they are immediately transported to the laboratory.
- After taking the swab, the eyes are regularly cleansed with normal saline.
- Inform the paediatrician, or GP in the community, and ensure the baby is examined and treated as a matter of urgency.
- The nasopharynx is also likely to be infected, which may lead to pneumonia unless promptly treated with systemic antibiotics.
- It is important to diagnose and treat any baby with chlamydial infection.
- It is thought that the baby who is affected by chlamydia pneumonia is more likely to develop obstructive lung disease and asthma than those with pneumonia from other causes.
- It may be up to 7 months before chlamydia infection becomes apparent and cultures from the pharynx, middle ear, vagina, and rectum of the baby are positive.
- Knowledge about the prevalence in the community and the effects on both mother and baby should encourage the midwife to take a sexual health history, be proactive in chlamydia testing and offer routine testing to all pregnant women in her care.

Useful websites

British Association for Sexual Health and HIV. Available at: ✍ www.bashh.org.uk.

Chlamydia. Available at: ✍ www.healthcarea2z.org/ditem_print.aspx/315/Chlamydia (accessed 2.5.10).

National Chlamydia Screening Programme. Available at: ✍ www.chlamydiascreening.nhs.uk/ps/index.html.

Neonatal Conjunctivitis and Pneumonia due to C. trachomatis. Available at: ✍ www.chlamydiae.com/restricted/docs/infections/ophth_neonat.asp (accessed 2.5.10).

Further reading

Brocklehurst P, Rooney G (2009). Interventions for treating genital chlamydia trachomatis infection in pregnancy. *Cochrane Database of Systematic Reviews* **4**, CD000054.

Dapaah S, Dapaah V (2009). Sexually transmissible and reproductive tract infections in pregnancy. In: Fraser D, Cooper M (eds) *Myles Textbook for Midwives*. 15th edn. London: Churchill Livingstone, pp. 415–32.

1 *British National Formulary* (2010). Available at: ✍ www.bnf.org (accessed 2.5.10).

Genital warts

- Genital warts are caused by the human papilloma virus, types 6 and 11.
- Sexual transmission is the most usual mode of infection.
- The incidence of genital warts diagnosed has steadily been rising over the past 10 years and the highest rates are seen in the female 16–24-year age group.
- They are not only uncomfortable, but also psychologically distressing.
- They are difficult and time-consuming to treat and may reoccur months or years later.
- Refer a woman who has genital warts to a specialist sexual health clinic for treatment and further investigation for other STIs.
- A colposcopy may be performed to exclude warts on the cervix.
- Although most genital warts are benign, it is important that an annual liquid-based cytology screen is recommended, as human papillomavirus (HPV) types 16, 18, 31, 33, and 35 are strongly associated with development of cervical cancer.
- The midwife has an important role in sexual health promotion, encouraging safer sex and promoting participation in the cervical screening programme, particularly if the woman is over 25 and not yet had her first screening test.

Genital warts in pregnancy

- Genital warts are caused by HPV.
- In pregnancy the warts may increase considerably in size and have a cauliflower-like appearance.
- Occasionally they are so large and widespread that they may obstruct the vulva and lower vagina and prevent a vaginal birth, therefore requiring a caesarean section.
- The normal treatment is drug contraindicated in pregnancy, because of possible teratogenic effects, therefore pharmacological treatment is not given until after the birth.
- Cryo-cautery is the only treatment possible during pregnancy, done at a specialist sexual health clinic.

Fetal and neonatal infection

- Babies and young children may develop laryngeal papilloma after being infected by maternal genital warts during vaginal birth.

Useful websites

British Association for Sexual Health and HIV. Available at: ℗ www.bashh.org.uk. (accessed 2.5.10)

Further reading

Dapaah S, Dapaah V (2009). Sexually transmissible and reproductive tract infections in pregnancy. In: Fraser D, Cooper M (eds) *Myles Textbook for Midwives*. 15th edn. London: Churchill Livingstone, pp. 415–32.

Gonorrhoea

- Gonorrhoea is the second most common STI in the UK.
- Prevalence is highest among sexually active adults under 25 years.
- It is a bacterial infection, caused by *Neisseria gonorrhoeae*.
- The organism adheres to mucous membranes and is more prevalent on columnar rather than squamous epithelium.
- The primary sites of infection are the mucus membranes of the urethra, endocervix, rectum, pharynx, and conjunctiva.
- Importantly, gonorrhoea frequently co-exists with other genital mucosal infections, such as those caused by *Chlamydia trachomatis*, *Trichomonas vaginalis*, and *Candida albicans*.
- Many areas are now also testing for gonorrhoea on the Chlamydia Screening Programme urine samples, because of the prevalence of co-infection. Be aware of the testing procedures in your own area.
- Up to 80% of PID in women under 26 is caused by gonorrhoea or chlamydia or both.
- The consequences of untreated gonorrhoea leading to PID include infertility, ectopic pregnancy, and chronic pelvic pain. Although uncommon, it may also cause disseminated general disease and arthritis—Reiter's syndrome.
- 50% of women may be asymptomatic.
- The most common symptom is increased or altered vaginal discharge (penile discharge in men).
- Other symptoms include lower abdominal pain, dysuria, dyspareunia, intermenstrual uterine bleeding, and menorrhagia.
- It is also good practice to screen the male partner(s) and to refer both partners to the local sexual health service for further STI screening, contact tracing, and follow-up.

Gonorrhoea in pregnancy

- The incidence of 1–5% is small, but the incidence of gonorrhoea nationally is rising, particularly in big cities. Midwives must, therefore, be vigilant, as there is evidence that it is detrimental in pregnancy.
- Gonorrhoea is associated with spontaneous abortion, chorioamnionitis, preterm rupture of the membranes, preterm labour, and very low birthweight. Postnatally, it can cause endometritis and pelvic sepsis, which may be severe.
- A Cochrane systematic review of interventions for treating gonorrhoea in pregnancy has concluded that the well-established treatment with penicillin and probenecid is effective.[1] However, antibiotic resistant strains are now becoming apparent and making treatment more difficult.

Fetal and neonatal infection

- The most common mode of transmission to the baby is through the infected cervix during vaginal birth.
- It may also be transmitted in utero, following prolonged rupture of the membranes.
- The risk of vertical transmission from an infected mother is 30–50%.

- The most usual manifestation of neonatal infection is gonococcal ophthalmia neonatorum.
- A profuse, purulent discharge from red and swollen eyes appears usually within 48h of birth.
- **It can permanently affect vision and can even cause blindness**, through corneal ulceration and perforation.
- The midwife must take swabs from both eyes, for gonococcal infection and general culture and sensitivity, and ensure they are immediately transported to the laboratory. The swabs are normally specially designated, containing a transport medium to keep the gonococcus alive until it reaches the laboratory.
- After taking the swab, the eyes are regularly cleansed with normal saline.
- Inform the paediatrician, or GP in the community, and ensure the baby is examined and treated with systemic antibiotics as a matter of urgency.
- The mother and her sexual partner(s) must be screened for infection and treated.

Useful websites

British Association for Sexual Health and HIV. Available at: ✍ www.bashh.org.uk.

Jatia KK (2009). *Neonatal Conjunctivitis*. Available at: ✍ http://emedicine.medscape.com/article/1192190-overview (accessed 2.5.10).

Further reading

Dapaah S, Dapaah V (2009). Sexually transmissible and reproductive tract infections in pregnancy. In: Fraser D, Cooper M (eds) *Myles Textbook for Midwives*. 15th edn. London: Churchill Livingstone, pp. 415–32.

1 Brocklehurst P (2001). Interventions for treating gonorrhoea in pregnancy (Cochrane review). In: *The Cochrane Library*, Issue 3. Oxford: Update Software,

Hepatitis B

- The hepatitis B virus (HBV) is the most commonly transmitted blood-borne virus worldwide and a major public health problem.
- It is an important cause of both mortality and morbidity from acute infection and chronic long-term sequelae, including cirrhosis of the liver and primary liver cancer.
- The virus can be transmitted both sexually and parenterally through infected blood and blood products.
- Other body fluids, such as saliva, menstruation, and vaginal discharge, seminal fluid, breast milk, and serous exudates have been implicated, but infection via these routes is far less common.
- Unsterilized equipment, such as that associated with injecting drug users sharing equipment, tattooing, and acupuncture is a source of infection.
- Importantly, healthcare workers may be infected through needlestick injury and must follow local policy for reporting such injuries and subsequent testing. In the UK, all healthcare workers at any risk are required to be immunized against HBV.
- Although the initial acute phase is characterized by a flu-like illness, followed by a phase characterized by jaundice, loss of appetite, nausea and fatigue, it may be asymptomatic in 10–50%.
- In chronic infection there are often no physical signs or symptoms, but there may be signs of chronic liver disease.
- The midwife has an important health promotion role, in careful history taking, detecting risk factors, giving evidence-based information and encouraging women to participate in antenatal HBV testing.

Hepatitis B in pregnancy

- If a woman is a carrier of HBV, she has an 85% risk of transmission of the virus to her infant.
- Acute HBV infection occurring during pregnancy is associated with an increased risk of spontaneous abortion and preterm labour and birth.
- The objective of offering HBV screening to pregnant women, and immunization of babies born to infected mothers, is to reduce the perinatal transmission of this infection.
- All women are offered screening for HBV during early pregnancy.

Fetal and neonatal infection

- If the mother tests positive for HBV, her baby will be vaccinated shortly after birth.
- Obtain consent for the baby's immunization prior to birth, and give the first dose as early as possible, but always within 24h.
- If the mother became infected during pregnancy or does not have the HBe antibodies, the baby should receive hepatitis B-specific immunoglobulin (HB1g) at birth, injected at a different site to the vaccine. This will give immediate immunity and reduces vertical transmission by 90%.
- Encourage and support breastfeeding, as there is no additional risk of virus transmission to the baby.

- Further doses of the vaccine should be given at 1 month and 6 months of age, and a booster dose at 12 months.
- Give the mother and the GP written information about the number of injections the baby requires, when the injections should be given, and who will be responsible for the administration of each dose.
- Stress the importance of completing the full course of immunization.
- In almost all cases of babies and children being infected it is almost always asymptomatic.

Useful website

British Association for Sexual Health and HIV. Available at: www.bashh.org.uk.

Further reading

Dapaah S, Dapaah V (2009). Sexually transmissible and reproductive tract infections in pregnancy. In: Fraser D, Cooper M (eds) *Myles Textbook for Midwives*. 15th edn. London: Churchill Livingstone, pp. 415–432.

Hepatitis C

- The hepatitis C virus occurs throughout the world and is mainly transmitted by infected blood, blood products and inoculation through the skin.
- With screening of all blood donors in the UK for the past 20 years, the incidence of transmission via infected blood and blood products is virtually nil, however this may not be true elsewhere.
- In intravenous drug users the infection rate is over 60%, by contamination from sharing needles and syringes.
- Sexual transmission rates are very low.
- The midwife has an important health promotion role in encouraging positive sexual health.

Hepatitis C in pregnancy

- Careful sexual health and intravenous drug taking history will indicate possible risk factors for infection.
- As with all other blood borne viruses it is important to follow universal safe precautions when handling blood and body fluids, to avoid possible health care worker infection.
- Find out what special precautions and handling of blood and body fluids are to be taken locally for a person known to be hepatitis C positive.
- The vertical transmission rate is 5% or less, but may be increased in a mother who is also HIV positive.
- Currently, there is no way of preventing vertical transmission, but avoiding unnecessary procedures, such as rupturing the membranes or applying a fetal scalp electrode will help.

Fetal and neonatal infection

- Encourage and support breastfeeding, as there is no evidence that breastfeeding increases the risk of transmission, unless the mother is symptomatic and has a high viral load.
- Encourage high standards of personal hygiene in the mother and the importance of hand washing when handling her baby.

Useful website

British Association for Sexual Health and HIV. Available at: ✆ www.bashh.org.uk.

Further reading

Dapaah S, Dapaah V (2009). Sexually transmissible and reproductive tract infections in pregnancy. In: Fraser D, Cooper M (eds) *Myles Textbook for Midwives*. 15th edn. London: Churchill Livingstone, pp. 415–432.

Herpes simplex virus

- There are two types of the herpes simplex virus (HSV).
- HSV1 is usually acquired in childhood or as a young adult coming into contact with infected oral secretions and causes 'cold sores'.
- HSV2 is sexually transmitted and the most common cause of genital herpes.
- Once acquired, HSV remains in the body for life and will cause frequent infection.
- The chance of becoming infected is increased with factors such as early age of initiation of sexual activity, the number of sexual partners, and previous genital infections.
- If the individual already has HSV1 virus, the symptoms of HSV2 first infection may be less severe.
- Commonly, the infection causes painful, vesicular, or ulcerative lesions of the skin and mucous membranes. Dysuria and an increased vaginal discharge may also occur. These are more pronounced in first infection.
- Systemic infection characterized by high temperature and myalgia may occur.
- Occasionally, the infection may be asymptomatic in adults.

Definitions

- *First episode primary infection:* is the first infection with either HSV1 or HSV2 virus. The symptoms tend to be pronounced and the lesions may last 2–3 weeks.
- *First episode non-primary infection:* the first infection with either HSV1 or HSV2, but the person already has pre-existing antibodies to the other type.
- *Recurrent infection:* recurrence of clinical symptoms.

Diagnosis

- Viral cultures from open lesions, with a special viral swab, are the easiest and one of the best methods of diagnosing infection. The swab should be sent to the laboratory immediately.
- Other specialist tests may be carried out in a sexual health clinic, where the woman should be referred for treatment.

HSV in pregnancy

- The effects of the first or recurrent infection, as discussed above, on the mother, will be treated as in the non-pregnant state and includes antiviral therapy, analgesia, saline baths, and topical anaesthetic gel to soothe the pain and discomfort.
- If the mother acquires primary infection in the first or second trimester oral antiviral therapy, aciclovir, will be commenced. Occasionally, the clinical manifestation may warrant intravenous therapy to reduce virus shedding and promote healing. Although not licensed for use in pregnancy, the clinical evidence is that its use is safe.
- If the mother is immunocompromised, as in HIV, the dose will need to be increased.

- From 36 weeks onwards continuous aciclovir therapy will reduce the risk of clinical risk of recurrence at the time of birth and allow a normal vaginal birth.
- A woman with active lesions after 34 weeks is delivered by caesarean section.
- Caesarean section is not indicated unless active genital lesions or symptoms of impending infection are present.

Fetal and neonatal infection

- The main danger of primary HSV infection in early pregnancy is congenital herpes that causes severe abnormalities, similar to those caused by rubella, toxoplasmosis, and cytomegalovirus.
- Active primary infection at the time of birth has a 40% risk of transmission to the newborn.
- Recurrent infection at the time of birth has a transmission risk of <5%, while virtually nil with asymptomatic virus shedding.

Useful website

British Association for Sexual Health and HIV. Available at: 🖱 www.bashh.org.uk.

Further reading

Dapaah S, Dapaah V (2009). Sexually transmissible and reproductive tract infections in pregnancy. In: Fraser D, Cooper M (eds) *Myles Textbook for Midwives*. 15th edn. London: Churchill Livingstone, pp. 415–32.

Syphilis

- Although rare in the UK, syphilis remains a high cause of fetal and neonatal loss in developing countries, particularly Africa.
- The overall number of cases of infectious syphilis has increased substantially in 16–34-year old females in the UK in recent years.[1] Congenital syphilis has therefore re-emerged.
- It caused by the bacterium *Treponema pallidum* and usually acquired by sexual contact.
- Infection causes a complex systemic disease that can involve almost every organ in the body.
- It can be congenitally transmitted across the placenta.
- Because of the increased incidence and its devastating effects it is still routinely screened for in early pregnancy in the UK (☐ see Screening for syphilis, p. 58).
- The midwife has a responsibility for effective sexual health promotion and encouraging effective long-term contraception for at least two years after this pregnancy. Both the woman's contraception and sexual health needs are best dealt with by the local specialist contraception and sexual health clinic.

Stage of the infection

Early infectious stage:
- *Primary*: occurs 9–90 days after exposure (average 21 days)
- *Secondary*: 6 weeks to 6 months after exposure (4–8 weeks after primary lesion)
- *Early latent*: 2 years after exposure.

Late non-infectious stage:
- *Late latent*: more than 2 years after exposure with no signs or symptoms
- *Neurosyphilis, cardiovascular syphilis, gummatous syphilis*: 3–20 years after exposure.

Syphilis in pregnancy

- Untreated syphilis may result in spontaneous abortion, preterm birth, stillbirth, or neonatal death.
- If the infant survives and, dependent on the stage of the infection in the mother, there is high risk of infant or childhood morbidity.
- Congenital transmission will occur from 4 months onwards and the highest risk is from 6 months onwards, once the Langhan's layer of the early placenta has completely atrophied, which was the protective mechanism.
- A woman diagnosed in pregnancy is likely to have early infectious syphilis and early treatment will prevent congenital infection.
- Treatment is usually with a course of intramuscular penicillin. For a woman with penicillin allergy, erythromycin is the drug of choice. Tetracycline is contraindicated in pregnancy.

- Treatment, follow-up, and contact tracing will usually be led by a consultant in genitourinary medicine, to whom the woman should be immediately referred.
- If untreated, up to one-third of pregnancies will result in stillbirth and 70–100% of babies will be infected.

Congenital syphilis

- Although the incidence of congenital syphilis is estimated at 70 per million births, this is likely to increase, while the overall increase in the incidence in the childbearing age group continues.
- Classification will depend on the stage of disease reached, with approximately two-thirds of liveborn infected babies showing no signs or symptoms at birth.
- Lesions will develop from 4 months onwards.
- Serology at birth is unreliable, because of the presence of passive transfer from the mother; the treponemal-specific IgM light test is unreliable and can give false positive or negative results.
- The baby should be further serologically tested at 6 weeks and 3 months of age, allowing time for passive maternal antibodies to disappear.
- In subsequent pregnancies, even if the mother has been followed up for 2 years and discharged, the baby should be tested at 3 months of age, in case any trepenomes have persisted in the maternal circulation.
- If the mother is still being followed up when she becomes pregnant again she should be immediately referred to the genitourinary medicine (GUM) clinic for investigation and management.

Useful website

British Association for Sexual Health and HIV. Available at: ℘ www.bashh.org.uk.

Further reading

Dapaah S, Dapaah V (2009). Sexually transmissible and reproductive tract infections in pregnancy. In: Fraser D, Cooper M (eds) *Myles Textbook for Midwives*. 15th edn. London: Churchill Livingstone, pp. 415–432.

---

1 Health Protection Agency (2009). *Syphilis and Lymphogranuloma venereum: Resurgent STI Infections in the UK*. Available at: ℘ www.hpa.org.uk/web/HPAwebfile/HPAweb_C1245581513523 (accessed 2.5.10).

Vaginal infections

During pregnancy an increased vaginal discharge is commonly experienced and is the result of normal physiological changes related to increased blood flow in the reproductive organs, and a decrease in the acidity of the vaginal discharge. Investigation should be considered if the woman reports itching, soreness, offensive smell, or pain on passing urine.

It is important to remember that *Chlamydia trachomatis* is the most common cause of infection and 70–80% of infected women are asymptomatic. All women should be offered a routine urine-based screening test in early pregnancy and at any other time, as required.

For specific infections see the relevant chapters in this section.

Obtaining a vaginal swab

- There are two methods to obtain a vaginal swab; high vaginal and introital.
- Usually even though significant vaginal discharge will be apparent, it will possibly be contaminated so obtaining the swab from deeper in the vagina will yield a more accurate result from laboratory investigation.
- A self taken swab is as effective. Tell the woman to count to 60 while rotating the swab in the vagina.
- A high vaginal swab is obtained by viewing the upper vagina with a speculum.
- Having consented to the procedure and removed the necessary undergarments, the client should lie on an examination couch, bend her knees, and with her heels together let her knees fall apart. Lighting should be adjusted to give a good view of the vulva and perineum.
- The speculum should be warmed (if of metal construction) and lubricated, and inserted gently into the vagina with closed blades orientated in the same direction as the vaginal opening. Once inserted, the blades should be slowly rotated until they are horizontal and opened slowly, bringing the cervix into view.
- The swab can now be taken from the fornices of the upper vagina, avoiding contamination from the vaginal entrance.
- Swabs for GBS are obtained from just inside the vaginal opening. At the same time a rectal swab is usually taken. There is less emphasis on avoiding contamination, as the organism inhabits both the rectum and lower genital tract.

Antenatal care

Confirmation of pregnancy

There are a number of options for women wishing to confirm their pregnancy. A range of home pregnancy testing kits are available from pharmacies, and most pharmacies will carry out a test for a small charge. GP surgeries also provide this service.

The tests are based on detecting the presence of β-human chorionic gonadotrophin (β-hCG), in the woman's urine or blood. This hormone is secreted by trophoblast or placental tissue from around 7–10 days after conception.

Other signs of pregnancy are:

- **Amenorrhoea**: absence of menstrual periods in a woman who normally experiences menstruation.
- **Nausea and vomiting**: common in the first trimester from 6 weeks' gestation, peaking at around 10 weeks' gestation and diminishing as the pregnancy reaches 12 weeks and beyond. It persists throughout pregnancy in some women.
- **Frequency of micturition**: increased urine production and pressure on the bladder due to the growing uterus.
- **Tiredness**: increased metabolic activity and rapid growth of uterine and placental tissue.
- **Breast tenderness/changes**: hormonal effects of oestrogen and progesterone. The breasts enlarge, become tender, and heavier.
- **Fetal movements**: these are a late sign, appearing in the second trimester as the fetus grows and the uterus becomes a larger abdominal organ. Early movements feel like fluttering or bursting bubbles. First-time mothers notice these later (18–20 weeks) than those undergoing a second or subsequent pregnancy (16–18 weeks).
- **Pica**: or craving for unusual foods, or combinations of foods— hormonal influences on the gastrointestinal tract alter the mother's perception of taste.

Dating the pregnancy

Ascertain the following:

- The first day of the LMP. This may be difficult to ascertain accurately, unless the woman is in the habit of recording this.
- The length of the menstrual cycle in days and its regularity.
- The number of days of bleeding and if the LMP was a normal bleed.
- The woman's usual method of contraception, and when this was stopped. If the LMP was a withdrawal bleed after oral contraceptive, this date is unreliable.

Calculate the EDD for a 28-day cycle by adding 7 days and 9 months to date of the LMP. Make adjustments for shorter or longer cycles. 📖 See also Taking a menstrual history, p. 16.

Confirm the dates by ultrasound scan. Most women will be offered a scan at around 14 weeks' gestation to coincide with serum fetal screening tests.

The earlier the scan the more accurate the estimation of fetal age. If the results differ from the menstrual date by more than 2 weeks, the scan date should be accepted as the correct date and the EDD adjusted accordingly.

Having accurate dates allows for correct interpretation of fetal screening tests and prevents unnecessary induction of labour for post-maturity.

Adaptation to pregnancy

Increasing amounts of circulating hormones bring about pregnancy changes throughout the body, and all body systems are affected to a greater or lesser degree. The changes allow the fetus to develop and grow, prepare the woman for labour and delivery, and prepare her body for lactation.

The reproductive system

- Most of the changes take place in the uterus, which undergoes hypertrophy and hyperplasia of the myometrium. The decidua also becomes thicker and more vascular.
- Progesterone causes the endocervical cells to secrete thick mucus, which forms a plug, called the operculum, in the cervical canal, protecting the pregnancy from ascending infection.
- Muscles in the vagina hypertrophy and become more elastic to allow distension during the second stage of labour.

The cardiovascular system

- Due to the increasing workload the heart enlarges.
- Cardiac output increases to accommodate the increasing circulating blood volume.
- Peripheral resistance is lowered, due to the relaxing effect of progesterone on the smooth muscle of the blood vessels, leading to a fall in blood pressure.
- To avoid aorto-caval compression, as the arterial walls are more relaxed, it is important to avoid placing the woman in an unattended supine position during the third trimester.
- Blood flow increases in the uterus, skin, breasts, and kidneys, and blood volume increases by 20–50%, varying according to size, parity, and whether the pregnancy is singleton or multiple.

The respiratory system

- Oxygen consumption increases by 15–20% at term.
- Tidal volume increases by 40%.
- Residual volume decreases by 20%.
- Alveolar ventilation increases by 5–8L/min, four times greater than oxygen consumption, resulting in enhanced gaseous exchange.
- The amount of air inspired over 1min increases by 26%, resulting in hyperventilation of pregnancy, causing CO_2 to be removed from the lungs with greater efficiency.
- Oxygen transfer to, and CO_2 transfer from, the fetus are facilitated by changes in the maternal blood pH and partial pressure of CO_2 (pCO_2).

The urinary system

- Renal blood flow increases by 70–80% by the second trimester.
- The glomerular filtration rate increases by 45% by 8 weeks' gestation.
- Creatinine, urea, and uric acid clearance are increased.
- Glycosuria occurs as a result of the increased glomerular filtration rate and is not usually related to increased blood glucose.

- The ureters relax under the influence of progesterone and become dilated. Compression of the ureters against the pelvic brim can lead to urinary stasis, bacteriuria, and infection of the urinary tract.
- As the fetal head engages at the end of pregnancy the bladder may become displaced upwards.

The gastrointestinal system

- Nausea is experienced by 70% of pregnant women, beginning at around 4–6 weeks and continuing until 12–14 weeks.
- Most women notice increased appetite and increased thirst in pregnancy.
- Reflux of acid into the oesophagus, resulting in heartburn, is common.
- Transit of food through the intestines is much slower and there is increased absorption of water from the colon, leading to an increased tendency to constipation.

Skeletal changes

- Pelvic ligaments relax under the influence of relaxin and oestrogen, with the maximum effect in the last weeks of pregnancy.
- This allows the pelvis to increase its capacity to accommodate the presenting part during the latter stage of pregnancy and during labour.
- The symphysis pubis widens and the sacro-coccygeal joint loosens, allowing the coccyx to be displaced.
- While these changes facilitate vaginal delivery, they are likely to be the cause of backache and ligament pain.

Skin changes

- Increased pigmentation of the areola, abdominal midline, perineum, and axillae due to a rise in pituitary melanin-stimulating hormone.
- The 'mask of pregnancy', or chloasma, a deeper colouring of the face, develops in 50–70% of women, is more common in dark-haired women, and is exacerbated by sun exposure.
- Striae gravidarum, commonly called stretch marks, occur as the collagen layer of the skin stretches over areas of fat deposition, e.g. breasts, abdomen, and thighs.
- The stretch marks appear as red stripes and change to silvery white lines within 6 months of delivery.
- Scalp, facial, and body hair become thicker. The excess is shed in the postnatal period.

The breasts

- Breast changes are one of the first signs of pregnancy noticed by the mother. From around 3–4 weeks' gestation there is increased blood flow and tenderness, veins become more prominent, and the breasts feel warm.
- Under the influence of oestrogen, fat is deposited in the breasts, increasing their size. The lactiferous tubules and ducts enlarge.
- The pigmented area around the nipple darkens.

- Progesterone causes growth of the lobules and alveoli, and develops the secretory ability of these structures, ready for lactation.
- Prolactin stimulates the production of colostrum from the second trimester onwards, and after delivery is responsible for the initiation of milk production.

The endocrine system

All the endocrine organs are influenced by secretion of placental hormones during pregnancy.

- *Pituitary hormones*: prolactin, adrenocorticotropic hormone (ACTH), thyroid hormone, and melanocyte stimulating hormone (MSH) increase. Follicle-stimulating hormone (FSH) and luteinizing hormone (LH) are inhibited. Oxytocin is released throughout pregnancy and increases at term, stimulating uterine contractions.
- *Thyroid hormones*: total thyroxine levels rise sharply from the second month of pregnancy. The basal metabolic rate is increased.
- *Adrenal hormones*: cortisol levels increase, leading to insulin resistance and a corresponding rise in blood glucose, particularly after meals. This makes more glucose available for the fetus.
- *Pancreas*: due to increasing insulin resistance, the β cells are stimulated to increase insulin production by up to four times during pregnancy. In women with borderline pancreatic function, this may result in the development of gestational diabetes, affecting 3–12% of pregnant women.

Blood values in pregnancy

Table 4.1 summarizes the main components of the blood and shows the values prior to pregnancy and the changes as a result of the maternal adaptation to pregnancy.
- The main feature is physiological anaemia due to increased plasma volume despite a rise in the red cell mass.
- Decreasing plasma protein concentrations lead to lower osmotic pressure contributing to the oedema seen in the lower limbs during pregnancy. Moderate oedema when not associated with disease is an indicator of a favourable pregnancy outcome.

Table 4.1 The main components of blood

Component	Non-pregnant	Change in pregnancy
Plasma volume	2600mL	3850mL at 40 weeks
Red cell mass	1400mL	1650mL at 40 weeks
Total blood volume	4000mL	5500mL at 40 weeks
Haematocrit (PCV)	35%	30% at 40 weeks
Haemoglobin	12.5–13.9g/dL	11.0–12.2g/dL at 40 weeks
Protein	65–85g/L	55–75g/L at 20 weeks
Albumin	35–48g/L	25–38g/L at 20 weeks
Fibrinogen	15–36g/L	25–46g/L at 20 weeks
Platelets	$150–400 \times 10^{3+}/mm^3$	Slight decrease
Clotting time	12min	8min
White cell count	$9 \times 10^9/L$	$10–15 \times 10^9/L$
Red cell count	$4.7 \times 10^{12}/L$	$3.8 \times 10^{12}/L$ at 30 weeks

The booking interview

The booking interview is a holistic assessment of the woman's social, health, educational, and psychological needs and identifies those needing additional care. The purpose of the interview is to obtain a history and exchange information so that future care during pregnancy and birth can be planned. Both verbal and written information is given to enable parents to make informed decisions about screening tests.

The following is a guide to the information given and obtained, and the investigations that can be performed during this appointment. All the information gained and given should be carefully recorded. As the interview proceeds it will be possible to establish a rapport and judge when it is appropriate to ask some of the more sensitive questions.

Social considerations

- Confirm the woman's name, age, and other relevant biographical details.
- Is she in a stable supportive relationship?
- What is her (and/or her partner's) occupation?
- Sensitive enquiry about whether she has experienced domestic abuse and if she is still in that relationship.

Emotional and psychological considerations

- Is the pregnancy planned?
- Is she happy to be pregnant?
- Has she any history of mental health problems?
- Has she any concerns about her health or her pregnancy?

Health considerations

- Ask about present health and the current pregnancy, are there any problems?
- Ask about previous obstetric history, number of pregnancies and births (gravida and parity), and whether these were normal.
- Are her previous children healthy?
- Ask about menstrual history and calculate the EDD.
- Ask about previous medical and family history such as twins, diabetes, epilepsy, hypertension, mental health issues, previous operations, and blood transfusions.
- Verify the blood group and rhesus (Rh) status.
- Measure the body mass index (BMI) and blood pressure, and test the urine for proteinuria.

Educational considerations

Information and discussion to obtain consent for the following:
- Offer screening for anaemia, red cell antibodies, hepatitis B, HIV, Rubella antibodies, and syphilis.
- Offer screening for asymptomatic bacteriuria.
- Offer screening for Down's syndrome.
- Offer an early ultrasound scan for gestational age assessment.
- Offer ultrasound screening for structural anomalies.
- Ask about lifestyle issues, diet, alcohol consumption, smoking, and any medications. Give advice and information as appropriate.

Taking a sexual history

- Unprotected sexual intercourse resulting in pregnancy may also put a woman at risk of contracting an STI.
- Sensitive discussion about her past and current sexual health will determine the need for STI testing.
- It is important to raise the issue of sexual health and STIs early in pregnancy to initiate diagnostic testing, appropriate referral to the sexual health service and sexual health promotion, if applicable.
- The rates of STIs in the UK have risen sharply in the past decade. The highest rates are found in women, gay men, teenagers, young adults, and black and ethnic minority groups.[1]
- While a programme of chlamydia screening in the 16–24-year age group has been instituted in the UK, this common STI is by no means limited to this age group and it is good practice to offer every pregnant woman urine-based screening, as a prevention for her ongoing, long-term sexual health and to prevent vertical transmission to her baby during vaginal birth.
- Unrecognized/untreated STIs may be vertically transmitted to the baby following rupture of the membranes and vaginal birth. 📖 See Chapter 3 for more specific discussion on individual infections.

The discussion should include:

- Length of current relationship
- Number of sexual partners in the past 12 months.

Symptoms

- Change in vaginal discharge
- Vulval/vaginal soreness or irritation
- Intermenstrual bleeding
- Postcoital bleeding
- Pain during sex (dyspareunia)
- Abdominal pain
- Contact of STI
- Past history of STI
- Contraceptive method(s)
- Condom use
- Is she an intravenous drug user past or present?
- Has she had sex with an intravenous drug user?
- Has she been paid for sex?
- Is her partner bisexual?
- Has any partner been of non-UK origin, in this country or abroad?

Investigations

Investigations may include:

Chlamydia

- Endocervical swab
- Self-taken swab
- Urine test (first catch).

Gonorrhoea
- Endocervical swab: high vaginal swab: candidiasis ('thrush'), *Trichomonas vaginalis*, bacterial vaginosis
- Viral culture swab: herpes, HPV.

Blood testing
- Syphilis
- HIV
- Hepatitis A
- Hepatitis B
- Hepatitis C.

Other
- Cervical screening:
  - Has the woman been called for screening at all? This will depend on the country she resides in and the age at which the screening programme commences.
  - If appropriate, has she been screened at all and when was her last test?
  - Has she ever been asked to attend for repeat testing within the normal recall time and has she ever had an abnormal result?
- Has she had a colposcopy examination and, if so, what was the outcome?

1 Health Protection Agency (2010). *Health Protection Report: HIV/Sexually Transmitted Infections.* Available at www.hpa.org.uk/hpr/infections/hiv_sti.htm (accessed 2.4.10)

Principles of antenatal screening

As science and technology advance, we are able to elicit more information about pregnancy, the mother, and the fetus than ever before. The scrutiny with which we examine every aspect of pregnancy has never been more detailed. It is very likely that further advances in these techniques will expose women to increasingly difficult choices and dilemmas. The midwife will need to be well prepared and informed to guide her clients through this process.

A range of activities come under the banner of 'antenatal screening'. Certain activities are a fundamental part of midwifery practice, e.g. measuring the fundal height, listening to the fetal heart, and the routine blood tests, including full blood count, group and Rh factor, and maternal serum for rubella antibodies. We may classify these as low intervention, unlikely to cause any ethical concern. Other types of screening, such as those undertaken to detect fetal abnormality, can lead to much moral difficulty.

The aims of screening

The whole pregnant population is screened because, although collectively this population has a low risk of abnormality, screening aims to identify those at a higher risk, so that more specific diagnostic tests can be applied.

Benefits of screening and diagnosis

- Reduce fetal abnormality.
- Reduce genetic reoccurrence.
- Reduce the incidence of mental handicap.
- Reduce the burden on family and society.
- Increase resources for those disabled individuals who are not detected before birth.

Adverse effects of screening and diagnosis

- Anxiety provoked by screening procedures.
- Psychological sequelae for parents.
- Risks of diagnostic tests to woman and fetus.
- Risks to the woman of a late termination of pregnancy.
- Risk of aborting a normal fetus.
- Long-term effects on society's attitude to the disabled.

Implications

- Inadequate counselling at the time of the test could mean that clients are not prepared for adverse outcomes, such as being recalled with a high-risk result, or giving birth to an affected child after having a low-risk result from the screening test.[1]
- No matter how good a test is technically, screening uninformed, unsupported clients by unprepared staff is a recipe for, at best, confusion and, at worst, great distress. This is avoidable.[2]

Consent and counselling

- Screening tests other than those performed in normal midwifery care are likely to reveal information that parents need to be prepared for, and to result in decisions being made about the future of the pregnancy.
- If, on consideration, parents decide not to take up the offer of tests, then this should be respected.
- In practice, it is difficult to ensure that clients are aware of all the ramifications of tests, especially when so many are on offer.
- Where informed consent has not been obtained, and a positive result to a screening test is returned, the practitioner is vulnerable to litigation.
- If a client's language barrier or intellect makes understanding difficult, it may not be professionally acceptable to go ahead with tests.
- The use of interpreters is problematic, but there is usually a protocol, and advice can be sought from a specialist midwife.
- If the client is not mentally competent, then she cannot effectively give consent as an autonomous person. The principle of beneficence could be invoked to provide care that is in the best interests of the client. Paternalism may be justified in any number of circumstances, notwithstanding the limited mental capacity of the client.

1 Grayson A (1996). Fetal screening. The triple test decision. *Modern Midwife* **6**(8), 16–19.

2 Marteau TM, Drake H. (1995). Attributions for disability: the influence of genetic screening. *Social Science and Medicine* **40**(8), 1127–32.

Screening for risk in pregnancy

Risk screening during pregnancy aims to identify those women at risk, so that a suitable pattern of care can be planned for the pregnancy with the appropriate professional.

For women deemed to be healthy and at low risk, midwife or midwife/GP care, based in the community, is a suitable alternative to consultant- or hospital-based care programmes.

Assessment of risk should be ongoing, so that deviations from the normal or the development of complications can be identified at any stage of pregnancy and referral to appropriate care arranged. This assessment starts at the booking interview or initial appointment. For many women this takes place in their own home and is conducted by the community midwife.

Women with any of the following need care over and above that recommended for low-risk healthy women by the NICE guidelines:[1]

- Cardiac disease including hypertension
- Renal disease
- Endocrine disorder or diabetes requiring insulin
- Psychiatric disorder (on medication)
- Haematological disorder (including thrombo-embolic disease)
- Epilepsy requiring anticonvulsant medication
- Malignant disease
- Severe asthma
- Drug misuse (heroin, cocaine, ecstasy)
- HIV or hepatitis B
- Autoimmune disorders
- Obesity: BMI 30kg/m^2 or above (or underweight – BMI <18kg/m$^{2)}$
- Women at higher risk, e.g. age >40 or <14 years
- Women who are particularly vulnerable or who lack social support.

Women who have experienced any of the following in previous pregnancies are at higher risk:

- Recurrent miscarriage (three or more)
- Preterm birth
- Severe pre-eclampsia, eclampsia, or HELLP syndrome
- Rh isoimmunization or other significant blood group antibodies
- Uterine surgery—caesarean section, myomectomy, or cone biopsy
- Ante- or postpartum haemorrhage on two occasions
- Puerperal psychosis
- Grand multiparity (>6)
- A stillbirth or neonatal death
- A small for gestational age infant (<5th centile)
- A large for gestational age infant (>95th centile)
- A baby weighing <2.5kg or >4.5kg
- A baby with a congenital anomaly (structural or chromosomal).

1 National Institute for Health and Clinical Excellence (2008). Antenatal care: Routine care for the healthy pregnant mother. Clinical guideline 62. London: NICE. Available at: ꙮ www.nice.org.uk/cg62.

Antenatal screening

The Department of Health has published standards to support the UK Antenatal Screening Programme on screening for infectious diseases in pregnancy.[1] These standards are both generic and specific and are part of a wider initiative to establish a quality assured national screening programme. Responsibilities in the trust/strategic health authority, clinic, or laboratory are clarified in the standards. The information below concentrates on the responsibilities at clinical level.

Generic standards for infectious diseases

All pregnant women are offered screening for rubella antibody, syphilis, HIV, and hepatitis B as an integral part of their antenatal care during their first and all subsequent pregnancies. Repeat testing during pregnancy is not usually necessary. The women have a right to decline screening.

Pregnant women arriving in labour who have not had antenatal care elsewhere are to be offered screening, priority being given to HIV and hepatitis B, and presumptive action is taken on a preliminary positive result until such time as the result is confirmed. If an HIV test result will not be available in time, appropriate preventive measures should be offered. Use of rapid test devices may be appropriate in this context.

Screening is only performed with documented consent, though this does not require a signature from the patient and the usual standards of confidentiality apply.

Screening for rubella antibodies

- Congenital rubella syndrome was first described in 1941.
- If the rubella virus is contracted during the first 8 weeks of pregnancy there is an 80% risk of malformations, microcephaly, and severe learning difficulties.
- If the virus is contracted after 9 weeks of gestation there is a 20% risk of deafness and brain damage. Handicap is rare after the 16th week.
- In order to prevent congenital rubella syndrome all children are offered protection from the virus with the measles, mumps, rubella (MMR) vaccine.
- Women are screened during early pregnancy, usually at the time of the other routine blood tests, to record their immune status.
- All non-immune women, and women with an antibody titre <10IU are recommended a further vaccine dose in the early postnatal period.
- If a pregnant woman reports recent contact with an infected individual her immune status is confirmed. A titre >10IU suggests immunity.
- If the titre is <10IU the test is repeated 2–3 weeks later. A fourfold increase in the titre suggests a recent infection.
- If a woman presents more than 10–14 days after exposure a high IgM titre indicates viraemia in the last 4 weeks.
- If infected in early pregnancy with a high risk of abnormality, termination of pregnancy would be offered.

1 Department of Health (2003). Screening for infectious diseases in pregnancy: Standards to support the UK Antenatal Screening Programme. Available at: ℘ www.dh.gov.uk (accessed 2.4.10).

Screening for syphilis

Syphilis can seriously complicate pregnancy and result in spontaneous abortion (commonly at around 18–20 weeks' gestation), stillbirth, intrauterine growth restriction, and perinatal death.

- Antenatal screening for syphilis is well established, forming part of the routine screening of all pregnant women during the first or early second trimester.
  - As the prevalence of this infection is very low, continuation of the screening programme has recently been questioned, notably by Kiss et al.[1] whose survey of the prevalence in Austria seemed to suggest no economic benefit from universal antenatal screening.
  - Connor et al.[2] carried out an epidemiological survey in the UK which suggested that targeting the screening to at-risk groups or stopping the screening programme would save relatively little money, and recommended that the current universal antenatal screening for syphilis should continue.
- Women who are at risk will be retested in the late second to early third trimester, as infection acquired during pregnancy still poses a significant risk to the fetus.
- Women who screen positive for the Venereal Disease Research Laboratory (VDRL) test will have this result confirmed by retesting with a *Treponema*-specific assay (*Treponema pallidum* haemagglutination test, TPHA test) and will be treated with antibiotics such as amoxycillin.

1 Kiss H, Widhalm A, Geusau A, Husslein P (2004). Universal antenatal screening for syphilis: is it still justified economically? A 10-year retrospective analysis. *Eur J Obstet Gynecol Reprod Biol* **112**(1): 24–8.

2 Connor N, Roberts J, Nicoll A (2000). Strategic options for antenatal screening for syphilis in the United Kingdom: a cost effectiveness analysis. *J Med Screen* **7**(1): 7–13.

HIV screening

Pregnant women should be offered screening for HIV infection early in antenatal care because appropriate antenatal interventions can reduce mother-to-child transmission of HIV infection. A system of clear referral paths should be established in each unit or department so that pregnant women who are diagnosed with an HIV infection are managed and treated by the appropriate specialist teams.[1] The Department of Health[2] has produced guidelines for the management of HIV screening during pregnancy and the following information is taken from this report.

- Most HIV infected children in this country have acquired the infection from their mothers. There are now interventions that can reduce the risk of mother-to-child transmission of HIV from 25% to 2%. In order to take advantage of these it is vital to diagnose the infection before birth.
- HIV prevalence varies across the UK but antenatal screening and the chance to offer treatment to affected women remains a cost-effective screening strategy.
- Information about the test is given to the woman during the booking interview. Pre- and post-test counselling should be offered. The nature of the test and how she will receive the results is explained.
- The implications of a positive result need to be explored. The woman is informed personally if the result is positive and she will be offered specialist counselling and support which is available for partners and family if requested.
- Women found to be positive are referred for specialist HIV treatment and advice about how to manage their own infection and interventions to reduce the risk of vertical and sexual transmission.
- Discussions cover the use of anti-retrovirals and caesarean section, early treatment and care for the child, and decisions about breastfeeding.
- The implications of a negative result and general sexual health are discussed. This is also an opportunity to discuss the dangers of becoming infected during pregnancy or lactation.
- Women who refuse an HIV test at booking should be re-offered a test, and should they decline again a third offer of a test should be made at 36 weeks. Women presenting to services for the first time in labour should be offered a point of care test (POCT).[3] A POCT test may also be considered for the infant of a woman who refuses testing antenatally.[3]
- In areas of higher seroprevalence, or where there are other risk factors, women who are HIV negative at booking may be offered a routine second test at 34–36 weeks' gestation as recommended in the British HIV Association (BHIVA) pregnancy guidelines.[4]

1 National Institute for Health and Clinical Excellence (2008). Antenatal care: Routine care for the healthy pregnant mother. Clinical guideline 62. London: NICE. Available at: ℘ www.nice.org.uk/cg62.

2 Department of Health (2003). Screening for infectious diseases in pregnancy: Standards to support the UK Antenatal Screening Programme. Available at: ℘ www.dh.gov.uk (3.5.10).

3 Department of Health (2008). UK National Guidelines for HIV testing. London: DH.

4 British HIV Association (2008). Management of HIV infection in pregnant women. Available at: www.bhiva.org/PregnantWomen2008.aspx (accessed 3.5.10).

The full blood count

- A full blood count (FBC) obtained in the first trimester acts as a baseline against which all other measurements can be compared.
- A FBC should be repeated at 28 weeks' gestation to allow for correction of anaemia prior to term.
- As pregnancy progresses, plasma volume expansion is greater than the corresponding rise in the red cell count, this leads to a haemodilution effect and the haematocrit falls, along with the haemoglobin (Hb) level. This is called physiological anaemia.
- Apparent anaemia can be a sign of an excellent adaptation to pregnancy. The effect is greatest at around 30–32 weeks' gestation.
- Lower mean Hb concentrations are associated with higher mean birth-weights, and higher mean Hb concentrations are associated with an increase in pre-term delivery and low birth-weight babies.
- Hb levels outside the normal UK range for pregnancy should be investigated and iron supplementation considered if indicated.
- The levels are 11g/dL at first contact and 10.5g/dL at 28 weeks' gestation.
- In order to correctly assess for anaemia the impact of gestational age on plasma volume should be considered. Use of haemoglobin level as a sole indicator of anaemia is not recommended.
- Serum ferritin is the most sensitive single screening test to detect adequate iron stores. Using a cut-off point of 30micrograms/L a sensitivity of 90% has been reported.[1]

1 National Institute for Health and Clinical Excellence (2008). Antenatal care: Routine care for the healthy pregnant mother. Clinical guideline 62. London: NICE. Available at: ✆ www.nice.org. uk/cg62.

ABO blood group and rhesus factor: anti-D prophylaxis for the Rh-negative mother

At the initial appointment as well as obtaining a full medical and obstetric history from the woman, venous blood is obtained so that blood group, Rh factor, and the presence of red cell antibodies can be determined. This test will identify women who are Rh-negative and who therefore require further antibody testing during pregnancy.

Recording the blood group is necessary for future reference if the mother needs a blood transfusion around the time of birth. Group O is the most common blood type in the UK; 85% of individuals will also have the Rh factor and will therefore be Rh-positive.

What is the Rh factor?

- The Rh factor is a complex protein antigen carried on the surface of the red blood cell. It is inherited from three pairs of genes called cde/CDE. It is the pair named D that makes an individual Rh-positive and is likely to cause Rh iso-immunization.
- Rh-negative women who carry an RhD positive fetus may produce antibodies to the fetal RhD antigens after a feto-maternal haemorrhage. These antibodies may cross the placenta in future pregnancies causing haemolytic disease of the newborn (HDN) if the fetus is RhD-positive.
- HDN can range in severity from stillbirth, severe disabilities, or death, to anaemia and jaundice in the neonate. To prevent this occurring, Rh-negative women who have experienced a suspected or known sensitizing event during pregnancy are given an intramuscular injection of anti-D immunoglobulin (anti-D Ig) to prevent antibody production.
- The anti-D Ig works by coating the fetal red cells that have escaped into the mother's circulation so that they cannot be recognized by her immune system. This prevents maternal antibody formation, and thus protects the RhD-positive fetus of any subsequent pregnancy.

What is a sensitizing event?

Very occasionally Rh-negative women may produce antibodies as a result of a mismatched blood transfusion, but fetal red cells from the RhD-positive fetus can cross the placenta and enter the woman's circulation at any time during the pregnancy, particularly if events cause bleeding from the placental site.

▶▶The most important cause of RhD immunization is during pregnancy where there has been no overt sensitizing event. Sensitizing events include:

- Threatened abortion, and abortion after 12 weeks' gestation
- Chorion villus sampling
- Threatened abortion, spontaneous abortion, termination of pregnancy
- Amniocentesis
- Antepartum haemorrhage
- Abdominal trauma
- Hypertension

- Eclampsia
- Traumatic delivery, including caesarean section
- Placental separation during the third stage of labour
- Manual removal of the placenta.

In the Rh-negative woman these events should be followed by prophylactic administration of anti-D immunoglobulin. NICE has reviewed the advice that recommends that all Rh-negative women receive prophylactic anti-D.[1]

- The treatment regimen may vary according to local costs. For instance being able to offer a one visit option, staff costs of administration and the cost of the immunoglobulin.
- The options are 500IU, at 28 and 34 weeks' gestation.
- 1000–1650IU at 28 and 34 weeks' gestation.
- A single dose of 1500IU at 28–30 weeks as well as cover for sensitizing events.
- If a sensitizing event is suspected, Kleihauer's test (on maternal venous blood) estimates the amount of fetal red cells in the maternal circulation, and a measured dose of anti-D can be administered. A 500IU dose is enough to deal with an 8mL transplacental transfusion of fetal blood. Prior to 20 weeks' gestation it is usual to give 250IU as a prophylactic dose.
- Blood samples are taken within one hour of delivery from the Rh-negative mother to test for maternal antibodies, and fetal cells (Kleihauer's).
- Also from the neonate, to discover its blood group and Rh factor. If the neonate is Rh-negative, then the mother requires no further anti-D Ig.

It is the midwife's responsibility to carry out tests during pregnancy to identify women who require anti-D prophylaxis. A full explanation should be given to the woman and her consent obtained for any tests or administration of anti-D Ig.

1 National Institute for Health and Clinical Excellence (2008). Routine antenatal anti-D prophylaxis for women who are rhesus D negative. Technical appraisal 156. London: NICE. Available at: ℘ www.nice.org.uk/ta156.

Screening for Down's syndrome risk

The incidence of Down's syndrome is approximately 1:600–1:700 across the age range of the childbearing population. There are variations in incidence according to maternal age:

- At 18 years of age the incidence is 1:2300
- At 35 years it is 1:200–350
- At 40 years it is 1:100
- At 45 years it is 1:45.

Taking age as the only risk factor would mean that <30% of affected fetuses would be detected by diagnostic testing, as it would not be appropriate to offer amniocentesis to all women.

Down's risk screening was developed in the 1980s to enable all pregnant women to be given an estimate of individual risk if they choose to be screened. The risk is calculated by examining a combination of the following factors:

- Maternal age
- Gestational age in completed weeks
- Maternal body weight
- Serum screening.

Maternal serum screening

- This enables examination of a combination of hormones and proteins present in the maternal bloodstream during early pregnancy.
- Levels vary according to fetal gestational age.
- Abnormally low or high levels are linked to genetic, chromosomal, and structural abnormalities of the fetus.
- High levels of α-fetoprotein (AFP) are associated with neural tube defects, and low levels with Down's syndrome.
- Neural tube defects can be confirmed by ultrasound scan and also amniocentesis.

Recommended screening: aims

- Screening for Down's syndrome should be performed by the end of the first trimester (13 weeks 6 days), but provision should be made to allow later screening (which could be as late as 20 weeks 0 days) for women booking later in pregnancy.
- The 'combined test' (nuchal translucency, β-hCG, pregnancy-associated plasma protein-A) should be offered to screen for Down's syndrome between 11 weeks 0 days and 13 weeks 6 days.
- For women who book later in pregnancy the most clinically and cost-effective serum screening test (triple or quadruple test) should be offered between 15 weeks 0 days and 20 weeks 0 days.
- When it is not possible to measure nuchal translucency, owing to fetal position or high BMI, women should be offered serum screening (triple or quadruple test) between 15 weeks 0 days and 20 weeks 0 days.

Sensitivity
- The sensitivity of the test is a measurement of how many affected fetuses are detected. This means that around 5% of women having the test will be recalled for further investigation.
- The false-positive rate is between 2.6% and 5%. This percent of women will be carrying a normal baby despite a high-risk screening result. About 60 women will be recalled for every affected baby diagnosed.
- The false-negative rate is 20%. This percent of women will be carrying an affected baby despite a low-risk screening result.

Results and consequences of screening
- Offer diagnostic testing if a woman's screen result is 1:10–1:210.
- If the result is 1:210+, then advise the woman that her screen result is low risk.
- Provide information about what the test involves, how the risk is calculated and what is meant by a risk factor.
- There needs to be understanding that low risk is not 'no risk' and that any woman could be the 'one' of the 1:800.
- Explain the nature of the diagnostic test and the risk of miscarriage from this test (1%).
- Discuss options following diagnosis of Down's syndrome, and provide non-directive support to the decision to choose termination or continuation of the pregnancy.

Further reading

National Institute for Health and Clinical Excellence (2008). Antenatal care: Routine care for the healthy pregnant mother. Clinical guideline 62. London: NICE. Available at: ℞ www.nice.org. uk/cg62.

Group B haemolytic streptococcus

Group B haemolytic streptococcus (GBS) is one of a number of common bacteria found in the gut of 30% of men and women. It is estimated that 25% of women carry this organism in the vaginal tract with no ill effect. Its significance is that it can be transmitted to the baby during delivery and is the most common cause of fatal bacterial infection in the early neonatal period.

Incidence

In the UK, approximately 1:2000 babies annually acquire GBS infection, presenting with septicaemia, pneumonia, or meningitis. A UK survey in 2001 identified 376 cases of early-onset GBS disease, 39 of which were fatal.

Presentation

There are two ways in which the infection will present:
- 90% of the infections are early onset, and 70% of babies are symptomatic at birth
- 10% are late onset, occurring after 48h and up to 3 months after birth.

Screening

There is little organized antenatal screening for GBS carriage in the UK at present and most maternity units rely on risk factor estimation to identify carriers and situations where the infection may be transmitted to the neonate.

Risk factors
- Previous baby affected by GBS.
- GBS bacteriuria detected in the present pregnancy.
- Pre-term labour.
- Prolonged rupture of the membranes.
- Pyrexia during labour.

Intrapartum antibiotic prophylaxis (IAP) is offered to women who have any of these risk factors. This approach differs from that in the USA, where all pregnant women are offered bacteriological screening at 35–37 weeks' gestation. This involves taking vaginal and rectal swabs, and all women who carry GBS are offered IAP. This results in 27% of all pregnant women being offered IAP during labour and a reduction in early onset GBS disease of 86%.

Royal College of Obstetrics and Gynaecology recommendations

The Royal College of Obstetrics and Gynaecology (RCOG)[1] has made the following recommendations in the absence of clinical trials and recent data on the prevalence of GBS carriage in the UK.
- Routine antenatal screening is not recommended.
- Antenatal treatment with penicillin is not recommended if GBS is detected incidentally.
- IAP should be considered if GBS is detected incidentally.
- There is no good evidence to support IAP in women who carried GBS in a previous pregnancy.
- IAP should be offered to women who had a previous baby with GBS disease.

- The argument for IAP is stronger in the presence of two or more risk factors.
- IAP should be offered, after discussion, to women with GBS bacteriuria.
- Antibiotic prophylaxis is not required for women undergoing elective caesarean section in the absence of labour and with intact membranes.
- Antibiotic prophylaxis is unnecessary for women with pre-term rupture of membranes unless they are in established labour.
- Penicillin should be administered as soon as possible after the onset of labour. Clindamycin should be given in the event of penicillin allergy.

1 Royal College of Obstetrics and Gynaecology (2007). *Preventing Group B Streptococcus Infection in Newborn Babies*. London: RCOG.

Sickle cell anaemia

Haemoglobin is a complex molecule with the ability to absorb oxygen easily and reversibly. The molecule is composed of iron and protein. The protein structure is inherited and is the part affected in haemoglobino-pathies, being either abnormal or partly missing.

A normal red blood cell (RBC) in an adult is filled with adult haemoglobin. Everyone inherits their haemoglobin type from their parents, half the responsible gene copies from each, and the usual type is HbAA.

Sickle cell trait

- Sickle haemoglobin (abbreviated HbS) has an abnormality of the protein part of the molecule.
- An individual inheriting HbS from one parent and HbA from the other will have haemoglobin type HbSA.
- This is known as the sickle-cell trait.
- The RBCs of such individuals will function normally and they will have few, if any, symptoms.
- However, these individuals have a 50% chance of passing this type of haemoglobin on to their children.
- This condition confers immunity from the malaria parasite, which explains the prevalence of the condition in areas where malaria infection is endemic.
- Due to population movement, individuals can inherit this type of haemoglobin even if their ancestry is from malaria-free areas.

Sickle cell anaemia

- In this case, the individual inherits HbS from both parents, so the haemoglobin type is HbSS.
- RBCs containing only HbSS react to hypoxia, acidosis, or dehydration by changing shape, from the usual bi-concave disc to a crescent or sickle shape.
- These RBCs are more fragile, easily damaged, and will clump together, blocking capillaries.
- Painful crises are provoked by the blockage of small blood vessels.
- The overall effect is that the RBCs are haemolysed, rapidly causing chronic haemolytic anaemia.

Effects on childbearing

- Subfertility
- Impaired placental function
- Increased risk of pregnancy-induced hypertension
- Pulmonary and renal problems
- Phlebitis
- Women with this type of anaemia need to be well hydrated during labour and need careful monitoring to avoid hypoxia should an anaesthetic be required.

Screening
- Information about screening for sickle cell diseases and thalassaemias, including carrier status and the implications of these, should be given to pregnant women at the first contact with a healthcare professional.
- Screening for sickle cell diseases and thalassaemias should be offered to all women as early as possible in pregnancy (ideally by 10 weeks). The type of screening depends upon the prevalence and can be carried out in either primary or secondary care.

Further reading

National Institute for Health and Clinical Excellence (2008). Antenatal care: Routine care for the healthy pregnant mother. Clinical guideline 62. London: NICE. Available at: ℘ www.nice.org. uk/cg62.

Thalassaemia

In this recessively inherited condition part of the haemoglobin protein is missing. The protein is made from structures called α and β chains. As several genes are responsible for the structure of these chains, it is possible to have varying degrees of the condition.

β-thalassaemia minor

The individual inherits one normal gene from one parent and one affected gene from the other parent. This is a carrier state, and has little effect on health other than mild anaemia. Affected individuals can pass on the defective gene to their children.

β-thalassaemia major

The individual inherits defective genes from both parents and can make no, or very few, β chains, so does not produce sufficient haemoglobin. This results in severe anaemia requiring regular blood transfusions and therapy to remove excess iron from the blood.

α-thalassaemia

People with normal haemoglobin carry four α globin genes, two from each parent. α-thalassaemia results from the deletion of one or more of these genes. Table 4.2 shows the result of deletions of one or more of the genes and the effect on the type of haemoglobin produced.

Table 4.2 Effect of gene deletions

Gene deletions	Diagnosis	Adult blood
$(\alpha\alpha/-\alpha)$	α^2 thalassaemia	Normal
$(\alpha\alpha/- -)$ or $(\alpha-/\alpha-)$	α^1 thalassaemia	Small red blood cells
$(-\alpha/- -)$	Hb H disease	Moderate anaemia
$(- -/- -)$	Hydrops fetalis	Not compatible with life

Screening for thalassaemia

- As with sickle cell anaemia, antenatal screening should be offered to all pregnant women as recommended.[1]
- A routine FBC will identify women with hypochromic, microcytic anaemia. Haemoglobin electrophoresis will then identify the underlying haemoglobinopathy.
- Knowing the carrier state of each parent allows counselling about the risks to the fetus of being a carrier or having the disease.
- Haemoglobinopathy screening is carried out on newborns as part of the neonatal blood spot test.

Impact of maternal thalassaemia major on pregnancy

- Depends on the degree of chronic anaemia and the oxygen deprivation that results from this.
- If the woman cannot adequately meet her own oxygen needs the fetus becomes progressively hypoxic.
- Fetal survival may be threatened with spontaneous abortion, intrauterine growth restriction, preterm birth, or intrauterine death.
- Women who are carriers (α- and β-thalassaemia trait) may be only mildly anaemic and require only supportive care.

Management of thalassaemia major during pregnancy

- Specialist medical and obstetric supervision is required.
- Blood transfusion therapy continues.
- Use of iron chelation therapy is not without risk and needs to be individualized.
- Iron deposition in the pancreas and thyroid increases the risk of the woman developing diabetes, so a glucose tolerance test would be indicated.
- Blood transfusion while vital increases the risk of cardiac failure, which in turn, increases the risk of maternal mortality by as much as 50%.

Women who are asymptomatic before pregnancy may find the added stresses of pregnancy can cause deterioration of their health status. The more severe the syndrome, the more significant are the consequences for the woman and fetus.

1 National Institute for Health and Clinical Excellence (2008). Antenatal care: Routine care for the healthy pregnant mother. Clinical guideline 62. London: NICE. Available at: ℬ www.nice.org. uk/cg62.

Antenatal examination

The purpose of the antenatal examination depends on the length of gestation at which it takes place.

NICE has published guidelines for the routine care of women who are experiencing a healthy, low-risk pregnancy.[1] The recommended number of scheduled appointments is determined by parity and the function of the appointment. For the primigravida with an uncomplicated pregnancy, 10 visits are adequate; and for the parous woman with an uncomplicated pregnancy, seven visits should be adequate.

Throughout the antenatal period, be alert to the signs and symptoms of conditions that affect the health of the mother and fetus, such as pre-eclampsia, diabetes, and domestic abuse.

- After the first appointment or booking visit, use the next visit to review, discuss, and document the results of all the screening tests undertaken earlier, and to identify women who need additional care.
- Arrange further investigations for a woman with a haemoglobin level of less than 11g/dL and offer iron supplementation.
- At each visit, measure the blood pressure and test the urine for protein.
- At each visit, be prepared to ask questions, give information and discuss issues about the woman's physical and emotional/psychological well-being; and to use the available time to provide education, supported by antenatal classes and written information.
- After 20 weeks, measure and plot the symphysis–fundal height to detect small or large for dates pregnancies.
- If requested by the mother, auscultate the fetal heart sounds by hand-held ultrasound.
- Offer anti-D prophylaxis to Rhesus-negative women at 28 and 34 weeks' gestation.
- Offer a second screening for anaemia and atypical red cell antibodies at 28 weeks' gestation. Investigate a haemoglobin level of less than 10.5g/dL and provide iron supplementation if necessary.
- At 36–37 weeks' gestation, confirm the lie and presentation of the fetus, and offer external cephalic version for women whose babies are in the breech position.
- If an earlier report showed the placenta extending over the internal cervical os, a further scan should be arranged and reviewed at 36 weeks.
- A further appointment should be arranged for women who have not given birth by 41 weeks, to offer a membrane sweep and induction of labour if this is unsuccessful.

1 National Institute for Health and Clinical Excellence (2008). Antenatal care: Routine care for the healthy pregnant woman. Clinical guideline 62. London: NICE. Available at: ℘ www.nice.org.uk/cg62.

Abdominal examination

An abdominal examination can be carried out at any stage of pregnancy and is used to determine the progress of pregnancy or labour and fetal well-being.

The examination is in three parts: inspection, palpation, and auscultation.

Ask for the woman's consent before the examination. Make her comfortable on the examination couch, lying supine with her head supported by one pillow. Her arms should be relaxed by her sides. Expose her abdomen but use a sheet or towel to cover her pelvic area and legs, preserving her privacy and dignity.

Inspection

- Inspect the abdomen for size and shape. In the primigravida the shape is oval, due to abdominal muscle tone. In the parous client, the shape may be more rounded.
- There may be a saucer-shaped depression below the umbilicus if the fetus is presenting in an occipito-posterior position.
- A heart-shaped uterus may indicate a transverse lie.
- The umbilicus may protrude and the linea nigra, which is the pigmented midline of the rectus sheath, may be apparent.
- Other abdominal scars may be apparent, as will striae gravidarum or stretch marks, which are pink at first turning to a silvery white as they age.
- Size should indicate the stage of pregnancy, which will be confirmed by measuring the symphysis–fundal height.
- Observe for fetal movements—this confirms a live fetus.

Palpation

- Locate the fundus and measure and plot its height above the symphysis pubis (in centimetres).
- The measurement in centimetres should approximately correspond to the number of weeks' gestation after 20 weeks. However, there is a wide variation of normal, due to maternal height, weight, and the length of the maternal abdomen. This does not have a proven predictive value in detecting small for gestational age fetuses.[1]
- The lie of the fetus is normally longitudinal, with the long axis of the fetus lying along the long axis of the mother.
- The presenting part is normally the fetal head. Breech presentation occurs in approximately 3% of pregnancies at term.
- Determine the position of the fetus:
  - The position of the occiput can be found by locating the fetal back, which feels smooth and firm and will lie anteriorly in the left or right side of the uterus if the occiput is anterior.
  - In posterior positions, the back may be felt in the left or right flank, or it may not be palpable. If fetal limbs are felt on both sides of the midline it is likely that the fetus is lying in an occipito-posterior position.
- Establish the relationship of the presenting part to the pelvic brim. The fetal head is engaged in the pelvis when the widest diameter of the fetal head has entered the pelvic brim.

Auscultation

- Hearing the fetal heart will confirm that the fetus is alive, but it does not have any proven predictive value. Routine listening is not recommended but, if the mother requests it, auscultation may provide reassurance.[1]
- Explain the findings of the examination to the mother and record them in her notes.

1 National Institute for Health and Clinical Excellence (2008). Antenatal care: Routine care for the healthy pregnant mother. Clinical guideline 62. London: NICE. Available at: ℛ www.nice.org. uk/cg62.

Monitoring fetal growth and well-being

As part of the overall antenatal assessment, the midwife is responsible for monitoring the growth and well-being of the fetus. Maternal well-being is the best indicator of fetal well-being, so evaluate the mother closely, looking for any problems that are likely to affect the fetus; for example, hypertension, infection, diabetes, and environmental factors, such as smoking, substance misuse, and dietary inadequacies.[1]

- Ask about fetal patterns of movement and activity. All fetuses are active at some stage during a 24h period. The standard is to ask whether there are 10 movements in a 12h period. Ask about strength of movements. This may change towards the end of pregnancy as the fetus has less room to move about. Determine whether the mother is aware of all of the fetal activity.
- Most mothers tend to know their baby's activity pattern well. Ask them to report any concerns, such as reduced activity especially after 40 weeks' gestation.
- If, during an antenatal visit, a mother reports diminished or absent movements, listen to the fetal heart with a Pinard's stethoscope or ultrasound transducer, and reassure the mother. (*Intrauterine death is an uncommon but possible occurrence. If you do not hear the fetal heart, explain this in an honest and sensitive way and make arrangements to confirm the absence of the heartbeat by ultrasound scan.*)
- If a mother seeks advice over the telephone, you may want to arrange a cardiotocograph (CTG) of the fetal heart. This would be carried out in hospital and a non-reassuring trace referred to the obstetrician.
- Carry out abdominal examination at prescribed times, according to whether the mother has been assessed as low or high risk. A more accurate assessment of fetal growth can be obtained if the same person examines the mother on each occasion.
- Overall growth of the uterus is estimated and the fundal height measured in centimetres. This should correspond roughly to the number of weeks' gestation, taking into account maternal height and build.
- Assess the volume of amniotic fluid surrounding the fetus and note increased or diminished amounts. Each pregnancy is assessed on its individual merits and over- or underproduction of amniotic fluid may be pathological or entirely innocent. If you are concerned, refer the woman to an obstetrician.
- When intrauterine growth restriction or large for gestational age fetuses are suspected, decide whether to refer for further investigation.
- A large for dates uterus may be due to a multiple pregnancy. The advent of routine dating scans has meant that multiple pregnancy is now diagnosed early unless there has been operator error or the woman has declined a scan.
- An ultrasound scan may be arranged, but take care not to make the mother overanxious. These conditions are often overdiagnosed, leading to much unnecessary worry for mothers.

- A scan to measure head:abdomen ratio, performed on more than one occasion, will distinguish between symmetrical and asymmetrical growth restriction.
- Scans estimating fetal weight are not reliable enough to predict an accurate birth weight, but they do provide a reasonable estimate to within 500g either side of a given figure.

1 National Institute for Health and Clinical Excellence (2008). Antenatal care: Routine care for the healthy pregnant mother. Clinical guideline 62. London: NICE. Available at: ℘ www.nice.org.uk/cg62.

Health advice in pregnancy

Smoking

As smoking is a potentially preventable activity it is a significant public health issue in pregnancy. There are a number of risks associated with smoking during pregnancy. Although the risks are well known, many women still require specific information about the effects and support to give up or reduce the number of cigarettes smoked. It is estimated that 25% of pregnant women who smoke stop before their first antenatal appointment, and 27% of women report that they are current smokers at the time of the birth of their baby.[1]

- Cigarette smoke contains carbon monoxide and nicotine. The haemoglobin in RBCs combines with oxygen but if carbon monoxide is present this replaces the oxygen in the cell.
- During gaseous exchange in the placenta the oxygen levels are reduced while the cigarette is being smoked and less oxygen is transferred to the fetus.
- Each time a cigarette is smoked the fetus can become hypoxic.
- Nicotine acts on the blood vessels making them narrow. This decreases the blood flow, reducing oxygen and nutrient supply in the body.
- Blood vessels in the placenta will be affected at the same time reducing oxygen and nutrient supply to the fetus.

These effects cause damage in several ways:
- Low birth weight due to reduced nutrition
- Preterm birth
- Stillbirth.
  Babies born to smokers may have the following problems:
- Decreased physical growth
- Decreased intellectual development
- Increased risk of sudden infant death syndrome
- Behavioural problems
- Asthma and respiratory problems
- Poor lung development.

The mother may also experience problems during pregnancy as a result of smoking:
- Increased risk of early miscarriage
- Placental complications such as placenta praevia and placental abruption
- Preterm labour
- Intrauterine infection.

The midwife is in a unique position to offer information and support to the mother who smokes. If the mother is able to give up early in pregnancy she will greatly increase her chances of a delivering a healthy baby. Many localities now have a midwife dedicated to smoking cessation support and mothers can be referred to this service to receive the help they need. Women who are unable to quit should be encouraged to reduce smoking.

Women who smoke should be offered:

- Advice about the specific risks of smoking during pregnancy
- Encouragement to use the NHS Stop Smoking Services and the NHS pregnancy smoking helpline (0800 169 9 169)
- Group support
- Discussion of the risks and benefits of nicotine replacement therapy (NRT). For those women who use NRT patches advice should be given on the importance of removing them before going to bed.

1 National Institute for Health and Clinical Excellence (2008). *Antenatal Care: Routine Care for the Healthy Pregnant Woman.* London: RCOG Press, p. 100.

Alcohol

When alcohol consumption is either occasional or moderate, it is recognized as a socially acceptable behaviour. Over 90% of the population consumes alcohol, but the quantity and frequency of alcohol consumption in women of reproductive age is increasing.

The consequences of alcohol consumption on pregnancy are difficult to study, due to confounding variables such as smoking, diet, socio-economic status, and other substance misuse. The effect of alcohol consumption on the developing fetus depends on:
• The timing in relation to the period of gestation
• The amount of alcohol consumed.
Effects can range from organ damage in the first trimester of pregnancy to growth restriction and inhibited neuro-behavioural development in the second and third trimesters.

Fetal alcohol syndrome describes the complete form of the condition and has become recognized as the foremost preventable, non-genetic cause of intellectual impairment. Another term used to describe various types of this condition is 'alcohol-related birth defects' (ARBD).

NICE[1] states that there is no conclusive evidence of adverse effects on either fetal growth or childhood IQ at levels of consumption below 1–2 units of alcohol once or twice per week, but recommends that women should avoid alcohol if planning a pregnancy and in the first trimester.

There is uncertainty about what constitutes a safe level of alcohol consumption during pregnancy but women should be informed that getting drunk, or binge drinking (5 drinks/7.5 units on a single occasion) may be harmful to the unborn baby.

One unit of alcohol equates to approximately 8g of absolute alcohol. The following measures are used as guides when discussing alcohol consumption (although it is recognized that 'home measures' are often larger than pub measures):
• 1 unit alcohol = 10g alcohol
• 1 unit alcohol = 1 pub measure of spirits
• 1 unit alcohol = ½ pint ordinary strength beer/lager
• 1 unit alcohol = 1 small glass red or white wine.

1 National Institute for Health and Clinical Excellence (2008). *Antenatal Care: Routine Care for the Healthy Pregnant Woman*. London: RCOG Press, p. 99.

Nutrition during pregnancy

Good nutrition is essential for a successful and healthy pregnancy, as poor nutrition is associated with adverse pregnancy outcomes. Increases in specific nutrients are recommended during pregnancy, but these are not difficult to attain in a well-balanced diet. The estimated average requirement (EAR) for energy during pregnancy is 2000kcal/day in the last trimester only,[1] therefore it is not necessary for a woman to 'eat for two'. Nutritional requirements also vary due to changes in basal metabolic rate, which varies widely, increasing in some women and decreasing in others.

Calcium

Calcium needs are highest during the last trimester. Calcium absorption is more efficient during pregnancy but it is still important to eat plenty of calcium-rich foods. The best sources are dairy products such as milk, cheese, yoghurt, dark-green vegetables, sardines, pulses, tofu, nuts, and seeds.

Iron

Iron is needed by the fetus and mother as a reserve for blood loss during pregnancy. Needs are normally met by an increase in absorption and absence of menstruation. Good maternal iron stores and a good dietary intake are needed throughout pregnancy. Lean red meat, chicken to a lesser extent, and fish are the best sources. Iron from animal sources is better absorbed than that from green vegetables, fortified breakfast cereals, bread, pulses, and dried fruit. Vitamin C helps the absorption of iron if taken at the same time.

Zinc

Zinc is involved in over 200 enzyme reactions in the body, including a key role in stabilizing the structure of DNA and RNA, therefore in conjunction with folic acid it helps to prevent neural tube defects. It is also an important mineral for fertility in both men and women. Although zinc is widespread in many foods it may be deficient in some diets due to a high consumption of highly processed foods.

Essential fatty acids

Essential fatty acids are particularly important during periods of rapid fetal brain growth and in early neonatal life. During pregnancy they are responsible for the production of prostaglandins and steroid hormones. Dietary sources include vegetable oils, oily fish (mackerel, tuna, and sardines) and lean red meat.

Vitamin D

Vitamin D is produced within the skin in response to sunlight. The majority of women have no difficulty in maintaining their own vitamin D levels but for vulnerable groups which include women whose cultural practices include covering the head and body, vitamin D synthesis may be reduced. For these women a 10micrograms/day supplement is recommended.

Vitamin B$_{12}$

Vitamin B$_{12}$ stores are not usually depleted as a result of pregnancy and lactation, but they can be impaired in vegetarians as vitamin B$_{12}$ is exclusively of animal origin. Vitamin B$_{12}$ levels can be maintained by consuming fortified products such as Marmite®, breakfast cereals, and soya products.

1 Department of Health (1991). *Report on Health and Social Subjects 41. Dietary Reference Values for Food Energy and Nutrients for the United Kingdom. Dietary reference values for the United Kingdom.* London: HMSO.

Weight gain in pregnancy and body mass index

Weight gain during pregnancy is extremely variable and can be influenced by factors such as maternal age, parity, BMR, diet, smoking, pre-pregnancy weight, size of the fetus, and maternal illness such as diabetes. The weight gain is distributed between the fetus, placenta, membranes, amniotic fluid, and the physiological development of maternal organs, e.g. uterus and breasts (blood and fat deposition in preparation for lactation). Most healthy women in the UK gain between 11 and 16kg, although young mothers and primigravidae usually gain more than older mothers and multigravidae.[1]

An optimal weight gain of 12.5kg is the figure used for an average pregnancy. This is associated with the lowest risk of complications during pregnancy and labour and of low birthweight babies.[2] Maternal weight gain tends to be more rapid from 20 weeks onwards, although excessive weight gain during pregnancy is associated with postpartum weight retention, as is increased weight gain in early pregnancy compared with late pregnancy. Weight gains above 12.5kg in women of normal pre-pregnancy BMI are unlikely to reflect an increase in fetal weight, maternal lean tissue, or water.

Perinatal outcome has a complex relationship with maternal pre-pregnancy BMI, as well as with antenatal weight gain. Calculating the BMI is a method of estimating the amount of body fat, based on weight and height. The index is calculated by dividing the individual's weight in kilograms by the square of his or her height in metres. Many charts are available for instant grading (Table 5.1).

Table 5.1 Grading of weight by BMI

BMI	Interpretation
<20	Underweight
20–24.9	Desirable
25–29.9	Overweight
>30	Obese

Appropriate weight gain for individual women should be based on their pre-pregnancy BMI (Table 5.2), as lower perinatal mortality rates are associated with underweight women who achieve high weight gains and overweight women who achieve low gains. The number of women in the obese category of BMI is escalating and rapidly becoming a major public health problem within maternity care.[3] Maternal and perinatal complications are much more prevalent, such as an increased risk of gestational diabetes, pre-eclampsia, macrosomia, and perinatal mortality.[3,4]

Table 5.2 Weight gain in pregnancy and BMI

Pre-pregnancy body mass index [weight (kg)/height (m^2)]	Recommended weight gain	
	kg	lb
Low (<19.8)	12.5–18.0	28–40
Normal (19.8–26)	11.5–16.0	25–35
High (26.0–29.0)	7–11.5	15–25
Obese (>29)[1]	6 (min.)	14 (max.)

Recommended reading

Webster-Gandy J, Madden A, Holdsworth M (2006). *Oxford Handbook of Nutrition and Dietetics*. Oxford: Oxford University Press.

1 Hytten FE (1991). Weight gain in pregnancy. In Hytten FE and Chamberlain G (eds) *Clinical Pathology in Obstetrics*. London, Blackwell Scientific: 173–203.

2 Goldberg GR (2000). Nutrition in pregnancy. *Advisa Medica*, London, **1**(2): 1–3.

3 Veerareddy S, Khalil A, O'Brien P (2009). Obesity implications for labour and the puerperium. *British Journal of Midwifery*, **17**(6): 360–362.

4 Stewart FM, Ramsay JE, Greer IA (2009). Obesity: impact on obstetric practice and outcome. *Obstetrician and Gynaecologist*, **11**(1): 25–31.

Food safety

Listeriosis

Listeria monocytogenes is a Gram-positive bacterium that is normally found in soil and water, on plants, and in sewage. The incidence of listeriosis in adults is 0.5:100 000 and the mortality rate is about 26% in vulnerable groups such as babies, the elderly, immunocompromised individuals (such as those with acquired immune deficiency syndrome (AIDS)), and during pregnancy. Infection is usually asymptomatic in healthy adults.

Currently it is thought to affect approximately 1 in 20 000 pregnancies and, due to the suppressed immune response in pregnancy, the bacteria can cross the placenta. Infection during pregnancy is serious and can lead to spontaneous abortion, stillbirth, preterm labour, congenital infection, or infection after birth. Affected babies often develop pneumonia, septicaemia, or meningitis, depending on when the infection occurred. Case studies of pregnancies complicated by listeriosis report a history of having had a flu-like illness up to 2 weeks before the onset of labour, and of eating soft French cheeses, pre-packaged salads, or pre-cooked chicken.

Advice from the Department of Health[1] for vulnerable groups includes the following:

- Avoid mould-ripened cheeses, such as Brie and Camembert, and blue-veined cheeses, such as Danish Blue or Stilton.
- Avoid meat, fish, or vegetable pâté, unless it is tinned or marked pasteurised.
- Thoroughly re-heat cook-chill foods and ready-cooked poultry.

Toxoplasmosis

Toxoplasmosis is an infection caused by the parasite *Toxoplasma gondii*, a microscopic, single-celled organism that can be found in raw and inadequately cooked/cured meat, cat faeces, the soil where cats defecate, and unpasteurized goats' milk. Infection is often asymptomatic, although if symptoms do present, they are of a mild flu-like illness. Infection produces lifelong immunity. It is predicted that 30% of people will have had toxoplasmosis by the age of 30 years.

Vulnerable groups are babies, the elderly, immunocompromised individuals, and pregnant women. The risk of vertical transmission ranges from 15% in the first trimester to 65% in the third trimester.[2] If the infection is contracted during the first trimester of pregnancy, then severe fetal damage is likely and may result in miscarriage or stillbirth. If it is contracted during the third trimester, then the risk of the fetus being infected is higher. Babies with congenital toxoplasmosis may develop encephalitis, cerebral calcification, convulsions, and chorioretinitis.

Immune status can be determined by serological screening, although routine testing in the UK is not offered, as it is predicted that 80% of women would be negative.[3] If infection during pregnancy is suspected, blood tests for antibodies will be able to detect whether the infection is recent, and amniocentesis or cordocentesis will determine whether the fetus is affected. Management may include antibiotic therapy. Termination of pregnancy may be offered when there is evidence of fetal damage or infection.

Avoiding the infection is the simplest and best way to prevent congenital toxoplasmosis; therefore the following advice should be given to pregnant women:

- Only eat well-cooked meat which has been cooked thoroughly right through (i.e. no traces of blood or pinkness).
- Avoid cured meats such as Parma ham.
- Wash hands and all cooking utensils thoroughly after preparing raw meat.
- Wash fruit and vegetables thoroughly to remove all traces of soil.
- Take care with hygiene when handling dirty cat litter. Wear rubber gloves when clearing out cat litter and wash hands and gloves afterwards. If possible, get someone else to do the job.
- Cover children's outdoor sandboxes to prevent cats from using them as litter boxes.
- Wear gloves when gardening and avoid hand-to-mouth contact. Wash hands afterwards.
- Avoid unpasteurized goats' milk or goats' milk products (although this route of transmission is rare).
- Avoid sheep that are lambing or have recently given birth.

There is no contraindication to breastfeeding by a woman who has, or is undergoing treatment for, toxoplasmosis.

Vitamin A

Vitamin A is a fat-soluble vitamin that is essential for embryogenesis, growth, and epithelial differentiation. The retinol form of vitamin A is found chiefly in dairy products such as milk, butter, cheese, and egg yolk, some fatty fish, and in the liver of farm animals and fish. Experiments in animals have shown that retinoids, but not carotenoids, can be teratogenic.[4]

A high dietary intake of vitamin A before the seventh week of pregnancy has produced an increased frequency of birth defects, including cleft lip; ventricular septal defect; multiple heart defects; transposition of the great vessels; hydrocephaly; and neural tube defects.

Retinol is given to animals as a growth promoter, and any excess is stored in the liver. Since 1990, women who are pregnant or planning a pregnancy have been advised to avoid eating liver and liver products such as pâté or liver sausage, as they contain large amounts of retinol.

Vitamin A deficiency is largely a problem of developing countries, and is relatively uncommon in the developed world in the absence of disease. In the UK, the reference nutrient intake (RNI) is 600micrograms/day, with a 100micrograms/day increase during pregnancy.[5] Most women in the UK have a vitamin A intake in excess of the RNI.

Cod liver oil supplements may contain large amounts of vitamin A and should not be taken during pregnancy, except on medical advice.

Caffeine

Caffeine is a methyl xanthine, a naturally occurring compound found in plants. It is present in tea, coffee, and chocolate, and acts as a stimulant. It is also added to some soft drinks and so-called 'energy' drinks, as well as over-the-counter anti-emetics and analgesics.[6] In pregnant women it is metabolized more slowly, and studies have suggested an association between the ingestion of caffeine and an increased risk of spontaneous abortion.[7] During breastfeeding an excessive intake can cause irritability and sleeplessness in both the mother and the baby.

The Committee on Toxicity of Chemicals in Food, Consumer Products and the Environment looked at the effects of caffeine on reproduction, and concluded that caffeine intakes above 200mg/day may be associated with low birthweight and, in some cases, miscarriage. Therefore, the Food Standards Agency[8] has issued advice to pregnant women to limit their intake of caffeine to less than the equivalent of two mugs of coffee a day.

It is not necessary for women to cut out caffeine in the diet completely, but it is important that they are aware of the risks, so they can ensure that they do not have more than the recommended amount. 200mg of caffeine is roughly equivalent to:

- 2 mugs of instant coffee (100mg each)
- 2½ cups of instant coffee (75mg each)
- 2 cups of brewed coffee (100mg each)
- 4 cups of tea (50mg each)
- 3 cans of cola (up to 80mg each)
- 4 (50g) bars of chocolate (up to 50mg each).

1 Food Standards Agency (2007). *Your questions answered: listeriosis.* Available at: ℘ www.food.gov.uk/multimedia/faq/anchorcatering (accessed 3 November 2009).

2 Tommy's The Baby Charity (2001). *Toxoplasmosis: A Hand Book for Health Professionals.* London: Tommy's. Available at: ℘ www.tommys-campaign.org/problems/ToxoAcquired.pdf (accessed 2.3.10).

3 Elsheikha HM (2008). Congenital toxoplasmosis: priorities for further health promotion action. *Public Health* **122**(4), 335–53.

4 Azais-Braesco V, Pascal G (2000). Vitamin A in pregnancy: requirements and safety limits. *American Journal of Nutrition* **71**(55), 1325S–335.

5 Department of Health (1991). *Report on Health and Social Subjects 41. Dietary Reference Values for Food Energy and Nutrients for the United Kingdom. Dietary Reference Values for the United Kingdom.* London: HMSO.

6 Jordan S (2002). *Pharmacology for Midwives The Evidence Base for Safe Practice.* Hampshire: Palgrave, p. 18.

7 Cnattingius S, Signorello LB, Anneren G, *et al.* (2000). Caffeine intake and the risk of first-trimester spontaneous abortion. *New England Journal of Medicine* **343**(25), 1839–45.

8 Food Standards Agency (2008). *Advice for Pregnant Women on Caffeine Consumption.* London: FSA. Available at: ℘ www.food.gov.uk/news/pressreleases/2008/nov/caffeineadvice (accessed 3 November 2009).

Folic acid

Folic acid is a water-soluble B vitamin that is necessary for DNA synthesis and has a key role in cell division and development. Folates are folic acid derivatives found naturally in foods. The richest sources are leafy green vegetables, potatoes, and other vegetables and pulses. Liver is one of the richest sources of folate but should not be consumed in pregnancy due to high levels of vitamin A (see Food safety, p. 88). A diet that is rich in other B vitamins and vitamin C is usually rich in folates. Folates are rapidly destroyed by heat and dissolve readily in water, therefore considerable losses can occur during cooking, keeping foods warm, and prolonged storage. Deficiency of folate can result in a megaloblastic or macrocytic anaemia, either through inadequate intake, malabsorption, or increased requirements, as in pregnancy or drug treatments with anticonvulsants and oral contraceptives. Requirements are increased in pregnancy due to increased cell turnover, and are particularly important around the time of conception and during early pregnancy.

The RNI for folate is 200micrograms/day for both males and females from the age of 11 years onwards. The Expert Advisory Group on Folic Acid and Neural Tube Defects (NTDs)[1] recommended that to reduce the risk of first occurrence of NTDs, women should increase their daily folate and folic acid intake by an additional 400micrograms (making a total of 600micrograms/day) prior to conception, or from the time they stop using contraception, and during the first 12 weeks of pregnancy. This can be achieved by:

- Eating more folate-rich foods
- Eating more fortified foods, such as bread and breakfast cereals
- Taking a daily folic acid supplement of 400micrograms.

These 400micrograms supplements are available on prescription, and are easily obtainable from pharmacies and health food shops. For women who have had a previously affected baby, a 5mg supplement is prescribed.

Some countries, for example the USA, have introduced mandatory fortification of flour used in food production with folic acid, in an effort to reduce the risk of NTDs even further. Such a strategy has been widely debated in the UK, but so far has been rejected on the grounds of masking the symptoms of vitamin B_{12} deficiency, issues for older people, technical aspects, and consumer choice.

1 Department of Health (1992). *Folic Acid and the Prevention of Neural Tube Defects: Report from an Expert Advisory Group.* London: DH.

Iron

Iron (Fe) is an essential mineral that has several important functions in the body. As an important component of the proteins haemoglobin and myoglobin, it carries oxygen to the tissues from the lungs; it is also a necessary component of some enzyme reactions. It is stored in the body in the form of the protein ferritin and haemosiderin; the amount of ferritin in serum is a useful indictor of body iron stores. Transferrin is an important protein involved in transporting iron within the body and delivering it to cells.

About 0.5–1mg/day is shed from the body in urine, faeces, sweat, and cells shed from the skin and gastrointestinal tract. High menstrual losses and increased requirements of pregnancy contribute to the higher incidence of iron deficiency in women of reproductive age. The body usually maintains iron balance by controlling the amount of iron absorbed from food.

There are two forms of iron in the diet: haem iron and non-haem iron. Haem iron in meat, fish, and poultry is absorbed very efficiently; this is not influenced by iron status. Non-haem iron, in cereals and pulses, is not as well absorbed as haem iron, but absorption is influenced by iron status and several other dietary factors. Approximately 10–15% of dietary iron is absorbed. Iron absorption follows a log linear response, in that when iron stores are high, absorption decreases, protecting against iron overload, and conversely, absorption increases when iron stores are low. Absorption is favoured by factors such as the acidity of the stomach, which maintains iron in a soluble form in the upper gut (in the ferrous form, Fe^{2+}, rather than the ferric form, Fe^{3+}). Non-haem iron absorption is improved significantly when meat proteins and vitamin C are present in the diet. Factors that can significantly inhibit iron absorption include calcium, phenolic compounds in tea, coffee, cocoa and some herbs, phytates in seeds, nuts, vegetables and fruit, and soya protein.

Demand for iron is increased during pregnancy because of the increased RBC mass and fetal growth. The need for iron is minimal in the first trimester but increases throughout pregnancy, with a substantial increase during the third trimester. The absence of menstruation, body stores, and increased absorption are believed to compensate for the increased demand.[1] Routine iron supplementation is no longer advocated, but supplementation may be necessary for women with low levels at the beginning of pregnancy.[2]

Iron deficiency results in a microcytic anaemia, and maternal anaemia during pregnancy is associated with an increased risk of preterm delivery.[3] The physiological changes in plasma volume and RBC mass make measurements of haemoglobin concentration unreliable in pregnancy; therefore, for the purposes of screening, serum ferritin is the best single indicator of storage iron, provided a cut-off point of 30micrograms/L is used.[4]

Recommended reading

Evans M (2008). Iron deficiency through the female life cycle—who should care? *MIDIRS Midwifery Digest* **18**(37), 404–8.

Webster-Gandy J, Madden A, Holdsworth M (2006). *Oxford Handbook of Nutrition and Dietetics.* Oxford: Oxford University Press.

1 Expert Group on Vitamins and Minerals (2003). *Risk Assessment Iron.* Available at: ⁂ www.food. gov.uk/multimedia/pdfs/evm_iron.pdf (accessed 4 August 2004).

2 Department of Health (1991). *Dietary Reference Values for Food Energy and Nutrients for the United Kingdom.* Report on health and social subjects 41. London: HMSO.

3 Scholl T, Reilly T (2000). Anemia, iron and pregnancy outcome. *Journal of Nutrition* **130**, 443S–7S.

4 Van den Broek NR, Letsky EA, White, SA Shenkin A (1998). Iron status in pregnant women: which measurements are valid? *British Journal Haematology* **103**(3), 817–24.

Peanut allergy

Peanut allergy is a serious adverse reaction to the proteins found in peanuts. The symptoms of peanut allergy vary from a mild, itchy rash or tingling around the mouth, to a severe, life-threatening situation that can include breathing difficulties and collapse. The number of individuals affected with peanut allergy is increasing, and it is suggested that the prevalence is around 1:200. Peanut allergy appears to be a lifelong condition, although the severity and nature of the symptoms may change, and approximately 25% of children with peanut allergy will grow out of it.

Peanuts (also called groundnuts or monkey nuts) are classified as a vegetable as they belong to the legume family (and are thus related to peas, beans, and lentils). They were introduced into the UK around the time of the Second World War and are now used in the manufacture of a wide range of foods. Cooking or roasting peanuts does not alter the allergenicity of these proteins, therefore both fresh and roasted peanuts may evoke a reaction. Many people have multiple allergies, therefore reactions to other legume proteins may occur, although this is less common. However, individuals allergic to peanuts do react more commonly to tree nuts, such as brazil, almond, and hazel.

The development of allergy or allergic disease is hereditary and known to occur more commonly in people who have other atopic conditions, such as eczema, asthma, or hay fever, or who have at least one close relative with such conditions.

Pregnancy, breastfeeding, and weaning

Although the research is inconclusive, it has been suggested that sensitization can occur *in utero* or through breastfeeding, as peanut protein has been detected in breast milk. However, the Department of Health's Committee on Toxicity of Chemicals in Food, Consumer Products and the Environment has recently completed a review and has concluded that there is no evidence that eating or refraining from eating peanuts has any bearing on a child acquiring peanut allergy. Therefore the revised advice is as follows:[1]

- Pregnant or breastfeeding women who wish to consume peanuts as part of a healthy diet may do so irrespective of any family history of allergies.[1]
- There is no reason for pregnant or nursing mothers who do not fall into this category to avoid eating peanuts, unless they themselves have a peanut allergy.
- The Department of Health recommends that all infants be exclusively breastfed for 6months. If a mother decides to introduce solid food before this time she should avoid peanuts or other allergic-type foods such as nuts, seeds, milk, eggs, wheat, and fish. When introduced, these foods should be given one at a time so that any allergic reaction is more easily identified.[2]

- If an infant has a known allergy or has been diagnosed with conditions such as eczema or there is a history of peanut allergy in the immediate family, the risk of developing an allergy is higher. For these infants it is advised that parents consult their GP or health visitor before giving peanuts or peanut-containing foods to their baby for the first time. There is no evidence to suggest that avoiding peanut consumption until 3 years of age will prevent peanut allergy.[1,2]

1 Department of Health (2009). *Revised Government Advice on Consumption of Peanut During Pregnancy, Breastfeeding and Early Life and Development of Peanut Allergy.* London: DH.

2 Committee on Toxicity (2009). *Statement on the Review of the 1998 COT Recommendations on Peanut Avoidance.* London: Food Standards Agency. Available at: http://cot.food.gov.uk/cotstatements/cotstatementsyrs/cotstatements2008/cot200807peanut (accessed 2.3.11).

Exercise

There are many benefits to be gained from taking exercise such as brisk walking, swimming, and gentle aerobic exercise during pregnancy:

- A more positive, healthy outlook during pregnancy.
- Greater ability to cope with the discomforts of pregnancy and labour.
- Less need for induction of labour, epidural analgesia, and caesarean section.
- The improvement in muscle tone, strength, and endurance resulting from regular exercise can prepare the woman for the physical stresses of labour and caring for the baby afterwards.
- After delivery, regaining the normal pre-pregnancy weight is easier.

Limiting factors

Certain situations that arise in pregnancy may limit the amount of exercise it is safe to take, or may make exercise contraindicated. The woman should seek medical advice prior to exercising if she has any of the following:

- Preterm rupture of the membranes
- Pregnancy-induced hypertension
- Antepartum haemorrhage
- History of premature labour or several miscarriages
- Muscle or joint problems
- Multiple pregnancy
- Low back pain
- Medical conditions, such as existing heart disease.

Advice

Provided there are no other problems and the woman is otherwise healthy, the following advice should be given regarding safe exercise during pregnancy.

For women who are used to regular exercise

- Drink water before, during, and after exercise.
- Do not undertake any exercise that results in becoming overheated. The fetus does not cool down as quickly as the mother and its oxygen requirements remain raised for longer.
- Start exercise gradually, as the body rapidly shifts oxygen and energy towards the working muscles. Lower the intensity of aerobic exercise and monitor her heart rate regularly throughout the exercise period.
- Avoid any exercise causing loss of balance and sports with a high risk of falling. Avoid bouncing and jerking movements and deep knee bends that put a strain on the hip and leg joints
- Stop immediately if any exercise causes dizziness, faintness, shortness of breath, nausea, contractions, vaginal bleeding, or fluid leakage.

If the mother is new to regular exercise

- Start very slowly, with a 10–15min period of gentle exercise.
- Gradually increase this to 30min as she becomes more familiar with the routine.

Most gyms and fitness clubs have trained attendants who can devise a programme for the pregnant and newly postnatal woman. It is safe to exercise for 30–40min, three times per week.

Employment

Many women want to continue to work during their pregnancy and there is legal protection for women who wish to do so.

A woman is not legally obliged to inform her employer of her pregnancy until she gives notice of the date she intends to start her maternity leave. That notification must be given by 15 weeks before the expected week of childbirth at the latest, i.e. when the woman is approximately 6 months pregnant.

It is advisable for the woman to inform her employer of her pregnancy, as she is entitled to certain rights:

- Protection under the Sex Discrimination Act against less favourable treatment
- Protection against being subjected to adverse working conditions and discrimination, or dismissed for a reason connected to pregnancy
- A right to paid time off for antenatal care
- Protection against being treated less favourably for taking time off for antenatal care
- A right to health and safety protection.

These rights are important, as adverse working conditions can affect the health of the mother and fetus.

There is a significant association between preterm births, small for gestational age infants, maternal hypertension, pre-eclampsia, and working conditions.

Advise women who work during pregnancy that the following may limit their ability to stay at work for the full pregnancy, unless their employer can rearrange their workload or responsibilities:

- Physically demanding work
- Long working hours
- Shift work
- Prolonged standing
- Heavy or repetitive lifting.

All employees are entitled to 52 weeks maternity leave regardless of length of service or number of hours worked. Maternity leave is divided into 26 weeks ordinary maternity leave and 26 weeks additional maternity leave. Factsheets are available from Working Families (℡ www.workingfamilies.org.uk).

Sexuality during pregnancy and beyond

Sexuality is one of the most difficult areas of human experience to define, as it is complex, varied, and contradictory. Defined simply, it is a person's capacity for sexual feelings, and childbirth is intrinsically linked with a woman's sexuality and sexual health. The changes that occur during pregnancy, childbirth, and the transition to motherhood are some of the most fundamental changes that a woman will encounter. Pregnancy is a normal life event that involves considerable adjustment by both the woman and her partner. A first pregnancy will bring the greatest changes. There are many contradictory and confusing aspects of pregnancy and sexuality, and it is a time surrounded by myths and misconceptions. It is the role of the midwife to dispel these myths and to provide sensitive support and information for the woman at all stages of pregnancy and childbirth.

Sexuality and pregnancy

How pregnancy affects sexuality will vary considerably from woman to woman. Women will be affected differently by physical and psychological changes that occur in pregnancy, as well as how they view their changing body image. Sexual desire may vary during pregnancy; it may decrease, increase, or remain unaltered, depending upon the stage of pregnancy and also upon other factors, which may include:
• Whether the pregnancy was planned or unplanned
• Whether the pregnancy was conceived naturally or with fertility treatment
• The response of others to the pregnancy
• Fears associated with pregnancy, e.g. harming the baby
• Stress, e.g. related to work, finances, etc.
• The woman's health and how tired she feels
• Her relationship with her partner.

Sexual intercourse is usually safe in pregnancy, provided both partners desire it and it does not cause discomfort. Sexual intercourse should be avoided in the relevant stage of pregnancy if there is:
• A history of recurrent miscarriages
• Vaginal bleeding
• Placenta praevia
• Premature dilation of the cervix
• Rupture of the membranes
• History of premature labour.

Some women may find penetrative sex uncomfortable during pregnancy and this could be due to any of the following physical factors:
• Pelvic vaso-congestion: pelvic floor exercises may help relieve this.
• Vaginal congestion and reduced lubrication: lubricants may help.
• Retroverted uterus: particularly in the first few week of pregnancy.
• Subluxation of the symphysis pubis and sacro-iliac joints.
• Weight of the partner on a gravid uterus later in pregnancy: alternative positions may be adopted.
• Deep engagement of the fetal head.
• Infections of the genital area: candida, *Trichomonas vaginalis*, genital herpes, or warts.

Psychosocial factors may include tiredness, anxiety and fear, low self-esteem, poor body image, sexual guilt, interpersonal problems between the woman and her partner.

Sexuality and labour

Some of the procedures and examinations performed during labour involve the exposure of the genital area and penetrative vaginal examination by either hand or a speculum. Many women find this very disturbing and difficult to cope with, not only because of the associated physical discomfort but also because of psychological feelings of vulnerability and powerlessness. This is especially relevant to women who have been sexually abused. There is an increased need for awareness of these factors by midwives and doctors, who often perform these examinations in a ritualistic manner and often without a sound rationale.

Obstetric procedures, including artificial rupture of the membranes, episiotomies, instrumental deliveries, and caesarean sections can also have a profound effect on a woman's sexuality. Many women find these procedures traumatic and they can have long-term consequences for sexual relationships.

The experience of seeing their partner in childbirth can affect men's sexuality. It can be a very powerful and overwhelming experience, which will bond the couple together, but it may also be a traumatic experience. The man may feel responsible for the pain and procedures his partner may be undergoing, or his reaction could be linked with feelings of inadequacy and powerlessness. In extreme cases this experience has been known to cause impotency.

Midwives and obstetricians need to be aware of the implications of obstetric procedures and the traumatic effects it can have on the lives of couples who have been in their care.

Sexuality postnatally

Sexuality following childbirth is a much neglected area that is inadequately addressed by many midwives and health professionals. Sexual behaviour and sexual health of women following childbirth has been shown to be influenced by profound psychological, interpersonal, social, and physical factors.[1] Many women are anxious about their bodies following the birth of a child and this is linked to perineal pain, soreness, and a decreased sense of attractiveness. Sexual activity and enjoyment following childbirth is usually diminished for up to 1 year.

Resuming sexual relations

There is no set time when to resume sexual intercourse. It is more important that it is the right time for both of the partners. It is advisable to wait 3 weeks before having penetrative sex. It is important to avoid deliberately blowing air into the vagina during oral sex during pregnancy and in the weeks following birth, as this may cause an air embolism. Contraception needs consideration before resuming sexual intercourse, as the woman will ovulate prior to menstruating. Some women will experience dyspareunia for a while following childbirth but if this does not resolve, they should be referred for medical advice.

Common causes of postnatal dyspareunia include:
- Decreased vaginal lubrication, either associated with breastfeeding or diminished sexual arousal
- Inflammation and infection
- Contracture and scaring of the perineum
- Sensitive hymenal or skin tags through malalignment of perineal repair.

Breastfeeding and sexuality

Women who breastfeed may find that they and their partners have a diminished sexual desire, while others may find it enhanced. The physiological and psychological experiences associated with breastfeeding may reduce sexual libido for the woman and also reduce vaginal lubrication. Tenderness of the breasts and leakage of milk may inhibit women from sexual activity while some men may find it off-putting.

It is normal for some women to feel sexual arousal while breastfeeding, this is a response to the oxytocin increase during breastfeeding.[2] Mothers will need reassurance as it may engender feelings of guilt and anxiety in the woman.

Many women will not menstruate while exclusively breastfeeding. Menstruation returns when the number of night-feeds decline or when the baby begins to have solid foods and breastfeeding is less frequent. Ovulation will occur before menstruation returns and the mother needs to ensure adequate contraception if another pregnancy is to be avoided.

Maternity care for lesbian mothers

When considering sexuality in relation to childbirth, it is important to acknowledge that some mothers are choosing to have babies outside of a heterosexual relationship and some will have a female partner. Many lesbian women have negative healthcare experiences and therefore it is important that midwives provide support and information in a non-judgmental, sensitive woman-centred approach that takes into to consideration the individual mother's needs. Specific considerations are:[3]
- Disclosure of sexual orientation should be confidential and not recorded in the notes
- Other health professionals should not be informed without the woman's expressed consent
- Provision of information should be appropriate to their needs
- The lesbian partners should be acknowledged as a couple and co-parents
- Creation of an atmosphere that acknowledges sexual diversity.

1 De Judicibus MA, McCabe MP (2002). Psychological factors and the sexuality of pregnant and postpartum women. *Journal of Sex Research* **39**(2), 94–103.

2 Convery KM (2009). Sexuality and breastfeeding: What do you know? *American Journal of Maternal/Child Nursing* **34**(4), 218–23.

3 Royal College of Midwives (2000). *Position Paper 22: Maternity Care for Lesbian Mothers.* Reviewed 2005. London: RCM.

Dealing with disability during pregnancy and beyond

Increasing numbers of women with disability are becoming users of maternity services, as they seek to live full and independent lives.[1] Often, simple measures can be taken by the midwife to enhance these women's experiences of maternity services. The Disability Discrimination Act, related to 'Access to goods, facilities and services', came into force in December 1996, making it unlawful for service providers to discriminate against people with disabilities by:

- Offering a lower standard of services
- Offering less favourable terms
- Failing to make alterations to enable disabled access
- This includes all hospitals and healthcare facilities.

Who are the disabled?

The World Health Organization has defined disability as: 'a restriction or inability to perform an activity in the manner or within the range considered normal for a human being, mostly resulting from impairment'.[2]

However, the definition of disability varies widely between different social groups and cultures, as do the meanings which are attached to a person being labelled as disabled.[3] In the UK it is very difficult to measure the number of disabled because, although local authorities must keep a record, disabled individuals are not required to register. Disability is also very subjective; not all people with impairments see themselves as disabled.

The problem is one of society, not of disabled people themselves. Disability is the result of:

- Stereotyping
- Discrimination
- Disadvantage
- Social exclusion.

Disability, sexuality, and pregnancy

- That disabled women might have sexual desires, have sex, or reproduce has provoked dispute.[4]
- Sexual performance for the disabled has been defined as a medical problem.[4]
- The disabled are capable of being, and entitled to become, parents.[5]

Women with disabilities are expected to forego mothering in the interest of the child, as some fears exist that:

- The disability will be handed on to the child
- The child will be psychologically harmed
- The child will be deprived
- The child will be burdened.

Disability and the midwifery services

Disabled women have reported the following difficulties encountered with maternity services:

- Lack of physical access

- Lack of accurate information about pregnancy and childbirth, especially in relation to their disability
- Lack of effective communication
- Ignorance of maternity professionals about both the medical and practical needs of disabled mothers
- Inflexibility in maternity services
- Language and attitudes which reflect prejudice
- Doubts about a disabled woman's ability to cope with motherhood
- Staff who do not respect a disabled woman's own knowledge of her disability[6]
- Negative attitudes from health professionals.[7]
  The RCM[8] supports the principle that:

'It is important that services reflect the needs of women who have disabilities and ensure that action is taken to overcome the obstacles which confront them. While physical obstructions are of course a frustrating problem, there are other equally daunting barriers resulting from prejudice and ignorance of able bodied professionals.'

Midwives and disabilities

Midwives must be aware of their own values and attitudes regarding the rights and responsibilities of childbearing.

Midwives have the potential to strengthen a woman in her ability to give birth and to be a parent in a society that may not be 100% supportive of her decision to do so.[7]

However, midwives have expressed concerns that:

- They do not always feel equipped to do this.
- There is a lack of a coordinated approach by health professionals and health authorities.
- Little is known about available information and resources.
- They are unsure about alternative support agencies.
- They feel that service provision is preventive rather than reactive.

General recommendations for practice

- Provide services in settings that are architecturally/physically accessible.
- Provide services that are psychologically accessible.
- Provide pre-conceptual care to assist the woman and her family prior to the decision to become pregnant.
- Provide pregnancy care that is sensitive, based on thorough assessment of physical and psychosocial needs, and well planned.
- One-to-one care and continuity are important.
- Plan for the special needs of labour and birth.
- Assist the mother to organize for the many needs of the postpartum period.[7]

Sensory impairment

Recommendations for women with visual impairment

- One-to-one care and continuity are important.
- Tactile models are helpful when describing aspects of the childbirth process, e.g. doll and pelvis, knitted uterus, cervical dilation chart which has holes representing the different stages of dilation.

- Teach and encourage the woman to palpate her own abdomen, focus in on fetal movements and listen to the fetal heart. This will enable her to know her infant antenatally.
- Familiarize the woman with the hospital prior to admission. If the woman requests the presence of her guide dog, organize this well in advance.
- All healthcare workers should introduce themselves verbally by name and function.
- Give full explanations before all procedures.
- Encourage immediate skin-to-skin contact following birth, to enable the woman to know her baby.
- Perform any examination of the baby with the woman present, giving a clear explanation of the procedure.
- Describe the baby's characteristics, expressions, movements, and behaviours.[7]

Recommendations for women with hearing impairment
- Determine the way in which the woman communicates most comfortably, e.g. writing, hearing aid, lip-reading, finger spelling, sign language, or interpreter.
- Provide one-to-one care or small classes for antenatal education.
- Make it clear in the records that the woman has a hearing impairment.
- If the woman is able to lip-read, obtain her attention before speaking, face the woman, do not over-mouth words, do not stand in shadows, and do not dim the room lights.
- Be patient, repeat and rephrase as required, avoid analgesia that causes drowsiness.
- Familiarize the woman with the hospital prior to admission. Choose a quiet room.
- Watch for facial expressions during procedures, the woman may not be able to communicate discomfort or concern.
- Wear a transparent mask if one is needed.
- Provide as much written literature as is available on all aspects of care.
- Provide early screening for babies at risk of either inherited or acquired deafness.
- Ensure that application for a baby alarm is made early in the antenatal period.
- Inform mothers about the RNID book *Pregnancy and Childbirth—a guide for deaf mothers.*[9]

Women with learning disabilities and perinatal mental health disorders
Recommendations for women with learning disabilities
Most parents with learning disabilities recognize that they need extra help and support. The support may be practical, emotional, or social, and mostly likely a combination of all three. In order to provide successful support, midwives need to recognize:
- That these parents are individuals who may have many skills and abilities on which to build
- Ways in which self-confidence and self-value can be increased

- That external influences will impact on the individuals.
  When teaching parenting skills, the midwife should:
- Break a task down into smaller sections, allow time, and be prepared to repeat the same information
- Avoid using long words or jargon
- Keep to the facts, avoid using abstract concepts
- Demonstrate the task alongside the parent, the parent then can watch the task and repeat the actions
- Allow the parents to complete as much of the task as they know before reminding them what comes next
- Always repeat the same prompt and the same set of instructions
- Write down training plans explicitly, showing verbal and physical prompts and at what stage of the task they occur
- Remember that the written word is not always the most effective or the best way to impart knowledge to parents. A variety of visual or audio tapes, photographs, or drawings may be more accessible, either on their own or accompanied by simple written information.
  When using written information:
- Avoid abbreviations
- Use simple words that are not too long
- Use large print; ask if they prefer capitals
- Highlight the main points
- Use lists or bullet points where possible.

Recommendations for perinatal mental health

The term 'perinatal mental health' is a term used increasingly to relate to the various mental health disorders experienced by women during pregnancy and the postnatal period. These include a previous history of mental disorder, signs and symptoms demonstrated in the antenatal period, along with the range of disorders that appear in the postnatal period.[10] Despite the high prevalence of postnatal depression (10–15%) such disturbances often go undetected.[11]

Midwives have a crucial role in reducing the effects of perinatal mental health disorders on the mother, her child, and the family.[12] Midwives should:

- Provide continuity of care and carer whenever possible
- Carry out a modified psychiatric history during the booking interview[12]
- Be alert to the increased likelihood of a woman relapsing or developing postnatal mental illness if she has a personal or family history of a psychiatric illness and/or a postpartum illness[13]
- Liaise swiftly and appropriately with the multidisciplinary team.

If the woman has a previous history of mental disorders, antenatal assessment by a psychiatrist is essential, along with a management plan for after delivery, and access to a perinatal mental health team.

Post-traumatic stress disorder

It has been suggested[14] that 3% of women may develop post-traumatic stress disorder. Midwives should be aware of:

- The trauma a woman may experience in childbirth
- The action that health professionals can take in order to prevent its occurrence

- The factors that can contribute to post-traumatic stress disorder, including:
  - Violent birth
  - Fear for the baby
  - Postpartum pain
  - Low energy levels
  - Sexual abuse before and during pregnancy
  - Excessive vomiting in pregnancy
  - Ectopic pregnancy
  - Hospital treatment for miscarriage
  - Macrosomia
  - Episodes of preterm labour although the mother gave birth at term[15]
- Post-traumatic stress disorder can result from loss of control and a sense of powerlessness in labour, lack of trust, and inadequate information.[16]

All women should have the opportunity to discuss with their midwife the care they received during childbirth.

Referral either to a postnatal listening service or to a 'Births after thoughts' programme should be available to all mothers, where they can talk to a midwife trained in this area.

Women with physical disabilities and chronic illness

Women may present with a wide range of physical disabilities and chronic illness during pregnancy, including multiple sclerosis, spinal cord injuries, cerebral palsy, amputees, and rheumatoid arthritis, to name but a few. The general recommendations for practice identified at the start of this section should be followed, together with the following:

- Caregivers should respect the woman as the primary source of information about how to proceed with care.
- Women with disabilities are very aware of their abilities and limitations, and all care should be discussed fully with them and their partners.
- Assist the woman to focus on her abilities and not her disabilities.
- Women with chronic illnesses will require information about the effect of their illness and drug therapy on the pregnancy, birth, postpartum period, and the newborn, as well as the possible effects of the pregnancy upon their condition.
- A multidisciplinary approach to care must be adopted to include the midwife, the obstetrician, the woman's disability and/or medical consultant, the physiotherapist and occupational therapist, etc.
- Help the woman to manage her own care regimes as much as possible.
- Take extra care to prevent skin breakdown if mobility is restricted.[7]

1 Fraser DM, Cooper MA (2009). *Myles: Textbook for Midwives*. Edinburgh: Churchill Livingstone.

2 World Health Organization (2001). Prevalence of impairments, disabilities, handicaps and quality of life in the general population: a review of recent literature. *Bulletin of the World Health Organisation* **79**(11), 1047–1055.

3 Helman CG (2007). *Culture, Health and Illness*, 5th edn. London: Arnold.

4 Kent J (2000). *Social Perspectives on Pregnancy and Childbirth for Midwives, Nurses and the Caring Professions*. Buckingham: Open University Press.

5 Thomas C (1998). Becoming a mother: Disabled women (can) do it too. *MIDIRS Midwifery Digest* **8**(3), 275–8.

6 Campion MK (1997). Disabled women and maternity services. *Modern Midwife* **7**(3), 23–5.

7 Carty E (1995). Disability, pregnancy and parenting. In: Alexander J, Levy V, Roch S (eds) *Aspects of Midwifery Practice: A Research Based Aapproach*. Basingstoke: Macmillan Press, pp. 571–4.

8 Royal College of Midwives (2000). *Maternity Care for Women with Disabilities*. Position Paper number 11a (reviewed 2005). London: RCM.

9 RNID (2004). *Pregnancy and Birth—A Guide for Deaf Women*. Peterborough: RNID in association with NCT.

10 Stewart C, Henshaw C (2002). Midwives and perinatal mental health. *British Journal of Midwifery* **10**(2), 117–21.

11 Cooper PJ, Murray L (1997). *Postpartum Depression and Child Development*. London: Guilford Press.

12 Lewis G (ed.) (2007). *The Confidential Enquiry into Maternal and Child Health (CEMACH). Saving Mothers' Live; Reviewing Maternal Deaths to Make Motherhood Safer—2003–2005*. The 7th Report on Confidential Enquires into Maternal Deaths in the United Kingdom. London: CEMACH.

13 Bates C, Paeglis C (2004). Motherhood and mental illness. *Midwives* **7**(7), 286–7.

14 Ayers S, Pickering AD (2001). Do women get post-traumatic stress disorder as a result of childbirth? *Birth* **28**, 630–63.

15 Seng JS, Oakley DJ, Sampselle CM, Killion C, Graham-Bermann S, Liberzon I (2001). Post-traumatic stress disorder and pregnancy complications. *Obstetrics and Gynaecology* **97**, 17–22.

16 Laing KG (2001). Post-traumatic stress disorder: myth or reality? *British Journal of Midwifery* **9**(7), 447–51.

Chapter 6

Minor disorders of pregnancy

Introduction

Minor disorders of pregnancy are a series of commonly experienced symptoms related to the effects of pregnancy hormones and the consequences of enlargement of the uterus as the fetus grows during pregnancy.

The conditions themselves pose no serious risk to the mother, but they are unpleasant and can affect her enjoyment of the pregnancy overall.

Close questioning of the mother is necessary to ascertain that the symptoms are not masking a more serious problem, and a sympathetic and helpful approach with prompt advice and treatment is needed.

Backache

Up to 90% of women may experience backache during their pregnancy making this the most common of the minor disorders of pregnancy. Obesity, a history of back problems, and greater parity increase the likelihood of backache occurring.

- During pregnancy ligaments become softer under the influence of the relaxin and stretch to prepare the body for labour.
- This is particularly focused on the pelvic joints and ligaments which become more supple to accommodate the baby at delivery.
- The effects can put a strain on the joints of the lower back and pelvis, which can cause backache.
- As the baby grows, the curve in the lumbar spine may increase as the abdomen is thrust forward and this may also cause backache.

The following advice can be given to the woman to alleviate backache:

- Avoid heavy lifting and use a good lifting technique, bending the knees and keeping the back straight when lifting or picking something up from the floor. The woman should take care when picking up a heavy older child.
- Heavy weights should be held close to the body.
- Any working surface used should be high enough to prevent stooping.
- When carrying loads such as shopping the weight should be equally balanced on both sides of the body.
- The woman can be shown how to sit and stand with her spine in a neutral position so that good posture is maintained.
- A firmer mattress gives better support during sleep. Using a bed board can make a soft mattress more supportive.
- Some women find relief from using pillows to support their pregnant abdomen while lying down.[1]
- Rest as much as possible as the pregnancy progresses.

If the backache is very painful and debilitating the woman can be referred to an obstetric physiotherapist for advice on lumbar support and helpful exercises.

---

1 Pennick V, Young G (2007). Interventions for preventing and treating pelvic and back pain in pregnancy. *Cochrane Database of Systematic Reviews* **2**, CD001139.

Constipation

Increased progesterone levels decrease gastrointestinal movement during pregnancy. A recent systematic review reported two studies, which showed that fibre supplements in the form of bran or wheat fibre increased the frequency of defecation and led to softer stools. It appeared that stimulant laxatives were more effective than bulk-forming laxatives, but may have caused more side-effects.[1]

Women who were constipated prior to pregnancy may find that this condition becomes more problematic when they become pregnant.

It may be due to displacement of the bowel by the growing uterus or a side-effect of oral iron therapy.

If possible, it is best to try to relieve constipation by natural means before resorting to medication during pregnancy, and the advice given by the midwife should reflect this.

Advice should include:
- Eating regular meals.
- Drinking extra water, fruit juice, or herbal tea. This should be up to 2L of fluid per day, more in hot weather.
- Eating five portions of fruit and vegetables per day.
- Eating foods containing a high fibre content, such as wholemeal bread, breakfast cereals, and prunes.
- Taking gentle exercise, 20–30min, three times per week.

A mild laxative, such as lactulose (15mL twice a day), may be prescribed if the above advice does not relieve the symptoms.

1 Jewell DJ, Young G (2007). Interventions for treating constipation in pregnancy. *Cochrane Database of Systematic Reviews* **2**, CD001142.

Frequency of micturition

Around 60% of women develop frequency of micturition early in pregnancy. This appears to be a more common symptom for nulliparas. The urgent need to empty the bladder, even small amounts, throughout the day and night is caused by pressure from the enlarging uterus on the bladder.

- Reassure women that this is normal as urine production in the kidney increases during pregnancy
- This generally improves by the 14th week as the uterus grows out of the pelvis
- Advise them not to drink a large amount before going to bed.

No treatment is needed for urinary frequency alone, but if micturition becomes painful, urinary infection should be excluded.

The symptoms may return during the last 4 weeks of pregnancy, when the presenting part enters the pelvis and creates pressure on the bladder, diminishing its overall capacity.

Pregnant women are also at risk of developing stress incontinence during pregnancy, related to physiological changes, hormonal influences and also mechanical stresses provoked by the enlarged uterus.

All pregnant women need to be taught how to perform pelvic floor exercises correctly, as improved pelvic floor tone prior to delivery can influence the return of good pelvic floor function after delivery.

- Explain how to locate the pubo-coccygeous (PC) muscle, by asking the woman to attempt to stop urine flow while urinating.
- Once the PC muscle is identified, the exercises should be carried out with an empty bladder.
- The initial exercise involves squeezing and holding the PC muscle for 3–5s, relaxing, and then repeating this until the muscle tires.
- The woman should attempt three sets of five squeezes once or twice a day for a week, then build up to three sets of 8, 10, 15, and then 20 squeezes.
- Once a routine is established, maintenance is achieved by attempting three sets four times a week.
- The exercise can be varied by including slow or rapid squeezes, and by exercising at different times of the day.

Indigestion and heartburn

During pregnancy, 30–50% of women experience indigestion or heart-burn. The discomfort is caused by acid reflux from the stomach through the oesophageal sphincter as a result of the relaxing effects of proges-terone. Later in pregnancy the growing uterus displaces the stomach, increasing intragastric pressure, which makes acid reflux more likely when lying down.

A Cochrane review[1] tried to assess the best interventions for heartburn during pregnancy. The authors were unable to draw conclusions about different treatments and recommended lifestyle changes first for mild heartburn in pregnancy women.

Advice should include:

• Eating several small meals a day
• Avoiding coffee, alcohol, and spicy foods
• Not to combine solid food with a drink, but take drinks separately from meals
• Sleeping with an extra pillow at night to raise the head and chest level above the level of the stomach
• Taking a calcium- or calcium-magnesium-based antacid to relieve symptoms
• Wearing loose clothing so that there is no undue pressure on the abdominal area.

1 Dowswell T, Neilson JP (2008). Intervention for heartburn in pregnancy. *Cochrane Database of Systematic Reviews* **4**, CD007065.

Nausea and vomiting

Nausea and vomiting are common in pregnancy, with about 80% of pregnant women experiencing anything from mild nausea on awakening, to nausea throughout the day with 50% experiencing some vomiting, during the first half of pregnancy.[1]

For many women, the symptoms subside after the 12th–14th week of pregnancy, coinciding with the ability of the placenta to take over support of the growing embryo.

The reasons for nausea are not known but it has been associated with:
- Increased levels of hCG
- Hypoglycaemia
- Increased metabolic demand
- The effects of progesterone on the digestive system.
  Advice to women should include:
- Have a few mouthfuls of something before getting up
- Have a snack ready at the bedside
- Get out of bed slowly
- Maintain a good fluid intake, and drink small amounts frequently throughout the day
- Eat little and often, every 2–3h during the day
- Have a rest in the middle of the day
- Eat plain crackers, small pieces of fruit, dry toast, or yoghurt
- Avoid alcohol, caffeine, spicy or fatty foods
- Ginger, in the form of tea or tablets, relieves nausea
- Eat a small snack before going to bed at night.
  A doctor should be consulted if:
- The woman is vomiting more than four times a day
- The above advice has not worked
- The woman is losing weight
- The woman is not keeping fluids down
- The woman requires anti-emetics
- The woman is experiencing dehydration. Hospital admission is advised for intravenous feeding, correction of electrolyte imbalance, and rehydration.

1 Annual Evidence Update on Antenatal Care (2007). *Nausea and Vomiting in Early Pregnancy.* NHS Evidence. Women's Health. Available at: ℘ www.library.nhs.uk//womenshealth/ViewResource.aspx?resID=269713 (accessed 20.3.10).

Varicose veins and haemorrhoids

Varicose veins are caused by weakening of the valves in the veins returning blood to the heart from the lower extremities, so they can occur in the legs, vulva, or rectum. Rectal varicosities are called haemorrhoids.

They can occur in any age group, but pregnant women are particularly prone if they have a family history of varicosities, are carrying twins, or have to sit or stand for long periods of time, for instance at work.

During pregnancy, the extra circulating blood volume increases pressure on the vessel walls and progesterone relaxes the blood vessel walls. The weight of the growing uterus creates back pressure in the pelvic and leg vessels. Constipation exacerbates haemorrhoids.

Signs and symptoms
- Legs ache and feel heavy.
- Throbbing sensation in the legs or vulva.
- Dilated surface veins in the vulva or legs.
- The vulva may be swollen and painful.
- Discomfort and itching round the anus and when opening the bowels.

Advice
- Avoid constipation and straining on the toilet.
- Ensure an adequate intake of fibre, e.g. fruit and also fluids.
- Avoid standing for prolonged periods of time.
- Wear graduated support tights to assist venous flow.
- Avoid constrictive clothing.
- Do not sit with the legs crossed.
- Take gentle exercise, such as walking, to help the circulation.
- Use vulval icepacks to reduce swelling.
- Proprietary haemorrhoid cream can be used safely during pregnancy.
- Be aware that iron supplements can cause constipation in some women and a liquid preparation may be preferable in this instance.

Teach the woman to recognize the signs and symptoms of deep vein thrombosis.

During delivery
- Promote a spontaneous normal delivery and use a non-directed pushing technique. Forceps or ventouse delivery may cause haemorrhoids to prolapse.
- Advise and encourage the woman to refrain from pushing during the second stage of labour until the vertex is visible, as this reduces straining efforts to a minimum.
- Avoid laceration to any vulval varicosities.

Chapter 7

Helping women cope with pregnancy: complementary therapies

Introduction

The use of complementary therapies (CTs) has escalated in recent years, with approximately two-thirds of the population accessing some kind of complementary therapy or treatment. This has been attributed to a change in people's expectations and choice, resulting in a desire for less dependency on drugs and invasive treatments that often involve adverse side-effects. Almost one-third of this group are pregnant women, so therefore many women choose to use CTs during pregnancy and childbirth.

It is therefore pertinent that midwives familiarize themselves with knowledge and the safety issues of CTs with regard to pregnancy and childbirth. Some midwives may choose to specialize in the use of CTs, while others will have received in-house training to use CTs in their practice. It is important that midwives encourage women to access reputable therapists who are dedicated to working with the special needs of pregnant women.

Although scientific evidence is sparse for many CTs, this is starting to change and mounting evidence from various sources worldwide is becoming established (☐ see Useful websites, p. 119). There is a plethora of anecdotal evidence that supports the safe use of CTs from European and Eastern cultures—such as Chinese medicine and herbal medicine. However, caution should always be exercised when using any form of treatment or therapy during pregnancy—expert advice is available and should be sought where there are any queries regarding the use of CTs for pregnant women (☐ see Recommended reading and Useful websites).

Some of the traditional elements of medical research make it difficult to measure some CTs where individual remedies or treatments are used e.g. homoeopathy, reflexology, acupuncture, thus the randomized clinical controlled trial is not truly evaluative, making it difficult to compare effectiveness with orthodox medicine. Qualitative research methods, case studies, surveys and audit are all useful means to explore the efficacy of CTs.

Recommended reading

Ernst E, Pittler M, Wider B (eds) (2006). *The Desktop Guide to Complementary and Alternative Medicine: An Evidence-based Approach*, 2nd edn. Edinburgh: Mosby.

Lewith G, Wayne JB, Walach H (eds) (2002). *Clinical Research in Complementary Therapies— Principles, Problems and Solutions*. London: Churchill Livingstone.

Mantle F, Tiran D (2009). *A-Z of Complementary and Alternative Medicine: A Guide for Health Professionals*. Edinburgh: Churchill Livingstone.

Miccozzi MS (2006). *Fundamentals of Complementary and Integrated Approach to Care*, 3rd edn. London: Elsevier.

Tiran D (2003). *Nausea and Vomiting in Pregnancy: An Integrated Approach to Care*. London: Elsevier.

Tiran D, Mack S (eds) (2000). *Complementary Therapies for Pregnancy and Childbirth*. Edinburgh: Churchill Livingstone.

Useful websites

Bach flower education, advice and courses: ℘ www.bachremedies.com or ℘ www.bachflowertraining.com.

Massage courses and educational site: ℘ www.childbirth-massage.co.uk.

Complementary Maternity Forum—a supportive network of midwives and complementary therapists who are dedicated to the safe use of CTs within maternity care: ℘ www.the-cma.org.uk (accessed 22.2.11).

Educational and research articles: ℘ www.essentialorc.com.

Educational Resource for Midwives and Complementary Therapists Providing Courses in CTs, Resource Materials, and Consultancy: ℘ www.expectancy.co.uk.

Books and journals on CTs: ℘ www.harcourt-international.com/journals.

International Federation of Professional Aromatherapists—the main professional organization for aromatherapy within the UK: ℘ www.ifparoma.org.

Aromatherapy Global Online Research Archives (AGORA) Index: ℘ www.users.erols.com/sisakson/pages/agoindex.htm.

Shiatsu Site—courses and consultancy for midwives and therapists: ℘ www.wellmother.org.

Natural Health website: ℘ www.winaturalhealth.com.

An excellent resource for papers and studies on complementary medicine is at: ℘ www.nccam.nih.gov/camonpubmed.

Homoeopathy

Homoeopathic remedies offer a gentle and safe alternative means of relieving some of the common ailments of pregnancy. Pregnancy is considered to be an acute state and therefore knowledgeable women may feel that they would want to self-medicate. However it is generally recommended that these women seek homoeopathic advice during pregnancy. Any pre-disposing, complex, or chronic conditions need to be treated by a qualified practitioner/midwife homeopath.

Morning sickness may well be treated with remedies that match the symptom picture of nauseous feelings in the morning, with minimal sickness or vomiting. However, women with long-term nausea and vomiting resulting in hyperemesis gravidarum would require input from a homoeopathic practitioner alongside conventional medical care.

General principles and administration

- Based on the theory of 'like cures like'—whereby matching the symptoms to the correct remedy profile is crucial.
- Tablets are taken sublingually, allowed to dissolve or chewed or sucked between meals to ensure optimum efficiency of the remedy.
- When taking homoeopathic remedies strong tastes should be avoided for at least 15min before and after taking the remedy. This applies to: smoking, alcohol, toothpaste, spicy foods, coffee, and some essential oils. These substances are said to act as an antidote to the effect of the remedies.
- Occasionally current symptoms can worsen before improvement is noted. This is usually only temporary and is an indication that the body has been stimulated into a healing response.
- Remedies should only be taken for when symptoms persist and then discontinued when they subside.
- Remedies should not be taken prophylactically
- It is safe to use homoeopathic remedies with orthodox medication, however, some drugs may have an antidoting effect. Preferably other medication should be avoided wherever possible to minimize this effect.
- Homoeopathic remedies cannot cause side effects due to the minute amount of the active substance used in their preparation.
- Homoeopathic remedies dosages come in a dilution factor—the higher the dilution the more potent the remedy. Common potencies for self-medication are 6c and 30c (centesimal = dilution of 1 part of original substance to 99 parts of dilutant). These are taken at frequent intervals until the symptoms subside. Potencies of 200c may also be used in which case only one or two doses are required.
- Homoeopathic remedies are prepared by a method of dilution and succussion (vigorous shaking) to the potency required. A 6c dilution is prepared as above followed by diluting 1 drop from the mother tincture with 99 parts of the dilutant (water and alcohol) and then succussed 100 times, this procedure is repeated another five times to arrive at a 6c (100) dilution.

- Minimal handling of remedies is important as the active ingredient of the remedy is on the outside of the tablet or pillule. Ideally the tablet should be tipped into the lid and then directly into the mouth.
- An important factor is that it is the amount of times the remedy is repeated which enhances the healing effect and not the strength of the remedy that is administered.

Example of treatment with homoeopathy

Constipation

Constipation is a common feature of pregnancy due to the effect of hormones in pregnancy, dietary changes, and may be the effect of iron therapy. Attention to diet is always important to help with the underlying cause. However, homoeopathic remedies have a lot to offer for relief of symptoms—in addition to physical symptoms the emotional disposition of the person is considered too:

- Nux vomica: frequent urge to pass stool, but is ineffectual. Passes only small amounts at a time, feels unfinished. Sensitive and irritable.
- Sepia: large, hard stool with much straining. Feels full with a sensation of a weight or ball in the anus that is not relieved by passing stool. Feels sluggish.
- Bryonia: large, hard, dry stool, which is difficult to pass. Headache, which is worse for movement. Irritability.
- Lycopodium: knotty, hard stool with ineffective attempt to expel stool. Rectal flatulence. Unfinished feeling. Tendency to be lacking in confidence and anxious.
- Kali carb: large hard stool with pain prior to expelling stool. Profuse micturition at night. Better for warm weather and during the day. Feels touchy, anxious, irritable and sluggish simultaneously.

Backache

Backache in pregnancy may be caused by physiological changes associated with the pregnant condition. Homoeopathy can be of benefit alongside other supportive treatments such as physiotherapy, transcutaneous nerve stimulation (TENS), chiropractic therapy and massage.

Heartburn

Homoeopathic remedies may provide an alternative to the conventional remedies for heartburn. Careful attention to matching individual symptoms to the most appropriate remedy is important. For example: when are the symptoms worse (after eating, first thing in the morning etc.); the abdominal sensations experienced (bloated, burning sensation, empty feeling etc.).

Arnica

This remedy is the most commonly used homoeopathic remedy for physical and emotional trauma. Excellent for soft tissue bruising, falls, concussion, and before and after surgery. It can also be applied topically to bruised areas, provided the skin is unbroken.

Aromatherapy

The use of essential oils during pregnancy and childbirth constitutes the most commonly used therapy within maternity care, possibly due to the subtle therapeutic effects of the oils themselves together with the nurturing aspects of some of the techniques used within aromatherapy.

Due respect to the potency of essential oils should be paramount at all times. Dilution, safety, and potential toxicity of essential oils is the key to safe administration in pregnancy. Some oils have diuretic and/or emmenagogic* properties which may limit the use of popular oils. Women should be encouraged to seek advice from their midwife or an aromatherapist if she wishes to use essential oils in pregnancy.

Many oils are contraindicated in pregnancy due to their strength and potential abortifacient properties, so when in doubt as to whether an oil is suitable, professional advice should be sought.

General principles

- Essential oils should never be taken internally.
- All essential oils should be diluted in some form prior to use, e.g. in a base oil or lotion, water, or vaporized or compress.
- Store in a dark locked cupboard away from children.
- Respect the storage and shelf life of essential oils.
- Adhere to recommended dosages for pregnancy.
- Adhere to cautions regarding pregnancy, epilepsy, hypertension, and other medical conditions.
- Use sound, respected sources of oils and carrier oils to ensure therapeutic quality.
- Always enquire about potential allergies prior to use, some oils may cause skin reactions if used neat or in high doses—therefore exercise caution with women who have sensitive skin or a history of allergies.
- Be aware of the woman's medical and obstetric history to ensure there are no contraindications to the use of essential oils or methods of administration.

Administration of essential oils

The two main routes for the administration of essential oils are the skin and the olfactory system. Studies have proved that traces of essential oils have been detected in blood, urine, sweat, and body tissues following therapy. The olfactory route is considered to be more quickly effective due to the chemical components of oils being taken directly to the limbic system via the olfactory bulbs. This also accounts for the effect oils have on the emotional aspects of well-being.

- The method of using oils will depend on the time available, the condition being treated, and the woman's preference (she may dislike touch).
- The amounts of essential oils used in therapy in this country are well below toxicity readings.
- To ensure extra safety to mother and fetus, the amounts used may be less than the normal adult dosage.

---

* Emmenagogue—an essential oil that contains properties which can induce or assist menstruation.

- The heightened sense of smell often experienced during pregnancy may also contribute to this reasoning.
- Dilutions for pregnancy 1–2% mix for massage—in 5mL carrier oil, a 2% blend would require two drops of essential oil in total. For a more dilute blend (1.5%) the amount of carrier is increased to 10mL and three drops of essential oil in total added.

Debate about the essential oils that are considered safe for pregnancy and childbirth continues. Table 7.1 is not an exhaustive list of essential oils but reflects the most common oils used for pregnancy and childbirth. Some practitioners may well have preferences for other oils not listed.

Table 7.1 Oils for pregnancy and childbirth

Essential oil	Properties	Comments
Chamomile (Roman—*Anthemisnobilis*) (German—*Matricariachamomilla*)	Antispasmodic antiseptic, calming, antifungal, analgesic, anti-inflammatory. Soothing for the skin, nervous, and digestive systems. Stimulates immune system	Avoid use of Roman chamomile until late pregnancy. German chamomile avoid in early pregnancy. German chamomile useful for sensitive skin
Clary sage (*Salvia sclerea*)	Anti-depressant, hypnotic, antiseptic, antispasmodic, anti-inflammatory, uterine tonic—assists contractions. Mainly used as a massage or compress	Do not use in pregnancy. May cause drowsiness, care with driving and alcohol. Oestrogenic properties. Reduces panic and lowers blood pressure
Eucalyptus (*Eucalyptus globulus*)	Nasal decongestant, antiseptic, pain relief, urinary tract infection. Inhalation, massage, compress	Avoid in epileptics and hypertension. May cause skin irritation. Clears head and cools emotions
Frankincense (*Boswellia carteri*)	Hysteria, hyperventilation, depression, genitourinary tract infections, decongestant	One drop inhaled from tissue/taper to relieve hyperventilation. Slight emmenagogue—low doses during pregnancy, calming oil for labour
Geranium (*Perlagonium graveolens*)	Balancing, analgesic, antispasmodic, decongestant, antiseptic, diuretic	Heavy aroma, check acceptability prior to use. Regulates hormone function. Eliminates waste and congestion. Useful for nervousness, fatigue, fluid retention varicose veins and cystitis

(Continued)

Table 7.1 (Contd.)

Essential oil	Properties	Comments
Grapefruit (*Citrus paradisi*)	Antiseptic, analgesic. Good for massage during pregnancy	Gentle safe oil, light refreshing aroma, photo toxic. Shelf life—3 months Relief of stress headaches. Useful for colds and flu
Jasmine (*Jasminium officinale*)	Analgesic, antispasmodic uterine tonic, pain, hormone balancing, sedative, aphrodisiac	Emmenagogue—not to be used until term. Very expensive. Aroma is over powering, caution with vaporizing, best used as massage in low doses. Regulates and deepens breathing
Lavender (*Lavendula angustifolia*)	Antiseptic, analgesic, pain relief, antispasmodic hypotensive First aid oil	Emmenagogue, use with caution in 1st trimester. Care with vaporization. May cause headaches or drowsiness.[1] Not to be used in combination with epidural anaesthesia or pethidine
Lemon (*Citrus limon*)	Anti-anaemic, antispasmodic bactericidal, circulatory tonic, skin tonic, immune system stimulant	Minimal phototoxic effect, short shelf life. Vaporization or in combination with other oils for massage. Headache, candida, cleansing action
Lime (*Citrus aurantifolia*)	Antiseptic, anti-viral anti-spasmodic, balances immune system, appetite regulator. Useful for sickness in pregnancy	Gentle, relaxing, safe oil, phototoxic
Mandarin (*Citrus reticulata*)	Antiseptic, analgesic, hormone balancing, flatulence, anxiety, nausea. Gentle uplifting effect	Good all round oil with pleasant aroma. Special affinity for women and children. Excellent for stretch marks
Neroli (*Citrus aurantium or bigaradia*)	Antispasmodic, aphrodisiac, induces peacefulness, uterine tonic, skin tonic	Very expensive. Stretch marks, stress, depression. Hypnotic effect—care with driving
Sweet orange (*Citrus sinesis*)	Antiseptic, skin tonic, relaxing, digestive disorders, anxiety	Phototoxic, possible skin irritation as with most citrus oils. Gentle versatile oil. Suitable for nausea, vomiting, stress, oedema, hypertension

Table 7.1 (Contd.)

Essential oil	Properties	Comments
Petitgrain (*Citrus bigaradia*)	Relaxing, stress, anxiety, nervous exhaustion, antioxidant, antispasmodic, skin tonic, antiseptic	Good for fear and panic. Insomnia, skin problems depression, digestive disorders
Rose (*Rosa centifolia or damascena*)	Antidepressant, antiseptic, antiviral aphrodisiac, vasoconstrictive, hormone balancing. Affinity with female reproductive system	Use for anxiety, insomnia constipation. Emmenagogue—preferably avoid until late pregnancy. Very expensive, but ideal oil for all women's needs. Ensure high quality oil used for therapeutic purposes
Sandalwood (*Santalum album*)	Calming, sedative, astringent, diuretic, decongestant, antiseptic, bactericidal	Suggested use varicose veins, cystitis, vaginal discharge, bronchitis, coughs, sore throats, heartburn, and nausea
Tea tree (*Melaleuca alternifolia*)	Strong antiseptic, antibacterial, antiviral antifungal, stimulates white blood cell production. Inhibits growth of many pathogenic bacteria	Effective for candida infection, acne (facial sauna). Prevention of infection, natural alternative to treat colds and influenza. Also effective as first aid treatment for mouth ulcers, bites, boils, burns, cold sores
Ylang ylang (*Cananga odorata*)	Aphrodisiac, sedative, tonic, antidepressant, hypotensive, antiseptic, emotionally balancing, stimulates the ovaries	Heady aroma. Use for anxiety, depression, panic, fear and shock. Regulates heart beat and slows breathing. Regulates flow of adrenaline

Routes of administration of essential oils

- Massage to parts of body (head, neck, back, feet) or whole body. (For dosage 🕮 see Administration of essential oils, p. 122).
- Bath: four to six drops suspended in milk or carrier oil and added after water has been run and then agitated to disperse oils evenly.
- Compress: three to four drops in hot or cold water. Flannel or sanitary pad is then immersed, wrung out and applied to the skin. Repeated once the flannel cools to body temperature.
- Footbath: three to four drops of essential oil added to warm water. Agitate and then soak for a minimum of 10min to gain benefit.
- Vulval wash: useful to help prevent infection, douches should not be used in the intrapartum period and postnatally. Use three drops of essential oil to 1L of warm water; agitate and pour over the vulval area.

- Room spray: 10 drops of oil to 200mL of water, preferably in a fine nozzle spray container.
- Tissue/cotton wool: one to two drops of essential oil and inhale as required.
- Taper: one drop of essential oil and waft under nostrils as required.
- Inhalation: traditional method of inhaling via a bowl containing hot water and oils with a towel over one's head. Safety precautions need to be exercised. Two drops of oil in the bowl and inhale for 10min. This procedure is not recommended for asthmatic people. This method may also be used as a facial sauna for skin conditions.
- Vaporizer or diffuser: naked flames are prohibited within maternity units, however electrical vaporizers are most suited and safe for institutional use. One to two drops of essential oil is used and the vaporizer switched on for no more than 10–15min per hour to prevent over intoxication of the oils chosen. Where women may wish to vaporize essential oils at home via a device with a naked flame they should be advised of the correct usage and safety implications.

Recommended reading

Price S, Price L (2003). *Aromatherapy for Health Professionals*. Edinburgh: Churchill Livingstone.

Tiran D (2000). *Clinical Aromatherapy for Pregnancy and Childbirth*, 2nd edn. Edinburgh: Churchill Livingstone, p.135.

Bach flower remedies

The Bach flower remedies (BFRs) were discovered by Dr Edward Bach in the 1930s. He believed that much ill health and suffering was a result of emotional distress and imbalance. When negative emotions are experienced, this also affects the proper functioning of the physical body. If negative emotions are left unresolved, then eventually ill health will occur. Dr Bach discovered 38 remedies, which he believed covered the full range of human emotions.

The Bach system is a simple self-help therapy that can be used safely by all groups of people, including pregnant women and babies. The BFRs can be used safely alongside orthodox medicine.

Using BFRs in pregnancy

Confirmation of pregnancy often brings a range of conflicting emotions—joy, shock, disbelief, feeling unprepared, anger, overexcitement, and anxiety. Untimely decisions may have to be made, and even breaking the news can be stressful. For all the many emotional states that may occur, the BFRs may help to bring balance and stability.

- *Walnut*: may help with adjusting to the physical, emotional, and mental changes of pregnancy.
- *Mimulus*: may help with worries about pregnancy, what people might think; fear of medical tests or needle phobia.
- *Honeysuckle*: may help when there are regrets and fears about past birthing experiences.
- *Elm*: may help if there is a sudden, overwhelming feeling of responsibilty to the prospect of motherhood.
- *Red chestnut*: may help when there is over-concern for the well-being of the fetus.
- *Olive*: may be useful for alleviating tiredness and exhaustion in early pregnancy.
- *Scleranthus*: may be helpful when there is difficulty in decision making, e.g. whether or not to have screening tests.
- *Crab apple*: for feeling unsightly or disgust of the pregnant state.
- *Pine*: for feelings of guilt, possibly harming the fetus in some way or neglecting other family members.
- *Willow*: if there is resentment about the pregnancy and the changes that are required, e.g. work, finances, etc.

As pregnancy starts to draw to a close, the woman may again experience conflicting emotions:

- Gratitude that the pregnancy and its physical discomforts will soon be finished
- Most will hope that they do not go past their due date
- Some may feel unhappy that the pregnancy is coming to an end, due to the special relationship they have developed with the fetus
- Others may be fearful of labour looming, how they will cope, how painful it will be, whether the baby will be alright, and how their partner will cope.

As a result many women find the final few weeks a time of anxiety and irritation.

- *Mimulus*: may be helpful for all the looming fears experienced.
- *Gentian*: may help if the woman feels despondent, particularly if she goes past her due dates.
- *White chestnut*: may be helpful if there are constant worrying thoughts.
- *Impatiens*: may help if there is irritability and impatience in the last few weeks, and especially if overdue.
- *Aspen*: for the mother who experiences a sense of uneasiness or unexplained fear.
- *Beech*: may be helpful if the woman is critical and irritated by people's company.
- *Agrimony*: for those who hide their fears and concerns behind a brave face.

Because of the very special relationship that develops between a mother and her unborn child, it is believed that the positive and negative experiences during her pregnancy may affect the fetus too. Therefore using BFRs in pregnancy to help cope with all the ups and downs of emotions may also result in a remedial effect on the fetus.

Rescue remedy

Rescue remedy is a combination of five of the 38 remedies that Dr Bach formulated, to be taken as an emotional first-aid remedy at times of stress and anxiety. Very often this remedy is the means by which people first become introduced to the remedies through friends, family, or colleagues. People commonly take the rescue remedy to cope with demanding situations, such as bereavement, going into hospital, visiting the dentist, medical procedures, interviews, driving tests, giving a presentation, stressful work or domestic situations, accidents, and operations.

The rescue remedy contains the following:
- *Star of Bethlehem*: for shock and trauma
- *Cherry plum*: for feeling out of control and irrational
- *Impatiens*: for irritability and impatience
- *Rock rose*: for extreme fear and panic
- *Clematis*: for dreaminess and detachment.

Administration of BFRs

The BFRs are extremely dilute, and all the flowers used are non-toxic. They are suspended in a weak alcohol solution bought as stock bottles. Drops are then diluted in fluid, ideally water or juice, and taken orally.

The remedies can be taken singularly or in combination of up to six remedies if several emotional states need to be addressed.
- Informed consent should be gained prior to administration of the BFRs and recorded in the maternal notes.
- Rescue remedy: put four drops into a glass of water or juice and sip at regular intervals as required.
- Individual remedies:
  - For day-to-day/short-term use: put two drops of each remedy chosen into a glass of water or juice and sip at regular intervals.
  - For long-term use: put two drops of each remedy chosen into a 30mL dropper bottle and fill with spring water. Take four drops on the tongue or in drinks at least four times daily. This should be used within 3 weeks.

Recommended reading

Ball S (2005). *The Bach Remedies Workbook: A Study Course in the Bach Flower Remedies*. London: Random House.

Howard J (1991). *The Bach Flower Remedies Step by Step*. Saffron Walden, England: CW Daniel Company.

Howard J (1992). *Bach Flower Remedies for Women*. Saffron Walden, England: CW Daniel Company.

Reflexology

Reflexology is an ancient therapeutic form of foot and hand massage that activates the body's natural healing responses. The feet and hands are seen as a miniature map of the whole body, and therefore can be utilized to treat various physical and emotional disorders. Reflexology is based on two main theories:

- The Chinese system of meridians and the circulation of Qi: reflexology provides a means of tapping into this energy system to unblock deficient, stagnant, or excessive flow of Qi.
- The Reflex Zone therapy approach recognizes that the feet are divided into 10 zones that correspond to specific bodily organs.

Benefits of reflexology in pregnancy

- Enhances the relaxation response, therefore reducing stress, which also has a positive effect on the fetus.
- Improves circulation, promoting the carriage of oxygen and nutrients to the cells.
- Stimulates the immune system.
- Improves nervous system function.
- Assists in the removal of toxins.
- Encourages the cooperation of all the organs in the body.

Reflexology may be used for many of the ailments experienced in pregnancy, or used alongside conventional treatments to provide extra support and reduce anxiety that often exacerbates physical disorders.

Pregnant women should be treated with reflexology by either a qualified reflexology practitioner with an understanding of the pathophysiology of pregnancy, or a midwife/reflexologist.

Contraindications to the use of reflexology in pregnancy

- Habitual miscarriage or unstable pregnancy
- Threatened abortion
- Vaginal bleeding
- Severe pregnancy-induced hypertension
- Deep vein thrombosis
- Ectopic pregnancy
- Low-lying placenta
- Placental abruption
- Preterm labour.

Recommended reading

Hall N (1994). *Reflexology for Women*. London: Thorsons.

Mackareth PA, Tiran D (2002). *Clinical Reflexology—A Guide for Health Professionals*. London: Churchill Livingstone.

Tiran D (2009). *Reflexology for Pregnancy and Childbirth: A Definitive Guide for Health Professionals*. London: Elsevier.

Oriental medicine

The Oriental approach to health is based on a holistic view of the individual, nature, and the universe. Illness is viewed as a process of energetic disharmony within the body, which eventually undermines emotional, physical, and spiritual health. Various therapeutic practices are employed, including: acupuncture, massage, herbal medicine, dietary reform, meditation, exercise, and breathing techniques. The therapies of acupuncture, reflexology, and shiatsu are the most commonly used in midwifery. These therapies are underpinned by the concepts of traditional Eastern philosophy:

- Qi (or Chi, universal energy that permeates the whole of nature, which may also be referred to as the life force, which is vital to health and well-being)
- Yin/Yang (the two apposing forces within nature that help to maintain balance and synthesis within the body and its functions)
- Meridians (a network of channels which transport Qi throughout the body).

Acupuncture points occur at intervals along the meridian lines, these can be described as miniature whirlpools or vortices that draw Qi deep into or out of the body's energy flow. These points serve as access points for the practitioner to needle (as in acupuncture) or for massage (reflexology and shiatsu) to produce therapeutic changes in the energy state of the patient.

Negative emotions are considered to have a debilitating effect on the flow of Qi throughout the body. The area of the body affected will depend on the type of emotion experienced; for example, anger will cause stagnation of liver Qi which, in turn, will lead to disorders such as diarrhoea, belching, and nausea.

Major shifts in the energetic patterns take place during pregnancy to support growth and development of the fetus. Pregnancy is considered to be a Yin state, which encourages an inward movement of energy. This reflects the woman's desire to reconsider values; to take more care of herself and focus on the fetus. Very often in Western culture it is difficult for women to foster this energetic pattern, due to their working and domestic environments. Therefore, many women are more Yang in nature; that is, they are focused externally from their pregnancies and a deeper nurturing experience. The resulting imbalance of Qi during pregnancy will result in various disorders.

Acupuncture

The systematic insertion of fine needles at specific acupuncture points to stimulate or balance the flow of Qi throughout the body. This therapy is based on empirical knowledge gained from the close observation of the effects of needling specific points, dating back at least 2500 years.

- During pregnancy, acupuncture treatment should always be carried out by an acupuncturist practitioner or a midwife acupuncturist.
- Acupuncture can be used for all the common ailments associated with pregnancy, e.g. backache, carpal tunnel syndrome, nausea, constipation.
- A full medical and obstetric history should be taken prior to commencing treatment.

- It is important to work closely with health practitioners involved in the woman's care, so that underlying medical conditions or problems arising as a result of pregnancy, where intervention may be necessary, can be initiated promptly, e.g. bleeding, severe sickness, abdominal pain.
- Certain acupuncture points are forbidden during pregnancy because they create a strong stimulating downwards force in the body. However, some of these points may be used for induction/augmentation of labour or to assist with delivery of the placenta.

Moxibustion

This is the use of heat (produced by burning moxa, the herb mugwort) to stimulate acupuncture points. Cigar-shaped sticks of dried moxa are lit and held closely to the skin over specific points. Attention to this alternative means of turning the breech followed on from a study in China of 260 primigravid women.[1]

The most common use for this in pregnancy is to turn breech babies from 33/34 weeks onwards:

- The point used is bladder 67 (at the lateral side of the base of the little toe nail), this point links to the uterine meridian. Stimulating this point with moxa heat is thought to enhance adrenocortical production, which in turn creates fetal movement within the uterus by stimulating placental oestrogens and prostaglandins.[2]
- Women can be taught to use this technique at home with the help of their partners (once or twice daily for 10–12 treatments).
- Research into the use of moxibustion suggests favourable outcomes and a safe alternative to external cephalic version (ECV)—the manual technique carried out by some obstetricians.
- Carrying out moxibustion at 33/34 weeks is questionable when the breech will often turn spontaneously before term or revert back to the breech position, However, taking these variables into consideration the moxa group still resulted in a larger amount of vaginal cephalic births.
- Moxa is a relatively safe, effective and easily administered method of turning a breech presentation and could be considered as a first option prior to ECV.[3]
- However, more research is needed to substantiate the success claims for moxibustion.
- The contra-indications are the same as for ECV.
- Other therapies that may be considered for turning the breech are: hypnosis, chiropractic, yoga, homoeopathy, and fetal acoustic stimulation.

Shiatsu

Shiatsu is an ancient form of massage used to aid relaxation and healing, also known as acupressure. Shiatsu means 'finger pressure', although hands, fists, and elbows, as well as fingers, may be used to apply pressure. Shiatsu follows the same principles as acupuncture, except that manual techniques, rather than needles, are applied to the acupuncture points. No drugs or oils are used, which makes it a safe therapy to use during pregnancy. The massage is undertaken over clothing.

Benefits of shiatsu

Shiatsu can:

- Help with the ailments of pregnancy
- Initiate a close relationship with the baby
- Help the woman tune in to her individual needs during pregnancy
- Encourage the woman to trust in the process of pregnancy and birth, and foster a positive approach
- Help the fetus to maintain optimal positioning, especially for labour
- Harness a positive and rewarding relationship with her partner, encouraging involvement during the process of pregnancy and childbirth.

Many midwives are discovering the many benefits of using the gentle, rewarding art of shiatsu in their practice. It:

- Is a relaxing therapy to perform
- Enhances the midwife–mother relationship
- Supports normality
- Enables the midwife to use hands-on skills
- Reduces the need for obstetric interventions
- Promotes responsibility for health.

Recommended reading

Cardini F, Marcolongo A (1993). Moxibustion for correction of breech presentation: a clinical study with retrospective control. *American Journal of Chinese Medicine* **21**(2), 133–8.

Kanakura Y, Kometani K, Nagata T, *et al.* (2001). Moxibustion treatment of breech presentation. *American Journal of Chinese Medicine* **29**(1), 37–45.

Neri I, De Pace V, Venturini P, Facchinetti F (2007). Effects of 3 different stimulations (acupuncture, moxibustion, acupuncture plus moxibustion) of BL. 67 acupoint at small toe on fetal behavior of breech presentation. *American Journal of Chinese Medicine* **35**(1), 27–33.

West Z (2001). *Acupuncture in Pregnancy and Childbirth.* London: Churchill Livingstone.

Yates S (2003). *Shiatsu for Midwives.* London: Elsevier.

1 Cardini F, Weixen H (1998). Moxibustion for the correction of breech presentation: a randomized controlled trial. *Journal of the American Medical Association* **280**(18), 1580–4.

2 Tiran D. (2004). Breech presentation: increasing maternal choice. *Complementary Therapies in Nursing and Midwifery* **10**(4), 233–8.

3 Ewies A, Olah K. (2002). Moxibustion in breech version—a descriptive review. *Acupuncture Medicine* **20**(1), 26–9.

Yoga

Pre-conception or pregnancy is the ideal time to start practising yoga as it encompasses physical, emotional, and spiritual preparation that will be helpful for this unique time in a woman's life. Many women experience deeper, instinctual, and nurturing feelings as they embark on their pregnancy, and may find that the gentle and relaxing practice of yoga provides fulfilment for them.

Many midwives are encouraging women to attend yoga classes during pregnancy, or may have undertaken training to provide this service themselves. Practitioners facilitating classes for pregnant women must have a thorough understanding of the pathophysiology of pregnancy with regard to yoga postures. Many postures are contraindicated, while others will require some modification due to the physical restrictions in pregnancy of the musculo-skeletal system. Particular care should be taken, especially if yoga is commenced during pregnancy due to the increased laxity of joints and muscles. Many yoga positions are contraindicated for symphysis pubis diastasis, particularly abductor movements. However, regular, gentle yoga practice may bring relief to many of the physiological discomforts of pregnancy including backache and provides tremendous benefits to enhance the experience of birth.

Physical benefits
- Increased suppleness, flexibility, and strength in the joints and important muscle groups that are used in labour and birth.
- Improved posture: helps the woman to cope with carrying the extra weight involved in pregnancy, and encourages the adoption of a favourable position for birth by the fetus, thus engagement of the fetus into the pelvis is more efficient.
- Helps to open up the pelvic outlet by simulating squatting and upright postures (squatting can open up the pelvic outlet by up to 30%).
- Pelvic floor muscles are strengthened and toned.
- Improved breathing and circulation; thus increased oxygen supply to the fetus.
- Elimination of toxins and waste material.
- Back pain related to pregnancy responds well to regular yoga practice.
- Other aches and pains and common ailments of pregnancy may be relieved.

Emotional/spiritual benefits
- Breathing awareness encourages relaxation, the release of tension, and better sleep patterns.
- Pregnancy is less tiring.
- The woman feels more energetic.
- The regular practice of relaxation during pregnancy enables the woman to tap into this sensation during labour, to help her cope better.
- The woman feels confident, empowered, and optimistic.
- Creates a more sensitive and receptive relationship with the fetus.

- Enhances nurturing and mothering instincts during pregnancy, in readiness for motherhood.
- Enables women to get in touch with their inner feelings and intuition.

A woman who practises yoga throughout pregnancy builds confidence in her body's ability to cope with the many adjustments that take place. She is more likely to take responsibility for her own health, and to work more harmoniously with her body during labour and birth.

Herbal medicine

Herbal medicine has its routes in history and folklore. In recent years it has regained popularity, however there is still much ignorance of its use amongst lay people. Self-medication with herbs may be appropriate using weaker doses in tablets and tinctures, however in pregnancy extreme caution should be used. Medicinal herbs are often quite potent and potentially toxic, so should only be prescribed by medical herbalists whose practice is subject to regulation.

Research has revealed that many herbal remedies may interact with conventional drugs, by either inhibiting or potentiating their effect. All herbal remedies should be discontinued at least 2 weeks prior to planned surgery as many may potentially affect blood clotting mechanisms.

Table 7.2 highlights the possible interactions of herbal medicines and conventional drugs that may be used during pregnancy.

Raspberry leaf tea

- Raspberry leaf tea is often recommended for pregnant women during pregnancy to tone the uterus and prepare for labour. It is known for its therapeutic properties as a uterine and circulatory tonic. Studies suggest that it may also have an antispasmodic effect.
- It is thought to aid ripening of the cervix, enhance uterine activity in labour, and promote involution, although this tends be anecdotal evidence rather than robust studies.
- It should not be taken throughout the whole of pregnancy, but commenced at about 32 weeks' gestation.
- Taken as a tea the amount is gradually increased, tablet form is also available.
- If Braxton Hicks contractions become strong and repetitive the dose should be reduced or discontinued.
- Raspberry leaf is contraindicated in the following conditions:
  - Uterine scar
  - History of preterm labour
  - Placenta praevia
  - Planned lower segment caesarean section (LSCS)
  - Bleeding from the genital tract.

Recommended reading

Mills S, Bone K. (2005) *The Essential Guide to Herbal Safety.* St Louis, Missouri: Elsevier.

Table 7.2 Interactions between herbal medicines and conventional drugs

Drugs—reason for use in pregnancy, labour and after the birth	Herbal remedies and dietary supplements to AVOID
Drugs used for severe morning sickness and for nausea in labour	Co-enzyme Q10; kava kava (withdrawn from sale in UK)
Aspirin for pain relief or to prevent problems of severe pre-eclampsia	Ginger; feverfew; gingko biloba
Ibuprofen and similar drugs used for pain relief	Ginger; feverfew
Contraceptive pill	St John's wort; ginseng; liquorice; chasteberry (*Vitex agnus castus*)
Steroids—used in premature labour to mature the baby's lungs	Chromium; liquorice; ginseng
Drugs to treat high blood pressure including pre-eclampsia	Ginseng; St John's wort
Anaesthetic drugs—stop all herbal remedies 2 weeks before surgery including planned Caesarean section	Ginger, gingko biloba, ginseng; liquorice
Antidepressants (MAOIs)	St John's wort; ginseng; kava kava (withdrawn from sale in UK)
Bromocriptine—may be used in infertility treatment	Chasteberry (*Vitex agnus castus*)
Blood-thinning/anticoagulant drugs (e.g. warfarin)—best to avoid herbal remedies completely except with expert advice	Dong quai; feverfew; garlic; ginger; gingko biloba; ginseng; papaya extract
Drugs to treat immune system problems—best to avoid herbal remedies completely	Echinacea; garlic; ginseng; St John's wort
Drugs to treat epilepsy—best to avoid herbal remedies completely except with expert advice	Grapefruit juice; echinecea; goldenseal; liquorice; St John's wort; evening primrose oil
Drugs used to treat diabetes—best to avoid herbal remedies completely	Gingko biloba; ginger; ginseng; co-enzyme Q10
Drugs to treat heart conditions—to avoid herbal remedies completely except with expert advice	St John's wort; ginger; motherwort; magnesium; ginseng; liquorice; black pepper essential oil; peppermint essential oil; passiflora (passion flower) co-enzyme Q10

From ℬ www.expectancy.co.uk. Copyright © Tiran D (2005), reprinted by permission of the publisher. MAOI, mono-amine oxidase inhibitor.

The need for
social support

Social support

Social support is a flexible concept which is consequently difficult to define. Schumaker and Brownell[1] define it as 'an exchange of resources between at least two individuals perceived by the provider or recipient to be intended to enhance the well-being of the recipient.' The three key components of social support are:

- Emotional support, this may be a warm and caring relationship, a presence or companionship, or a willingness to listen
- Informational support, which is the giving of good advice or information
- Practical or tangible support which may be financial or could be physical comfort support during labour.

Most social support is provided by friends, family, and community but social support by health professionals is important. It has been shown to have a positive impact on general health and well-being.

How does social support work?

- It works as a buffer against stress.
- It assists the development of coping strategies.
- It can influence behaviours that impact on health.
- It can facilitate recovery from illness.

Midwives and social support

Midwives have a key role in supporting women through pregnancy and childbirth. Key areas of midwifery support identified by women are:[2]

- Good communication
- Good listening skills
- Practical support
- Knowing their carers and being known by them
- Continuity of care and carer.[3]

Social support should be integral to maternity service.

Effects of social support

In pregnancy

- Reduces anxiety resulting in greater confidence, lack of nervousness, reduced fear, and positive feelings towards birth.
- Reduces psychological and physical morbidity.
- Can increase satisfaction with care and communications.
- Gives an increased sense of control.

In labour

It can reduce:[4]

- Duration of labour
- The amount of pain relief required
- Operative vaginal delivery
- The 5-min Apgar score of <7
- Reduce the likelihood of caesarean section where companions were not normally admitted.

There is also evidence of[3]:
- Greater satisfaction with birth
- Longer duration of breastfeeding
- Decrease in perineal trauma
- Less postnatal depression and less difficulty in mothering.

Considerations

- Social support may not be adequate to counter the effects of poverty and social disadvantage on health.
- Little is known as to which elements of social support are useful or effective.
- Doulas have been found helpful in providing social support especially in labour although they are not commonly present at birth in England.
- A wide range of interventions have been utilized in research and all are classified as social support.

1 Schumaker S, Brownell A (1984). Towards a theory of social support: closing conceptual gaps. *Journal of Social Issues.* **40**, 11–36.

2 McCourt C, Percival P (2000). Social support in childbirth. In: Page LA (ed.) *The New Midwifery: Science and Sensitivity.* Edinburgh: Churchill Livingstone.

3 Hodnett ED (2005). Continuity of caregivers for care during pregnancy and childbirth. *Cochrane Library,* Issue 2. Oxford: Update Software

4 Oakley A (1996). Giving support in pregnancy: the role of research midwives in a randomized controlled trial. In: Robinson S, Thomson A (eds) *Midwives, Research and Childbirth.* London: Chapman and Hall.

Screening for domestic abuse

- Domestic abuse refers to a wide range of physical, psychological, sexual, emotional, and financial abuse of people who are, or who have been, intimate partners regardless of gender or sexuality. It also covers issues that mainly concern women from minority ethnic backgrounds, i.e. forced marriage, female genital mutilation and 'honour crimes'.
- The Confidential Enquiry into Maternal and Child Health[1] highlights that 20% of women in England and Wales say they have been physically assaulted by a partner and more than 30% of cases first start during pregnancy.
- Women may also experience an increase in the extent and nature of physical abuse during pregnancy.
- Domestic abuse impacts on maternal and perinatal mortality and morbidity.[1]
- Domestic abuse is generally underreported. It has been found that women are more likely to disclose if asked specific questions by a midwife, than if left to disclose themselves.[2] This then enables opportunity for women to access help.

What do women need?

Women need to be:
- Asked
- Believed
- Treated with respect
- Given time
- Given information.
  Use RADAR, a mnemonic for professionals:
R = Routine enquiry
A = Ask direct questions
D = Document findings safely
A = Assess woman's safety
R = Resources; give women information on resources available and Respect their choices.

Routine enquiry

- Offer at a range of points throughout the childbirth experience.
- Women should be seen alone at least once during the antenatal period to enable disclosure more easily.
- Because disclosure can be difficult, asking at different times during the childbirth experience is recommended. Suggested times:
  - At booking
  - 15/16 weeks
  - 28 weeks
  - 36 weeks
  - During the postnatal period
  - At discharge
  - Or at any opportune time.
- To facilitate disclosure, the environment needs to be quiet and private and where confidentiality can be assured.

- Women whose first language is not English, or with other communication barriers, should have access to appropriately trained interpreters.
- It is important that the woman understands the limits of confidentiality with regard to the well-being and safety of any children in the household.

Ask direct questions
- Women should always be unaccompanied when being asked about domestic abuse.
- How to ask: 'Because abuse or violence is so common in women's lives, we now routinely ask about abuse in relationships so that we can give all women information about agencies that can help'.
- This can then be followed up by more specific questions, for example;
  - 'Have you ever been afraid of your partner's behaviour or are they verbally abusive?'
  - 'Have you ever been hurt by your partner—slapped, kicked or punched?'
  - 'Have you ever been forced to do something sexual that you didn't want to?'

Document findings safely
- Healthcare professionals have a duty of care to record domestic abuse. The records may form part of future protection for an abused woman.
- Where to record:
  - In the hospital notes, not in the hand-held notes.
- What to record:
  - Who accompanies the woman, with information regarding their behaviour.
  - Any disclosure.
  - Are there any children in the household?
- Try to obtain a safe correspondence address from the woman.

Assess woman's safety
- Does she feel safe?
- Is it safe for her to go home?
- You may need to help her with direct referral to support services.
- Discuss safety planning.

Resources
- Give women information and contacts for local services that provide support:
  - Wallet cards
  - Leaflets
  - Free phone National Domestic Abuse Helpline—0808 2000 247
  - Display information within the maternity unit
  - Wallet cards available in 'women only' areas, e.g. toilets.
- Routine enquiry about domestic abuse can help reduce the stigma associated with abuse and the hidden/taboo nature of domestic abuse.

- Your role within routine enquiry is to signpost the woman towards appropriate support services, rather than attempting to solve her problems. Find out how women and midwives can be supported in the area where you work; what are the local support services and how can they be accessed?

Recommended reading

Department of Health (2010). *Responding to domestic abuse: A handbook for health professionals,*. London: DH. Available at: ℘ www.dh.gov.uk/prod_consum_dh/groups/dh_digitalassets/dh/en/documents/digitalasset/dh4126619.pdf (accessed 18.2.11).

Tacket A (2004). *Tackling Domestic Violence: The Role of Healthcare Professionals.* 2nd edn. Home Office Development and Practice Report. London: Home Office Publications. Available at: ℘ www.homeoffice.gov.uk/rds (accessed 24.3.10).

1 Lewis, G (ed.) (2007). *The Confidential Enquiry into Maternal and Child Health (CEMACH). Saving Mothers' Lives: Reviewing Maternal Deaths to Make Motherhood Safer—2003–2005.* The 7th report on Confidential Enquires into Maternal Deaths in the United Kingdom. London: CEMACH.

2 Bacchus L Mezey G, Bewley S, *et al.* (2004). Prevalence of domestic violence when midwives routinely enquire in pregnancy. *British Journal of Obstetrics and Gynaecology,* **111**(5), 441.

Recognition of sexual abuse

It is important that midwives are open to the possibility that any woman they are caring for may have been sexually abused. It is difficult to estimate how many women have suffered sexual abuse, as statistics vary widely and it is often underreported. However, it is suggested that up to a quarter of all women may be subjected to unwanted sexual experiences.[1]

Consequences of sexual abuse for pregnancy and childbirth

- Increased risk of pregnancy.
- Increased risk of late booking.
- Increased anxiety about birth.
- Slower, more difficult birth.
- Increased risk of intervention.
- Increased difficulties with breastfeeding, bonding, and postnatal depression.

Recognition of sexual abuse survivors

Women who have a history of sexual abuse may present with a combination of any of the following:

- Little or no prenatal care
- Multiple unplanned pregnancies, many ending in abortion
- Repeat attendance at antenatal clinics, GP, or emergency departments for minor injuries or trivial or non-existent complaints
- Drug and alcohol abuse
- History of multiple sexually transmitted diseases
- Recoiling when touched
- Obsession with cleanliness
- Scars from self-mutilation
- Unusual fear of needles
- Insistence on female carers, unless cultural
- Extreme sensitivity about body fluids on under-pads, sheets, and gowns
- Unable to labour lying down
- Extreme concerns about exposure and nakedness during labour and with breastfeeding
- Refuses catheterization
- Intense gag reflex
- Refuses the taking of infant's temperature rectally.

Simple steps to prevent re-traumatization

- As part of routine antenatal care, ask all women sensitively if they have been sexually abused. Reassure that this is more common than many women realize, but certain events in childbirth can trigger memories and flashbacks.
- Consider what you would say and do if a woman discloses a sexual abuse history to you.
- Never trivialize or minimize the impact of sexual abuse. It is important to adopt non-judgemental and supportive responses to women who disclose.

- Give control to the woman, by telling her about the procedures, explain what is going to happen, ask for permission to proceed, and wait until it is given, at all stages antenatally, intranatally, and postnatally.
- Be alert to signs that might indicate a sexual abuse history.
- Ensure absolute privacy.
- Be alert to non-verbal communication and listen to what is not being said.
- Reassure and affirm to the woman that her body is working for her, that the pain is natural labour pain and explain what is happening to her body.

1 Barlow J, Birch L (2004). Midwifery practice and sexual abuse. *British Journal of Midwifery* **12**(2), 72–5.

Management of substance misuse

The use of illicit substances such as cocaine and heroin during pregnancy is associated with a number of unfavourable outcomes. Early referral to a specialist midwife will provide a more efficient coordination of care. This is particularly significant in view of the contribution of substance misuse to maternal mortality.[1]

Poor outcomes associated with substance misuse can range from:

- Prematurity
- Intrauterine growth restriction—reductions in birth weight are most marked in the infants of women who are multiple-drug users
- Premature rupture of the membranes
- Meconium stained amniotic fluid
- Fetal distress
- Opiates increase the likelihood of antepartum haemorrhage
- Cocaine has been associated with placental abruption particularly if taken around the time of delivery.[2]

Antenatal care is often inadequate because of late presentation, reluctance to have involvement with social services, and a chaotic lifestyle. In order to improve outcomes it is important to engage pregnant drug users early and some drug services have set up joint clinics with antenatal services and also liaise with labour wards.

The overall aim of antenatal care is to minimise harm and stabalize the woman's lifestyle. For women using opiates, substitution therapy with methadone is associated with greater success of antenatal care and better maternal and infant outcomes.

Methadone prescriptions are arranged using strict and detailed guidelines. Oral methadone is dispensed in 1mg/mL solution and the usual dose is between 10 and 20mg daily to be taken as a single dose. The dose is adjusted according to the degree of dependence.

It is recommended[2] that the midwife should aim to:

- Encourage the woman to attend antenatal care regularly
- Normalize the care as much as possible taking into account the social and medical problems associated with substance misuse
- Give accurate and honest advice on the risks of substance misuse
- Provide good communication between professionals so advice is consistent
- Provide an individualized multi-agency plan for each client.

Obtaining a history

All information disclosed is confidential and should only be recorded in the hospital notes, not the client-held notes. The following information should be documented:

- What drugs are being used with any additional substances such as alcohol or diazepam?
- The amount used daily in either dosage or monetary terms
- The method of use and whether clean equipment is used
- Length of time of use and what was being used at the time of conception

- Partner's drug use if any
- What social support is available including the involvement of any other agencies?

Investigations

The following investigations may be performed having first asked for consent.
- Hepatitis C
- HIV
- Drug screen.

The woman may be referred to a specialist drug liaison midwife to coordinate her antenatal care if one is available in the area and also to a medical social worker. The woman's health visitor may also be involved especially in follow-up care.

The notes need to have a paediatric alert documented for continuing care of the baby once delivered.

1 Lewis, G (ed.) (2007). *The Confidential Enquiry into Maternal and Child Health (CEMACH). Saving Mothers' Lives: Reviewing Maternal Deaths to Make Motherhood Safer—2003–2005.* The 7th report on Confidential Enquires into Maternal Deaths in the United Kingdom. London: CEMACH.

2 Department of Health (England) and the devolved administrations (2007). *Drug Misuse and Dependence: UK Guidelines on Clinical Management.* London: Department of Health (England).

Preparing the parents for birth

'Antenatal education is a crucial component of antenatal care, yet practice and research demonstrate that women and men now seek far more than the traditional approach of a birth and parenting program attended in the final weeks of pregnancy'.[1]

Many women having their first baby find themselves isolated from a social support network, having moved away from where they were brought up and working full time, which isolates them from neighbours and the surrounding community. Through attendance at antenatal classes, parents may benefit from meeting new friends who will be going through the same experiences.

Parent education classes can also provide an opportunity to discuss fears and worries and to exchange views with other parents-to-be, as well as providing information about aspects of pregnancy, labour, birth and the care of the baby. Special classes may be developed for instance for teenagers or women experiencing multiple pregnancies.

Parents attending antenatal classes need to:
- Obtain balanced, realistic information so they know what to expect
- Learn skills that will help them to cope during labour
- Know about the emotional and social aspects of birth and being a parent
- Learn about life after birth and caring for their new baby.

Antenatal class management

Managing an antenatal class requires practice, and experience can be gained from working alongside an experienced class leader. The main points for the midwife who facilitates a class to consider are listed below.
- It is important to have received good preparation in adult learning techniques and to have gained confidence in managing and leading small interactive learning groups.
- Continuity of course leadership is essential to avoid duplication or omission of content and, more importantly, because the leader has to earn the trust of the group, in order to build relationships that enable the group to reflect on and discuss sensitive issues.
- Lectures are of limited value; it is more important to give information in short sessions that allow the learning of practical skills and subsequent discussion.
- Parents need to have the opportunity to learn about and to try out self-help strategies for dealing with labour.
- Topics such as labour pain, crying babies, exhaustion, and postnatal mental health issues need to be given a realistic perspective.

1 Svensson J, Barclay L, Cooke M (2008). Effective antenatal education: strategies recommended by expectant and new parents. *Journal of Perinatal Education* **17**, 33–42.

The birth plan

Discuss the birth plan with the woman and take opportunities to support her in her choices for the birth at any point during pregnancy. As the birth becomes imminent, record her wishes and give her the opportunity to discuss any concerns in the last few weeks of the pregnancy.

A birth plan should be flexible enough to take into account the unexpected. Enable the woman to appreciate that labour does not always go to plan. The following are some suggestions of things a woman may wish to discuss for inclusion in her plan.

- The place of birth will have been organized early in pregnancy, but this may alter if significant changes occur such as the presentation and position of the fetus, or if the pregnancy goes beyond the due date by more than 1 week.
- Birth companion—name of who the woman wants to have with her in labour. This may be her partner, or a female relative, or friend.
- Positions for labour and birth. Provide explanations of the benefits of certain positions and remaining mobile for as long as possible.
- Pain relief. Explain the risks and benefits of methods of pain relief and their effect on labour and on the fetus, so the woman makes an informed choice about her preferences.
- Eating and drinking during labour. Preference within a range of suitable easily digested foods and drinks can be expressed, provided the mother remains at low risk during her labour.
- The third stage of labour. Discuss how this is to be managed and how this may need to change if her risk of haemorrhage alters.
- The need for perineal suturing. Small first-degree tears need not be sutured if they are not actively bleeding. There is limited evidence to support non-suturing of larger tears or of second-degree tears.[1]
- The first feed and skin-to-skin contact. If breast feeding, the baby will be encouraged to feed during the first hour after birth. All mothers should be offered the opportunity for early skin-to-skin contact with their baby.
- Discuss administration of prophylactic vitamin K for the prevention of haemorrhagic disease of the newborn.
- Discuss any cultural or religious customs the mother may wish to observe.

1 Kettle C, Tohill S (2008). Perineal care: non-suturing of muscle and skin in first- and second-degree tears. *British Medical Journal Clinical Evidence* (online). 2008 Sep 24: pii: 1401. Available at: http://ukpmc.ac.uk/backend/ptpmcrender.cgi?accid=pmc2907946&blobtype=pdf (accessed 18.2.11).

Preparation for infant feeding

All pregnant women should be informed about the benefits and management of breastfeeding.[1]

Recording a woman's feeding intention at booking is questionable because:

- She may feel that she cannot change this decision at a later date
- Subsequent discussion may be more difficult if she has stated an intention to bottle feed
- Discussing breastfeeding when a woman has stated an intention to bottle feed may seem unnecessary.

Preparation for breastfeeding

No special care of the breasts is required in preparation for breastfeeding, but the following may be helpful:

- Bathing in the normal way is all that is necessary to keep the breasts and nipples clean
- Using soap may cause irritation as it removes the natural antiseptic lubricants (sebum) secreted from Montgomery's tubercles
- It is useful to learn the skill of hand expression in the last month of pregnancy
- All women and their partners should have the opportunity to discuss breastfeeding during the antenatal period
- All women and their partners should have the opportunity to attend antenatal education classes/workshops related to breastfeeding.

Preparation for artificial feeding, i.e. with infant formulas

If a mother has chosen to artificially feed her infant, the midwife should support her, but it is important to ensure that the mother has made an informed choice and is aware of the benefits of breastfeeding both for the baby and for herself.

Women should not receive instruction on how to make up bottles of infant formula as part of their antenatal group sessions; however, they should:

- Have the opportunity to discuss infant feeding individually with a health professional[2]
- Receive information and instruction on how to make up bottles,[2] if required, on a one-to-one basis or one-to-two basis with an appropriately trained health professional
- Receive information and instruction on how to sterilize equipment used in the preparation of infant feeds
- Receive information on artificially feeding, for example, the different types of formulas.

---

1 Unicef (1998). *Implementing the Ten Steps to Successful Breastfeeding*. London: Unicef UK Baby Friendly Initiative.

2 National Institute for Health and Clinical Excellence (2006). Routine postnatal care of women and their babies. Clinical guideline 37. London: NICE. Available at: www.nice.org.uk/cg37.

Chapter 9

Recognizing and managing pregnancy complications

Bleeding in early pregnancy

Once a pregnancy has been confirmed, any vaginal bleeding should be reported as it could signal a potential complication. Around 15% of women experience bleeding early in pregnancy. This could be related to events such as:

- *Implantation bleed*—a small amount of blood escapes as the fertilized ovum embeds in the lining of the uterus.
- *Decidual bleed*—bleeding from the decidual lining at the time a menstrual period would be expected, before the enlarging gestation sac completely fills the uterine cavity.

There may be other causes of bleeding not related to the uterus, such as:

- Cervical erosion that bleeds on contact
- Vaginitis
- Cervical polyp
- Ectopic pregnancy—a pregnancy implanted outside the cavity of the uterus, commonly in the fallopian tubes
- Hydatidiform mole
- Cervical erosion that bleeds on contact—post-coital bleed.

The most significant cause of bleeding is spontaneous miscarriage, 80% of which occur in the first trimester. Spontaneous miscarriage can be classified as follows.

- *Threatened:* bleeding with no uterine contraction or pain and the cervix does not dilate.
- *Inevitable:* when the cervix dilates or the membranes rupture.
- *Complete:* the cervix closes and bleeding stops after the expulsion of the gestation sac.
- *Incomplete:* retained placental tissue causes persistent bleeding and uterine contractions; requires evacuation of the uterus under anaesthetic to prevent the development of infection.
- *Missed:* the retention of a dead pregnancy; chorionic tissue may survive and produce hCG which enables the pregnancy to be retained in the uterus.
- *Miscarriage with infection:* infection following expulsion of the gestation sac, commonly after incomplete abortion.
- *Recurrent:* loss of three or more early pregnancies.
- *Induced:* surgical or medical method.

The woman does not require any specific treatment if bleeding is minimal and resolves spontaneously; although she may wish to confirm that the pregnancy is still viable.

The National Service Framework[2] recommends provision of early pregnancy assessment units (EPAUs) where woman may be referred for a further pregnancy test and ultrasound scan to confirm whether or not the pregnancy is continuing.

Persistent bleeding with pain requires admission to hospital for assessment and management. Post-miscarriage bleeding may require further treatment. Occasionally, if no infection is present and the uterus is empty, bleeding will settle after administration of ergometrine.

1 Royal College of Obstetrics and Gynaecologists (2006). *Management of Early Pregnancy Loss.* Green-Top Guideline 25. London: RCOG Press.

2 Department of Health (2004). *National Service Framework for Children, Young People and Maternity Services.* Maternity Standard. London: DH, p. 25.

Antepartum haemorrhage

- *Definition*: bleeding from the genital tract after the 24th week of pregnancy and before the onset of labour.
- Antepartum haemorrhage (APH) complicates 2–5% of all pregnancies and is responsible for significant maternal mortality and morbidity.
- In the latest CEMACH report[1] five women died from APH.
- The most common causes are placenta praevia with an incidence of 31% and placental abruption with an incidence of 22%.[2]

Placenta praevia

As the placenta encroaches on the lower uterine segment, bleeding occurs as the uterus stretches and grows. The lower uterine segment forms from 28 weeks.

- Bleeding is painless and presents as a fresh loss.
- There is often persistent malpresentation of the fetal presenting part.
- There is a further risk of postpartum haemorrhage (PPH) as the retractive power of the lower segment is poor.

There are four grades of placenta praevia:

- *Grade 1.* The placental edge encroaches on the lower uterine segment, but does not reach the internal cervical os. Blood loss is usually minimal so the mother and fetus remain in good condition and vaginal delivery is possible.
- *Grade 2.* The placenta is partially in the lower uterine segment and reaches but does not cover the internal cervical os. Blood loss is moderate and fetal hypoxia is more likely to be present than maternal shock. Vaginal delivery is possible if the placenta is anterior.
- *Grade 3.* The placenta partially covers the internal cervical os but not in a central position. Bleeding is likely to be severe, particularly in late pregnancy when the cervix starts to efface and dilate. Vaginal delivery is not possible as the placenta precedes the fetus.
- *Grade 4.* The placenta is completely covers the internal cervical os and the risk of torrential haemorrhage makes caesarean section essential to save the mother and the fetus.

Management depends on the amount of bleeding and the gestation. Admit the mother to a consultant unit for her condition to be assessed.

Mild to moderate bleeding

- Abdominal examination.
- Cardiotocograph to monitor fetal condition.
- Commence intravenous infusion.
- FBC and cross-match units of blood as per protocol.
- Ultrasound to confirm fetal well-being and position of placental border.
- Timing and mode of delivery will depend on the general condition of the woman, the extent of bleeding and the gestation.

Profuse bleeding

- Commence intravenous fluid immediately and transfuse blood as soon as it becomes available.
- Once the woman's condition is stable, prepare her for emergency caesarean section.

Placental abruption
Causes
- Multiparity
- Pre-eclampsia and eclampsia
- Hypertension
- Abdominal trauma
- Multiple pregnancy
- Polyhydramnios
- Previous abruption
- Folate deficiency.

Presents as continuous abdominal pain, sometimes with uterine contractions superimposed, with or without vaginal bleeding. Bleeding may be concealed inside the uterus, apparent as vaginal loss or both.

There may be symptoms of severe shock, disproportionate to the amount of blood lost. The pain may be localized if the abruption is small, and is felt over the site of the abruption. The uterus is very tender on palpation and hard ridges may be felt. The fetal heart beat may be absent.

Pain is caused by:
- Intrauterine pressure
- Stretching of the peritoneum
- Tearing of the myometrium as blood is pushed back into the muscle layers of the uterus.

Management
- Depends on the degree of maternal shock and the condition of the fetus.
- Mild abruption may be treated conservatively with rest and careful monitoring of the fetal and maternal condition. An ultrasound scan will confirm the diagnosis and a FBC and Kleihauer test will assess the amount of bleeding.
- The mother may return to community care once the bleeding has stopped and if maternal and fetal condition is good. Follow-up antenatal care will be consultant led with more frequent attendance.
- For a more severe abruption:
  - Commence intravenous infusion
  - FBC and cross-match as per protocol
  - Commence blood transfusion as soon as blood is available
  - Provide pain relief
  - Perform a clotting screen and Kleihauer test
  - Perform cardiotocography to monitor the status of the fetus
  - Prepare for induction of labour or caesarean section as the fetal and maternal condition dictates.

Complications due to placental abruption are:
- Disseminated intravascular coagulation (DIC)
- Acute renal failure
- Anaemia
- Sepsis
- Fetal death
- Fetal hypoxia
- Prematurity.

1 Potdar N, Navti O, Konje JC (2009). Antepartum haemorrhage. In: Warren R, Arulkumaran S (eds) *Best Practice in Labour and Delivery*. Cambridge: Cambridge University Press, pp. 141–44.
2 Lewis, G (ed.) (2007). *The Confidential Enquiry into Maternal and Child Health (CEMACH). Saving Mothers' Lives: Reviewing Maternal Deaths to Make Motherhood Safer—2003–2005*. The 7th report on Confidential Enquires into Maternal Deaths in the United Kingdom. London: CEMACH.

Breech presentation

In this presentation the fetus is in a longitudinal lie with the buttocks entering the pelvis first.

Incidence
- At 20 weeks: 40%
- At 28 weeks: 15%
- At 34 weeks: 6%
- At 40 weeks: 3%.

Classification
- *Breech with extended legs:* 70%. The legs are straight and the feet may lie on either side of the head, acting as a splint and making it difficult to ballot the head.
- *Complete or flexed breech:* 25–29%. The knees are bent and ankles crossed so the feet lie close to the buttocks.
- *Footling breech:* rare. From the flexed breech one foot falls downwards to present over the cervical os. The foot may slip through as the cervix dilates in labour.
- *Knee presentation:* very rare. From the flexed breech one knee falls downwards over the cervical os.

Causes
- Preterm labour.
- Polyhydramnios.
- Multiple pregnancy—the second twin is often a breech presentation.
- Placenta praevia—the placenta takes up room in the lower uterus, leaving less space for the fetal head to present.
- Contracted pelvis—not enough room for the fetal head to engage in the pelvis.
- Multiparity.
- Fetal or uterine abnormality.

Antenatal diagnosis
- On abdominal palpation the head is felt at the top of the uterus and it ballots easily unless splinted by extended legs.
- The breech is smaller, softer, and more irregular than the hard smooth, rounded head.
- Fetal heart sounds are heard above the level of the maternal umbilicus.

Management
- If breech presentation is diagnosed at the 36-week antenatal visit, offer the mother external cephalic version to convert the breech to head presenting. This is arranged to take place as close to term as possible, commonly at 38 weeks' gestation.[1]
- A 50% success rate has been reported for the procedure, depending on the skill and experience of the operator.[2]
- External cephalic version should be performed by an obstetrician or specialist trained midwife in a hospital setting.

- The procedure should be explained to the mother with reasons and possible risks, so that she can give informed consent.
- Perform an ultrasound scan prior to the procedure to confirm the fetus is not compromised, locate the placenta and confirm fetal position, and afterwards monitor the fetal heart and the placenta, in case of accidental bleeding.
- Some hospitals use tocolysis to relax the uterus prior to and during the procedure.
- The mother should have an empty bladder, and it is sometimes helpful to elevate the foot of the bed.
- The obstetrician disengages the breech from the pelvis, locates the fetal head, and attempts to manoeuvre the fetus through a forward somersault towards the iliac fossa until the head is presenting. (Be careful not to pinch the mother's skin!)
- The procedure should be abandoned if the fetus does not turn easily.
- A cardiotocograph is used to monitor the fetal heart throughout the procedure.
- The woman stays in hospital for about 2h after the procedure and will be seen a week later to confirm the presentation.
- Anti-D immunoglobulin is offered if the woman is Rh-negative.
- If the procedure fails, or the presentation re-converts to breech, the woman has the option of attempted vaginal delivery or elective caesarean section at 39 weeks.

Contraindications

- Previous caesarean section
- Antepartum haemorrhage
- Placenta praevia
- Multiple pregnancy
- Small for gestational age fetus
- Hypertension
- Pre-eclampsia due to increased risk of placental separation
- Oligohydramnios
- Ruptured membranes.

1 Royal College of Obstetrics and Gynaecologists (2006). *External Cephalic Version and Reducing the Incidence of Breech Presentation.* Guideline 20a. London: RCOG Press.

2 Varma R (2002). Managing term breech deliveries: External cephalic version should be routine practice in the UK. *BMJ* **324**, 49–50.

Hyperemesis

Hyperemesis means excessive vomiting and this condition can occur in 3–20% of pregnancies. It is an extremely unpleasant condition and sufferers can become depressed and demoralized that the early stage of pregnancy makes them feel so ill.

Hyperemesis gravidarum should be considered when all other causes of persistent nausea and vomiting have been ruled out.

Pyelonephritis, pancreatitis, cholecystitis, hepatitis, appendicitis, gastroenteritis, peptic ulcer disease, thyrotoxicosis, and hyperthyroidism can present in similar fashions, with intractable nausea and vomiting, and are treatable conditions. Late presenters need also to be ruled out for HELLP syndrome and other causes of hepatic and central nervous system dysfunction.

It usually lasts anytime from the sixth to the 16th week of pregnancy and is characterized by:

• Vomiting several times a day
• Persistent nausea
• Dehydration
• Reduced urine output
• The appearance of ketones in the urine.

It can be a potentially life-threatening condition especially if the electrolyte or acid/base balance becomes disordered. In severe cases hospitalization becomes necessary in order to provide rest.

Intravenous fluid, up to 5–6L/day using the appropriate amounts of sodium, potassium, chloride, lactate or bicarbonate, glucose, and water, are primarily used in correcting the hypovolaemia, electrolyte and acid–base imbalances, and ketosis.

Anti-emetics can be prescribed in the short term, usually promethazine.

Fluids and diet are gradually reintroduced until a normal diet is tolerated. There are usually no ill-effects on the pregnancy and once the condition improves pregnancy proceeds normally.

Special consideration must be given to the risk of thromboembolism in women with this condition. If hospitalized women require bed rest, the application of thrombo-embolic deterrent stockings (TEDS) is recommended.

Recommended reading

Symonds I (2009). Abnormalities of early pregnancy. In: Fraser D, Cooper M. *Myles Textbook for Midwives*. 15th edn. London: Churchill Livingstone, pp. 225–6.

Infections

Coughs, colds, and flu

These common infections pose little threat to the fetus and symptom relief is all that is necessary. Advise fluids, rest, and paracetamol up to normal maximum doses, e.g. 1g four times a day. Inhaled decongestants are safe but cough linctus should be avoided.

A productive cough could be a sign of bacterial infection requiring antibiotic treatment and the woman should be referred to her GP.

Urinary tract infections

Women should be offered screening by mid-stream urine culture for asymptomatic bacteriuria early in pregnancy, as identification and treatment reduce the risk of preterm birth.[1]

Around 1 in 25 women develop a urinary tract infection during pregnancy. The symptoms are:
- Discomfort or burning sensation on micturition
- Pain in the bladder region/lower pelvis
- Frequency of micturition.

An ascending infection involving the kidneys or bloodstream may cause:
- Loin pain
- Vomiting
- Fever
- Uterine contractions—the symptoms of premature labour may mask a urinary tract infection and midstream urine should be obtained for culture to rule this out.

Mild infections are treated with oral antibiotics, but a more serious infection requires admission to hospital for intravenous antibiotic therapy and rest.

Bacterial infections

BV is present in up to 20% of pregnant women who are slightly more likely to deliver pre-term.[2] Treatment is with clindamycin orally or vaginally, or metronidazole gel. Reoccurrence is common.

Chlamydia affects 2–13% of pregnant women. It is associated with pre-term delivery, pre-labour rupture of the membranes, chorioamnionitis and post-partum endometritis.[3] Chlamydia screening is not offered routinely but this policy may change with the implementation of the opportunistic chlamydia screening programme. Treatment is with erythromycin.

GBS is the leading cause of serious neonatal infection in the UK. Approximately 40% of adults carry the bacteria in the gastrointestinal or reproductive tract. Pregnant women are not routinely screened but those who present with high risk factors for this infection are offered screening at 34–36 weeks' gestation so that intrapartum antibiotics (penicillin) can be administered.[4]

The risk factors are: pre-term delivery, prolonged rupture of the membranes, GBS cultured in a urine sample, known carriage of GBS or a history of GBS in a previous pregnancy.

Sexually transmitted diseases

Gonorrhea is rare but on the increase. It is associated with adverse pregnancy outcomes;[5] however the infection is treatable with penicillin or ciprofloxacin.

Syphilis is an acute or chronic infection screened for in early pregnancy. The incidence in the UK is low and it can be treated with penicillin.[6]

Viral infections

Genital herpes

Presents as a flu-like illness followed by an outbreak of vulval sores which are very painful. These usually heal after 7–10 days. This is sometimes mistaken for candidiasis as it seemingly responds to cream or pessaries. Occasionally it is symptomless.

The herpes virus then remains dormant in the spinal nerves and can be reactivated, causing a secondary attack. During pregnancy herpes causes most problems if a first attack occurs after 28 weeks' gestation. Secondary attacks are much less of a risk.

The main risk is transmission of the virus to the baby during birth. Herpes can also cause premature labour and affect fetal growth.[7]

An elective caesarean section at 38 weeks' gestation is usually advised if a primary attack occurs after 28 weeks' gestation, or in early labour if there are vulval sores present. Affected women may be offered treatment with aciclovir after 20 weeks' gestation.

Hepatitis B

All women are offered screening in early pregnancy. Hepatitis B during pregnancy does not increase maternal mortality or morbidity or the risk of fetal complications. Approximately 90% of the infants of HBsAg carrier mothers with positive hepatitis B e-antigen (HBeAg) will become carriers if no immunoprophylaxis is given.[8] Neonates given the Hepatitis B immunoglobulin within 24 hours of birth will be prevented from developing the infection and becoming carriers themselves.

Chickenpox

This is a fairly common infection and many women are exposed during pregnancy.

If a woman has already had chickenpox, there is no risk to the fetus, but if a woman has never had chickenpox and contracts it before 20 weeks' gestation, there is a risk of the fetus developing a severe infection—chickenpox syndrome.[9]

Varicella zoster immunoglobulin antibody treatment reduces the risk of chickenpox syndrome and should be given 10 days after the initial attack.

Between 20 weeks and term there is no risk to the baby as protective antibodies are produced which cross the placenta.

If a mother develops a rash within a week before delivery to 1 month afterwards, there will not have been time for the transfer of antibodies to take place and the baby is at risk of severe infection after the birth.

Toxoplasmosis

Toxoplasmosis is caused by the parasite *Toxoplasma gondii*, which is found in raw meat and in cats that eat raw meat and their faeces. It rarely causes illness in an adult, although it can present as a flu-like illness with swollen lymph glands (📖 see also Food safety, p. 88).

In pregnant women it is of concern as it can lead to fetal infection and the following potential problems:

- Miscarriage
- Stillbirth
- Growth problems
- Blindness
- Brain damage
- Epilepsy
- Deafness.

Prevention is the best strategy. Women may be offered pyrimethamine or sulfadiazine to limit transmission of the infection.

Advise pregnant women to:

- Cook all meat thoroughly until there are no pink areas and the juices are clear
- Wash hands, utensils, and surface areas after preparing raw meat
- Wash soil from fruit and vegetables before eating
- Always use gloves when gardening and wash hands afterwards
- Ask someone else to clean litter trays if a cat owner, or to wear gloves and wash hands thoroughly afterwards.

1 National Institute for Health and Clinical Excellence (2008). Antenatal care: routine care for the healthy pregnant woman. Clinical guideline 62. London: NICE. Available at: 🖱 http://guidance.nice.org.uk/CG62.

2 Guerra B, Ghi T, Quarta S, et al. (2006). Pregnancy outcome after early detection of bacterial vaginosis. *European Journal of Obstetrics and Gynecology and Reproductive Biology* **128**, 40–453.

3 Blas MM, Canchihuaman FA, Alva IE, Hawes SE (2007). Pregnancy outcomes in women infected with *Chlamydia trachomatis*: a population-based cohort study in Washington State. *Sexually Transmitted Infections* **83**, 314–18.

4 Pettersson K (2007). Perinatal infection with Group B streptococci. *Seminars in Fetal and Neonatal Medicine* **12**, 193–7.

5 Brocklehurst P (2002). Antibiotics for gonorrhoea in pregnancy. *Cochrane Database of Systematic Reviews* **2**, CD000098.

6 Walker GJA (2001). Antibiotics for syphilis diagnosed during pregnancy. *Cochrane Database of Systematic Reviews* 2001, **3**, CD001143.

7 Royal College of Obstetrics and Gynaecologists (2007). *Management of Genital Herpes in Pregnancy.* Green Top Guideline 30. London: RCOG Press.

8 Chang M-H (2007). Hepatitis B virus infection. *Seminars in Fetal and Neonatal Medicine* **12**, 160–7.

9 Royal College of Obstetrics and Gynaecologists (2007). *Chickenpox in Pregnancy.* Green Top Guideline 13. London: RCOG Press.

Intrauterine growth restriction

Growth restriction is failure of the fetus to reach normal growth parameters.[1] This refers to a fetus that is less than the 10th percentile for its gestational age. Clinical measurement is often unreliable but if growth restriction is suspected the mother should be referred to the obstetrician for confirmation.

Causes of intrauterine growth restriction

Maternal factors which might influence fetal growth

- Alcohol abuse
- Smoking
- Substance misuse
- Poor nutrition
- Hypertensive disorders
- Maternal cardiac or renal disease.

Pregnancy factors which might influence fetal growth

- Multiple pregnancies (twins, triplets, etc.)
- Placenta problems
- Preeclampsia or eclampsia
- Intrauterine infection
- High altitudes.

Monitoring growth

- In the third trimester, ultrasound scans can be used to measure growth of the fetus if the clinical findings give cause for concern.
- It is important to recognize large for gestational age as well as growth-restricted fetuses.
- The two most common measurements used in monitoring growth are the head and abdominal circumferences.
- The abdominal circumference is a useful when assessing growth, because of fat deposition in the fetal liver. This is reduced in growth-restricted fetuses and increased in macrosomic fetuses. The ratio between the head and abdominal circumference helps distinguish between the two types of growth restriction:
  - Asymmetrical growth restriction
  - Symmetrical growth restriction.

Asymmetrical growth restriction

- This is characterized by falling abdominal circumference measurements but the head circumference stays within normal limits.
- This is referred to as 'brain sparing', as the brain continues to receive nutrients and continues to develop while the fat and glycogen deposits in the liver dwindle as the fetus is compromised.
- It is usually apparent in the later stages of pregnancy and is due to placental insufficiency.
- This is a sign that the oxygen supply to the fetus will slow down in the near future.

Symmetrical growth restriction

- The fetus may be genetically small but otherwise normal, or may be suffering from such poor nutrition that both the brain and other organs are affected.
- The head and abdominal circumference have a close ratio and both measurements are reduced.
- The genetically small fetus will be apparent from the first scan, but this may also be due to external influences, such as maternal malnutrition, infection, or substance misuse, or to a congenital anomaly.

It is often difficult to distinguish between the growth restricted and merely small fetus. The cause may be attributed to incorrect dates and the woman given a revised date of delivery. Measurements taken from the early pregnancy scan are therefore essential to avoid induction of labour that is either too early or too late.

1 Baschat AA, Galan HL, Ross MG, Gabbe SG (2007). Intrauterine growth restriction. In: Gabbe SG, Niebyl JR, Simpson JL (eds) *Obstetrics: Normal and Problem Pregnancies.* 5th edn. Philadelphia, PA: Elsevier Churchill Livingstone.

Multiple pregnancy

Incidence

In natural conceptions 1:80 result in twin pregnancy. 1:6400 conceptions results in triplets, and 1:512 000 results in quadruplets. The incidence of multiple pregnancies overall is on the increase due to the impact of successful infertility treatment.

Where an average incidence of triplets in a maternity unit delivering 3000 babies a year might result in a triplet birth every 2 years, it is becoming more common to see two to three such births in a year.

Twin pregnancy has the highest incidence and can be divided into two types:

Monozygotic—sometimes referred to as identical twins. The incidence is 2.5–4 per 1000 births.
- Results from one ova and one spermatozoa.
- There is one chorion membrane and one placenta.
- There are two amnion, one for each twin.
- The babies are always the same sex, blood group, eye colour, etc.

Dizygotic or non-identical twins. The incidence is more frequent with hereditary factors from both the mother and father affecting the frequency.[1]
- Results from two ova and two spermatozoa.
- There are two chorion and two placenta though these may be so closely joined that they look like one.
- There are two amnion, one for each twin.
- The babies may be the same sex or one of each, and no more alike than any other family members.

Diagnosis is invariably made at the time of the dating scan early in the second trimester. By 20 weeks the uterus will be large for gestational age and this is obvious on palpation. If a mother is late booking or has not received antenatal care the diagnosis may be made quite late in pregnancy. It is rare nowadays to diagnose twins only once the mother is in labour.

Special considerations

Serum screening tests for fetal abnormality are unsuitable as the results will be unreliable. Nuchal translucency scans, placental biopsy or amniocentesis are options the mother may wish to consider.

During pregnancy the mother has a higher risk of complications developing such as:
- Miscarriage
- Exaggerated minor disorders of pregnancy
- Premature labour
- Pregnancy induced hypertension
- Anaemia—due to the demands of two fetuses.
- Polyhydramnios—excess amounts of amniotic fluid
- Placental abruption
- Placenta praevia
- Intrauterine growth restriction.

Antenatal management

- Early diagnosis so relevant information and support can be organized.
- Determination of whether the twins are identical or not (zygosity).
- Chorionicity—if the pregnancy has only one chorion there is a three- to fivefold higher risk of perinatal mortality. This can be determined from a scan in the first trimester.
- A multiple pregnancy can be shorter than a single pregnancy. The average is 37 weeks for twins, 34 weeks for triplets, and 32 weeks for quads.
- Identical or monochorionic twin pregnancies should have a scan every 2 weeks from diagnosis to look for discordant growth patterns; a sign of feto-fetal transfusion syndrome.
- Non-identical twin pregnancies should have a scan every 4 weeks to monitor growth.
- Regular measurement of maternal haemoglobin levels and iron supplements if needed.
- The mother needs additional support both to prepare her for the birth and also the care and feeding of the babies.
- The mother will need to pay particular attention to her dietary needs, the need for rest and the possibility that she may have to stop work earlier than intended.

1 Nair M, Kumar G (2009). Uncomplicated monochorionic diamniotic twin pregnancy. *Journal of Obstetrics and Gynaecology* **29**, 90–3.

Obstetric cholestasis

Obstetric cholestasis, also known as intra-hepatic cholestasis of pregnancy is a disorder of the liver where the flow of bile is reduced, resulting in increased levels of bile acids in the mother's bloodstream. This is thought to be caused by sensitivity to the hormone oestrogen and tends to affect up to 1% of pregnant women.[1]

Women with a family history of the disorder and those with multiple pregnancy are more at risk.

Symptoms

- Itching: due to the excess bile salts in the bloodstream, begins in the palms of the hands and soles of the feet then spreads to the limbs before becoming generalized.
- Jaundice: a rare symptom, indicating problems with the synthesis of bilirubin.
- Loss of appetite.
- Insomnia.
- Meconium staining in the amniotic fluid.
- Fetal heart rate changes: bradycardia or tachycardia.
- Preterm labour.
- Postnatal bleeding: due to underproduction of clotting factors by the liver.

Management

- Serum screening for bile acids and liver function tests.
- Ultrasound scan to exclude maternal gallstones that may be causing reduction of the flow of bile.
- Drug treatment may improve the condition, but the drug used, ursodeoxycholic acid, is unlicensed and can only be given with the woman's full consent and in the knowledge that the drug has *not* been tested on pregnant women.
- There is a small risk that babies whose mothers have cholestasis may be stillborn, and some obstetricians prefer to induce labour at 38 weeks' gestation or earlier if there are signs of fetal compromise. There is at present insufficient data to support or disprove the value of this intervention.
- The mother may be prescribed oral vitamin K daily until delivery to prevent postnatal bleeding.
- Betamethasone may be given to mature the fetal lungs if preterm delivery is anticipated.
- The baby will require vitamin K at delivery to prevent bleeding.
- The mother may be advised follow-up liver function tests and a further scan to exclude gallstones.
- She should make a full recovery with return of normal liver function.
- The condition may re-appear in subsequent pregnancies.

---

1 Royal College of Obstetrics and Gynaecologists (2006). *Obstetric Cholestasis*. Guideline 43. London: RCOG Press.

Pregnancy-induced hypertension

Hypertensive disorders of pregnancy affect 1 in 10 pregnancies overall and 1 in 50 severely. Pregnancy-induced hypertension (PIH) is the second leading cause of maternal death with 18 deaths in the latest CEMACH report.[1]

There is also an impact on perinatal mortality as the condition is associated with placental abruption, intrauterine growth restriction in otherwise normal fetuses, and preterm birth; 500–600 babies a year die as a result of PIH.

Aetiology

- Unknown, but thought to be linked to genetic and immunological influences.
- Begins in early pregnancy and is related to disorders of the developing placenta. The invading trophoblast cells of the fertilized ovum are normally able to restructure the maternal spiral arteries in the decidual lining of the uterus to create a low-pressure, high-flow blood supply to the developing fetus.
- Placental development is completed by around 18 weeks' gestation, and if this has not progressed normally, the spiral arteries supplying the placental bed remain narrow, and retain their responses, causing generalized vasospasm and ischaemia.
- After 20 weeks gestation the mother's blood pressure rises in response to this, causing generalized endothelial damage in her circulatory system, leading to vasoconstriction, platelet activation, and placental insufficiency.
- In the end stage of PIH, sometimes referred to as pre-eclampsia, end-organ damage affects the renal and hepatic systems, with symptoms such as proteinuria, disruption of the clotting mechanism, and disturbed fluid distribution, leading to generalized oedema.
- This is a progressive condition and multisystem disease, relieved only by delivery of the baby and placenta. Rarely, eclampsia develops, characterized by convulsions, loss of consciousness, and severe hypertension.

Diagnosis and clinical features

- Blood pressure: systolic >20–25mmHg over the baseline; diastolic >15mmHg over the baseline. These changes persist for two readings more than 4h apart.
- Proteinuria: >0.30g protein daily, or dipstick showing 2+ protein from clean-catch mid-stream urine sample (MSU).
- Oedema: rapid weight gain before oedema noted. The oedema will involve the upper extremities.

Severe: maternal criteria

- Systolic >160mmHg; diastolic >110mmHg
- >5g proteinuria in 24h (4+ on stick)
- Altered liver function—epigastric pain
- Persistent headache
- Hyperreflexia

- Thrombocytopenia
- Oliguria
- Pulmonary oedema.

Severe: fetal criteria
- Intrauterine growth restriction <5th centile
- Oligohydramnios.

Management

Midwives play a critical role in screening and identification of women who are developing pregnancy induced hypertension. During each antenatal care appointment the midwife measures the blood pressure, tests the woman's urine for protein, and observes for signs of excessive oedema.

If the midwife detects mild hypertension without proteinuria an increased level of surveillance will be required and the woman asked to attend more frequently to have her blood pressure and urine monitored. Collaborative care provides the most effective management and after referral to the consultant for investigation the woman can often resume her care in the community provided her condition does not deteriorate.

Once protein appears in the urine the woman should be referred to consultant led antenatal care and this may take place on an outpatient basis, in a day care setting or the woman may be referred to triage with a view to further management. Admission to hospital is required when the mother and fetus require more monitoring and evaluation than can be provided in a day care setting.

Antihypertensives may be prescribed mainly to prevent severe hypertension developing which protects the mother from the risk of cerebral haemorrhage. Methyldopa is a centrally acting antihypertensive safe for use in pregnancy in doses up to 1g daily. Labetalol, a β-blocking drug is also commonly used for this purpose.

The midwife's role is to provide whatever emotional and supportive care is appropriate for the practice setting. Once admitted to hospital the woman will have a daily antenatal examination including urinalysis and the condition of the fetus is monitored by daily cardiotocograph. Blood pressure recording will be undertaken at least every 4h during the day and if the mother wakes during the night.

FBC, renal and hepatic chemistry, plasma proteins, and clotting factors will be monitored closely and any deterioration in the maternal or fetal condition will lead to the decision to deliver the baby either by induction of labour or caesarean section.

1 Lewis, G (ed.) (2007). *The Confidential Enquiry into Maternal and Child Health (CEMACH). Saving Mothers' Lives: Reviewing Maternal Deaths to Make Motherhood Safer—2003–2005*. The 7th report on Confidential Enquires into Maternal Deaths in the United Kingdom. London: CEMACH.

The impact of obesity during pregnancy and beyond

Recent figures suggest that in the UK the rising rate of obesity within the general population will have a major impact on public health. For the childbearing population this is already having an impact. Obesity represents one of the greatest and growing overall threats to the childbearing population of the UK.

Obesity in pregnancy is usually defined as a BMI of 30kg/m^2 or greater at booking.[1] In the UK national statistics about the prevalence of obesity during pregnancy suggest that 50% of women of childbearing age are overweight or obese.[2]

The predominance of obese women among those who died from thromboembolism, sepsis, and cardiac disease recorded in the latest CEMACH report[3] means that early multidisciplinary planning regarding mode of delivery and use of thromboprophylaxis for these women is essential.

Pre-pregnancy counselling and weight loss, together with wider public health messages about optimum weight should help to reduce the number of obese women who become pregnant.

Risks of obesity in pregnancy

Obesity in pregnancy is associated with increased risks of complications for both mother and baby. Women with obesity in pregnancy also have higher rates of induction of labour, caesarean section and PPH and there is an increased risk of post-caesarean wound infection.[4]

There is also evidence that babies of obese women have significantly increased risks of adverse outcomes, including fetal congenital anomaly, prematurity, stillbirth and neonatal death.[4]

Risks for the mother
- Maternal death or severe morbidity
- Cardiac disease
- Spontaneous first trimester and recurrent miscarriage
- Pre-eclampsia
- Gestational diabetes
- Thromboembolism
- Post-caesarean wound infection
- Infection from other causes
- Postpartum haemorrhage
- Low breastfeeding rates.

Risks for the baby
- Stillbirth and neonatal death
- Congenital abnormalities
- Macrosomia
- Prematurity.

Pre-pregnancy care
- Women of childbearing age should have the opportunity to optimize their weight prior to pregnancy.

- Advice on weight and lifestyle plus regular monitoring of weight, BMI, and waist circumference should be offered during consultations for family planning or during pre-conception consultations.
  - Women of childbearing age with a BMI of 30kg/m² or above should receive information and advice about the risks of obesity during pregnancy and supported to lose weight before conception.[5]

Pregnancy care

- Women should have their BMI calculated at the booking visit and the result documented in the handheld and electronic record.
- Discuss her eating habits and how physically active she is. Find out if she has any concerns about diet and the amount of physical activity she does and try to address them.[5]
- Advise her that a healthy diet and being physically active will benefit both her and her unborn child during pregnancy and will also help her to achieve a healthy weight after giving birth. Advise her to seek information and advice on diet and activity from a reputable source.[5]
- Advise her on how to use Healthy Start vouchers to increase the fruit and vegetable intake of those eligible for the Healthy Start scheme (women <18 years and those who are receiving benefit payments).[5]
- Dispel any myths about what and how much to eat during pregnancy. For example, advise that there is no need to 'eat for two' or to drink full-fat milk. Explain that energy needs do not change in the first 6 months of pregnancy and increase only slightly in the last 3 months (and then only by around 200cal/day).[5]
- Advise her that moderate-intensity physical activity will not harm her or her unborn child. At least 30 minutes per day of moderate intensity activity is recommended.[5] Swimming or brisk walking is ideal and this should start slowly and build up for those who are not used to this level of activity.
- Pregnant women with a BMI of 40kg/m² or above should be referred for a consultation with an obstetric anaesthetist, so that difficulties with venous access, or regional or general anaesthesia can be identified. A management plan for labour should be discussed and documented.
- An appropriate size arm cuff should be used to measure blood pressure at antenatal visits and the cuff size recorded in the antenatal notes.
- Women with a BMI of 30kg/m² or above should be screened for gestational diabetes.
- Pregnant women with a BMI of 40kg/m² or above should have a third trimester assessment of their manual handling requirements.
- A risk assessment for thromboembolism should be carried out and both antenatal and post delivery thromboprophylaxis considered.

Care during labour

- Women with a BMI of 35kg/m² or above should give birth in a consultant led obstetric unit.
- An Obstetrician and Anaesthetist of appropriate seniority should be informed and available for care of a woman in labour with a BMI of 40kg/m² or above.

- Women with a BMI of 40kg/m² or above should have venous access established in early labour. These women should receive continuous midwifery care.
- Operating department staff should be informed early of any woman weighing greater than 120kgs who require operative delivery.
- Women with a BMI of 30kg/m² or above should have an actively managed third stage of labour.

Postnatal care

- Obesity is associated with low breastfeeding initiation and maintenance rates, so specialist advice and support should be offered both antenatally and postnatally.
- Early mobilization should be encouraged.
- Women with a BMI of 30kg/m² or above should continue to receive nutritional and physical activity advice with a view to weight reduction. The 6–8 week post natal assessment can be a useful time to offer further support. This can continue to be followed up at 6-monthly intervals by the GP or other appropriate health professional.[5]
- Women with a BMI of 30kg/m² should have regular follow up by their GP for the development of type 2 diabetes.
- Women who develop gestational diabetes should receive annual screening for cardio-metabolic risk factors and receive advice on nutrition and weight management.

Practical considerations

Maternity units should have guidelines in place to facilitate care of women with BMI of 30kg/m² or above with respect to referral criteria, facilities and equipment.
The following are required:
- Large blood pressure cuffs
- Sit-on weighing scale
- Large chairs and wheelchairs
- Ultrasound scan couches, ward and delivery beds
- Theatre trolleys and operating theatre tables
- Lifting and lateral transfer equipment.

1 Centre for Maternal and Child Enquiries and Royal College of Obstetricians and Gynaecologists (2010). *Management of Women with Obesity During Pregnancy.* London: RCOG Press.

2 NHS Information Centre (2008). *Health Survey for England 2006: CVD and Risk Factors: Adults, Obesity and Risk Factors Children.* London: NHS Information Centre. Available from: ℜ www. ic.nhs.uk (accessed 22.2.11).

3 Lewis, G (ed.) (2007). *The Confidential Enquiry into Maternal and Child Health (CEMACH). Saving Mothers' Lives: Reviewing Maternal Deaths to Make Motherhood Safer—2003–2005.* The 7th report on Confidential Enquires into Maternal Deaths in the United Kingdom. London: CEMACH.

4 Catalano PM (2007). Management of obesity in pregnancy. *Obstetrics and Gynecology* **109**, 419–33.

5 National Institute for Health and Clinical Excellence (2010). Dietary interventions and physical activity interventions for weight management before during and after pregnancy. Guideline PH27. London: NICE. Available at : ℜ http://guidance.nice.org.uk/PH27 (accessed 22.2.11).

Medical conditions during pregnancy

Asthma

Asthma is the most common chronic disease in children and young adults and is on the increase; 4–8% of pregnant women have asthma. The condition is often underrecognized and suboptimally treated.[1]

Effect of pregnancy on asthma

- Asthma tends to improve in pregnancy especially during the last 12 weeks but it can be very variable, with some remaining stable and others worsening.
- Breathlessness due to the increasing size of the uterus is sometimes mistaken for worsening asthma.
- Many women experience a worsening of their symptoms because they stop taking their asthma medication because of concerns about the effects on the fetus.
- Women who deteriorate during pregnancy tend to have the most severe asthma.

Effects of asthma on pregnancy

- Good control is essential for maternal and fetal well-being. Poor control is associated with pregnancy induced hypertension, pre-eclampsia, increased caesarean section, pre-term delivery, intrauterine growth restriction, and low birthweight.
- Asthma treatment during pregnancy is no different to that at other times and the inhaled medications are safe.
- Very little inhaled medication reaches the fetus.
- More harm is likely from withholding treatment than from continuing it.

Management of asthma during pregnancy

- Objective monitoring of lung function.
- Avoiding or controlling asthma triggers.
- Patient education and individualized pharmacological therapy.
- Those with persistent asthma should be monitored by peak expiratory flow rate, spirometry to measure the forced expiratory volume in 1s, or both.
- The ultimate goal of asthma therapy is maintaining adequate oxygenation of the fetus by prevention of hypoxic episodes in the mother.
- Asthma exacerbations should be aggressively managed, with a goal of alleviating asthma symptoms and attaining peak expiratory flow rate or forced expiratory volume in 1s of 70% predicted or more.
- Pregnancies complicated by moderate or severe asthma may benefit from ultrasound for fetal growth and accurate dating and antenatal assessment of fetal well-being.
- Asthma medications should be continued during labour, and the mother should be encouraged to breastfeed.

1 Dombroski MP (2006). Asthma and pregnancy. *Obstetrics and Gynecology* **108**, 667–81.

Cardiac conditions

Women with congenital heart disease are surviving to become pregnant in greater numbers due to advances in surgery and better management of care. Antenatal care is a complex issue and early referral to a specialist centre is advisable so that the specialist midwife, cardiologist, obstetrician, anaesthetist, fetal medicine specialist, haematologist, neonatologist and cardiac nurse can meet the woman to plan her care and review her progress regularly. This appointment should take place as early as possible as she is a high risk case and requires multidisciplinary care.

Significance of cardiac conditions

- Congenital heart disease occurs in 0.8% of newborns.
- Advances in medical treatment and surgery have resulted in 85% survival rates.
- Cardiac disease is the leading cause of maternal death in the UK with 48 deaths in the last triennium.[1]
- Cardiac conditions have many implications for pregnancy due to the normal associated cardiovascular changes:
  - Peripheral vasodilation which is the body's initial response to pregnancy.
  - Decreased peripheral resistance.
  - Increase in plasma volume by 50%.
  - Increase in RBCs of 20%—physiological haemodilution giving the impression of anaemia but is normal to pregnancy.
  - Cardiac output increases by 50%.

Assessment

This can be difficult as normal pregnancy symptoms mirror the symptoms of cardiac disease. The following are all associated with normal pregnancy, however the woman should be encouraged to report any new symptoms no matter how subtle:
- Shortness of breath—dyspnoea, at rest or on exertion
- Raised respiratory rate—tachypnoea
- Tiredness
- Dizziness
- Fainting—syncope.
  The woman should be examined at every visit for:
- Cyanosis
- Pallor
- Prominent neck veins
- Peripheral oedema
- Rapid weight gain
- Blood pressure, heart rate, and rhythm
- Auscultation of heart sounds to record type and grade of murmurs
- Auscultation of the lung bases to detect pulmonary oedema.

Investigations

- Electrocardiogram.
- Echocardiogram.
- 12 and 20 week scans.

- Fetal growth scans every 4 weeks.
- Exclude diabetes, avoid anaemia, and treat any infection.

Most maternal cardiac conditions present a high risk for intrauterine growth restriction (IUGR) and pre-eclampsia so the midwife should continue normal antenatal surveillance. Drug therapy will continue during the pregnancy and may involve the use of anticoagulants in some conditions. Regimens should be monitored closely with individual drugs considered for their likely effect on pregnancy and the fetus.

Recommended reading

Boyle M, Bothamley J (2009). Cardiac disorders: care during pregnancy, labour and the puerperium. *Midwives* **October/November**, 36–7.

1 Lewis, G (ed.) (2007). *The Confidential Enquiry into Maternal and Child Health (CEMACH). Saving Mothers' Lives: Reviewing Maternal Deaths to Make Motherhood Safer—2003–2005.* The 7th report on Confidential Enquires into Maternal Deaths in the United Kingdom. London: CEMACH.

Diabetes

- Diabetes during pregnancy can be classified into three forms:
  - Insulin-dependent diabetes, which is present prior to pregnancy (type 1 diabetes)
  - Non-insulin dependent diabetes (type 2 diabetes)
  - Gestational diabetes (GDM) or impaired glucose tolerance, which arises as a result of pregnancy and then resolves after the birth. The incidence is between 3% and 12% of the pregnant population. Overt diabetes will develop in 20–30% of women with GDM within 5 years.[1]
- Non-diabetic pregnant women are offered a glucose challenge screen to detect GDM if any two of the following risk factors are present:
  - Glycosuria on two occasions on testing at an antenatal visit (early morning sample)
  - History of diabetes in a close relative
  - Obesity, BMI >27
  - Previous baby weighing more than 4.5kg
  - Previous unexplained perinatal death
  - Previous baby with congenital malformations
  - Unexplained severe polyhydramnios (excess amniotic fluid in the uterus).
- Maternal complications which might arise in the pregnant diabetic client are related to poorly controlled glucose levels in the maternal serum:
  - Urinary tract infection
  - Vaginal infection
  - Polyhydramnios
  - Pregnancy-induced hypertension
  - Fetal macrosomia leading to shoulder dystocia.

Fetal complications

- Congenital abnormality—four times higher than in non-diabetic women
- Prematurity associated with delayed lung maturity
- Perinatal death (due to the above conditions)
- 1:100 risk of the child themselves becoming diabetic.

Carbohydrate metabolism during pregnancy (non diabetic)

- Pregnancy itself is said to be diabetogenic as a result of changes due to the action of the pregnancy hormones.
- The fetal/placental unit alters glucose metabolism in the following ways:
  - From the 10th week fasting blood sugar progressively falls from 4 to 3.6 mmol/L
  - The placenta produces a hormone called human placental lactogen, which increases the maternal tissue resistance to insulin
  - Blood glucose levels therefore are higher after meals and remain so for longer than in the non-pregnant state.
  - More insulin is required by the body and output of insulin in the pancreas increases by three to four times the normal rate.

- Extra demands on the pancreatic B cells precipitate glucose intolerance or overt diabetes in women whose capacity to produce insulin was only just adequate prior to pregnancy (GDM).
- Utilization of fat stores results in raised free fatty acid and glycerol levels, making the woman more readily ketotic.

Management of diabetes/GDM[2]

If the mother is already diabetic, her insulin requirements will be increased during pregnancy and her pregnancy will be monitored carefully. If it is safely achievable, women with diabetes should aim to keep fasting blood glucose between 3.5 and 5.9 mmol/L and 1h postprandial blood glucose <7.8 mmol/L during pregnancy.

Women with type 2 diabetes may form the largest population of pre-pregnancy diabetics and be exposed to the same levels of risk related to pregnancy outcomes. Their condition may indeed be diagnosed for the first time during pregnancy due to screening for GDM. Careful monitoring of glycaemic control, provision of insulin as a replacement or in addition to metformin therapy could improve outcomes.

For women who develop GDM a careful assessment of their insulin needs is required and therapy commenced in accordance with the need to control blood glucose levels in the prescribed range.

Women with insulin-treated diabetes should be advised of the risks of hypoglycaemia and hypoglycaemia unawareness in pregnancy, particularly in the first trimester. During pregnancy, women with insulin-treated diabetes should be provided with a concentrated glucose solution and women with type 1 diabetes should also be given glucagon; women and their partners or other family members should be instructed in their use.

General principles of care for women with diabetes in pregnancy

- Ensure as much as possible that pregnancies are planned.
- Early booking (before the 10th week of pregnancy).
- Joint care with an endocrinologist specializing in diabetes.
- Blood sugar profiles every 2 weeks and glycosylated haemoglobin monthly.
- Prevention of excessive maternal weight gain.
- Healthcare professionals should be aware that the rapid-acting insulin analogues (aspart and lispro) have advantages over soluble human insulin during pregnancy, and should consider their use.
- Pregnant women with pre-existing diabetes should be offered retinal assessment by digital imaging with mydriasis using tropicamide following their first antenatal clinic appointment and again at 28 weeks if the first assessment is normal. If any diabetic retinopathy is present, an additional retinal assessment should be performed at 16–20 weeks. If retinal assessment has not been performed in the preceding 12 months, it should be offered as soon as possible after the first contact in pregnancy in women with pre-existing diabetes.
- If renal assessment has not been undertaken in the preceding 12 months in women with preexisting diabetes, it should be arranged at the first contact in pregnancy. If serum creatinine is abnormal (120 micromol/L or more) or if total protein excretion exceeds 2g/day,

referral to a nephrologist should be considered (estimated glomerular filtration rate (eGFR) should not be used during pregnancy). Thrombo-prophylaxis should be considered for women with proteinuria above 5 g/day (macroalbuminuria).
- Careful screening for urinary tract and vaginal infection, with prompt treatment.
- Discuss the need for fetal anomaly scan in light of the increased risk of malformations.
- Careful monitoring of fetal growth by regular ultrasound scans.
- At 36 weeks' gestation a discussion will take place with the mother regarding mode of delivery and the options available. A recommendation of induction of labour or elective caesarean section will be made should the maternal or fetal condition warrant this.

1 Peters RK, Kjos SL., Xiang A., Buchanan TA (1996). Long-term diabetogenic effect of single pregnancy in women with previous gestational diabetes mellitus. *International Journal of Gynecology and Obstetrics* **54**, 213–13.

2 Royal College of Obstetricians and Gynaecologists (2008). *Diabetes in Pregnancy: Management of Diabetes and its Complications From Preconception to the Postnatal Period.* Commissioned by the National Institute for Health and Clinical Excellence. London: RCOG Press.

Epilepsy

It is estimated that 1 in 250 of all pregnancies in the UK are in women with epilepsy. These women face unique problems when it comes to controlling their epilepsy during a pregnancy.

Women with epilepsy taking antiepileptic drugs (AEDs) have a two to three times greater risk of having a child with a major congenital malformation than women without epilepsy. Nevertheless, it is still overwhelmingly likely that a woman with epilepsy will have a normal pregnancy and give birth to a healthy child.

The pregnancy should be identified early so adjustments to anticonvulsive therapy can be made and a higher dose of folic acid (5mg) can commence. Some AEDs have been associated with altered concentrations of folate and an increased incidence of neural tube defects.

The main problems in pregnancy are related to the number of seizures experienced. During pregnancy some women notice a reduction in the number of seizures, but others may experience an increase.

Generalized convulsive seizures may cause metabolic alterations in the mother's body, increase her blood pressure, and change her circulation pattern. There is also an increased risk of injury to the fetus from falls.

Management

Recommendations for management during pregnancy:[1,2]
- Continue folic acid 5mg daily until at least 12 weeks' gestation.
- Adjust anticonvulsant regime if necessary on clinical grounds.
- Offer serum screening at 16 weeks and a detailed anomaly scan at 18–22 weeks.
- For women on enzyme-inducing anticonvulsants, prescribe oral vitamin K 20mg daily from 36 weeks until delivery. Commence earlier if judged to be at risk of preterm delivery.
- Control prolonged seizures using IV diazepam to a maximum of 20mg (10mg bolus plus slow injection of further 2mg boluses if required).
- Rectal administration of the intravenous preparation is an option if intravenous access is unavailable.
- Postnatal care should include advice about the likelihood of breakthrough seizure in the postpartum period. This is related to hormonal change and lack of sleep. Bagshaw et al.[3] in a small cohort of 84 women stated that problems were associated with bathing the baby and taking the baby outside the home. Women need support and reassurance during this time.

1 Royal College of Obstetrics and Gynaecologists (1998). The management in pregnancy of women with epilepsy. Available at: ℛ http://www.nhshealthequality.org/nhsqis/files/maternityservices_pregnancywithepilepsy_spc6RH5_DEC97.pdf (accessed 22.2.11).

2 Stokes T, Shaw EJ, Juarez-Garcia A, Camosso-Stefinovic J, Baker R (2004). *Clinical guidelines and evidence review for the epilepsies: diagnosis and management in adults and children in primary and secondary care.* London: Royal College of General Practitioners.

3 Bagshaw J, Crawford P, Chappell B (2008). Problems that mother's with epilepsy experience when caring for their children. *Seizure* **17**, 42–8.

Thromboembolic disorders

Venous thromboembolism (VTE) is the obstruction of a blood vessel, usually a large vein, with thrombotic material carried in the blood from its site of origin to block another vessel.

Several factors are associated with an increased risk of VTE during pregnancy:

- Increasing maternal age
- Increasing parity
- Operative delivery
- Immobility and bed rest
- Obesity
- Dehydration
- Thrombophilia.

According to Lewis[1] it is particularly important to recognize the risk of VTE in the mother with a raised BMI of 30 or above. The risks are present from the first trimester onwards. In the years 2003–2005, 41 women died of VTE and 16 of these women had a BMI of 30 or over.[1]

Thromboembolic disorders can be categorized as:

- Superficial thrombophlebitis
- Deep-vein thrombosis
- Pulmonary embolism.

Superficial thrombophlebitis

- This is caused by the formation of a clot in a superficial varicose vein as a result of stasis and the hypercoagulable state of pregnancy.
- Varicose veins commonly occur in pregnancy because of increased venous pressure in the legs and the action of progesterone.
- A red, inflamed area appears over the vein, which feels firm on palpation.

Management

- Encourage the woman to mobilize wearing TEDS.
- Instruct her to raise her leg when sitting and give her exercises to be carried out daily.
- Local warming applications may provide additional comfort.
- The inflammation should subside within a few days and the clot in the superficial vein causes no immediate hazard.
- Observe the woman closely for signs of DVT.

Deep-vein thrombosis

- A less common but more serious condition.
- A clot forms in the deep vein of the calf, femoral, or iliac veins and there is a risk that fragments may break off and travel through the circulation, causing embolus.
- The woman will complain of pain in the leg and there may be oedema and a change in colour in the affected leg.
- The calf or leg is painful on palpation and dorsiflexion of the foot causes acute pain.

Management

- Commence anticoagulant therapy to prevent further clotting and reduce the risk of pulmonary embolus.
- Continue intravenous heparin via an infusion pump until the acute signs have resolved.
- Elevate the leg and give analgesia as required.
- When symptoms have improved, begin mobilization with the leg well supported.
- Continue anticoagulants for 6 weeks with self-administered subcutaneous low-dose heparin. During the postnatal period warfarin may be used. Breastfeeding is not affected by either therapy.

Pulmonary embolism

- This occurs when a clot becomes detached from a leg vein and is carried via the inferior vena cava through the heart and into the pulmonary artery.
- Small clots passing into the lung cause pulmonary infarction. If the artery is completely blocked, death occurs quickly. Pulmonary embolism occurs as a result of a DVT in the ileo-femoral veins. Most cases occur in the immediate postnatal period.
- This remains the leading direct cause of maternal death in the UK.[1]
- Symptoms include:
  - Acute chest pain due to ischaemia in the lungs
  - Difficulty breathing (dyspnoea)
  - Blue discoloration of the skin (cyanosis)
  - Coughing up blood (haemoptysis)
  - Pyrexia
  - Collapse.

Management

- Summon urgent medical assistance.
- Sit the woman upright and administer oxygen.
- Measure vital signs every 15min.
- If resuscitation is required, commence cardiac massage and artificial ventilation.
- Give anticoagulation with intravenous heparin and strong analgesia, such as morphine.
- If the woman survives, continue anticoagulation therapy and administer the thrombolytic drug streptokinase to accelerate the breakdown of the clot. Patients with a minor embolus may present with less specific symptoms, such as fever, cough, or pleuritic pain. Commence anticoagulant therapy and continue until symptoms resolve.

1 Lewis, G (ed.) (2007). *The Confidential Enquiry into Maternal and Child Health (CEMACH). Saving Mothers' Lives: Reviewing Maternal Deaths to Make Motherhood Safer—2003–2005.* The 7th report on Confidential Enquires into Maternal Deaths in the United Kingdom. London: CEMACH.

Principles of thromboprophylaxis

Following publication of the latest report of the Confidential Enquiries into Maternal Deaths in the UK in December 2007,[1] the recommendations of the RCOG on thromboprophylaxis in the antenatal, intranatal, and postnatal periods may be followed until new guidelines have been approved. A summary of the recommendations appears in the report and can also be found in RCOG guidelines.[2]

The risk factors for VTE include:
- Previous VTE
- Congenital or acquired thrombophilia
- Obesity (BMI 35 or above. Those with a BMI of 40 or above are at high risk)
- Parity of 4 or above
- Gross varicose veins
- Surgical procedures during pregnancy or the postnatal period
- Hyperemesis
- Dehydration
- Severe infection
- Pre-eclampsia
- Long-haul travel
- >4 days of bed rest.

The main recommendations for thrombo-prophylaxis are:[1]
- All women should be screened for risk factors for VTE in early pregnancy and again if admitted to hospital or on development of other problems
- Women with a previous VTE should be screened for thrombophilia
- In all pregnant women immobilization should be minimized and dehydration avoided
- Women with previous VTE should be offered thromboprophylaxis with low-molecular-weight heparin (LMWH) in the postnatal period.
- Women with recurrent VTE, or VTE with a family history of VTE in a first-degree relative, or with previous VTE and thrombophilia, should be offered LMWH antenatally and for 6 weeks post partum.
- Women with three or more persisting risk factors should be considered for LMWH for three to five days postnatally.

1 Lewis, G (ed.) (2007). *The Confidential Enquiry into Maternal and Child Health (CEMACH). Saving Mothers' Lives: Reviewing Maternal Deaths to Make Motherhood Safer—2003–2005.* The 7th report on Confidential Enquires into Maternal Deaths in the United Kingdom. London: CEMACH.

2 Royal College of Obstetricians and Gynaecologists (2009). *Thrombosis and Embolism during Pregnancy and the Pinerperium, Reducing the Risk.* Green Top 37. London: RCOG. Available from: http://www.rcog.org.uk/womens-health/clinical-guidance/reducing-risk-of-thrombosis-greentop37a. (accessed 22.2.11).

Thyroid disorders

Pregnancy makes special demands on the thyroid gland which enlarges due to the influence of oestrogen. The hormone hCG has thyroid stimulating properties and may even cause hyperthyroidism in excessive amounts.

There are four main disorders of the thyroid affecting pregnancy:

- Iodine deficiency
- Hypothyroidism
- Hyperthyroidism
- Postpartum thyroiditis.

Iodine deficiency

- Leads to a condition called goitre. In mothers who have goitre and are also hypothyroid, 30% of pregnancies will result in spontaneous abortion, stillbirth, or congenital abnormalities.
- This condition is rare in the UK as iodine is present in a variety of foods such as shellfish, saltwater fish, mushrooms, and soya beans.
- When iodine deficiency occurs in the first trimester this may lead to developmental failure of the central nervous system, resulting to severe learning difficulties, deafness, and spasticity.
- In the second and third trimester the iodine deficiency may lead to an infant being born with hypothyroidism. This consists of large tongue, dry coarse skin, umbilical hernia, and lethargy. The condition responds to iodine or thyroid hormone replacement and prognosis is related to when the condition first started.

Hypothyroidism

Symptoms

- Hypothermia and intolerance to cold
- Decreased appetite, weight gain, and constipation
- Dry rough flaky skin and hair loss
- Impaired concentration and memory
- Extreme fatigue.

Effects on pregnancy

- Spontaneous abortion and stillbirth rates are higher in this group.
- Symptoms should be observed for and thyroid function measured in any pregnant woman in whom there is a suspicion of dysfunction.
- If diagnosed, treatment with replacement thyroid hormone is prescribed.

Hyperthyroidism

Symptoms

- Increased temperature and heat intolerance
- Restlessness and insomnia
- Increased appetite, weight loss, and diarrhoea
- Exophthalmos—protrusion of the eyeball.

Effects on pregnancy
- A high fetal mortality rate.
- The condition should be suspected in any pregnant woman who fails to gain weight despite a good appetite or presents with any other features of the condition.
- Anti-thyroid drugs may be used with caution as they may cause hypothyroidism in the fetus.

Postnatal thyroiditis

Around 11–17% of women develop postnatal thyroid dysfunction between 1 and 3 months post delivery. It resolves spontaneously in two-thirds of those with this condition. The remainder pass into a hypothyroid state and although most recover, a small number continue to be hypothyroid.

Recommended reading

Casey BM, Leveno KJ (2006). Thyroid disease in pregnancy. *Obstetrics and Gynecology* **108**(5), 1283–92.

The Endocrine Society (2007). Management of thyroid dysfunction during pregnancy and postpartum: an Endocrine Society clinical practice guideline. *Journal of Clinical Endocrinology and Metabolism* **92**(8), S1–S47.

Nicholson WK, Robinson KA, Smallridge RC, Ladenson PW, Powe NR (2006). Prevalence of postpartum thyroid dysfunction: a quantitative review. *Thyroid* **16**(6), 573–82.

Renal conditions

There are a number of changes in the urinary tract as a result of pregnancy.
- Plasma volume expansion of 30–50% is conserved by the kidneys.
- There is an increased frequency of micturition in the first trimester due to the growing uterus compressing the bladder within the pelvis. This effect is noticed again in the third trimester as the bladder displaces when the fetal head engages.
- As a result of the hormonal effect on the renal tubules the renal threshold for glucose is lowered independently of blood glucose levels.
- There is dilation and enlargement of the ureters under the influence of progesterone leading to an increased risk of urinary stasis, obstructed urine flow and ascending infection.
- Pregnancy does not make renal function worsen in women who are normotensive and who have normal kidneys.
- Proteinuria, hypertension, or impaired renal function present at conception determines fetal prognosis.

Renal disorders in pregnancy can range from asymptomatic bacteriuria to end stage renal disease requiring dialysis. Every pregnant woman with renal disease should be classed as a high risk pregnancy especially when impaired renal function or hypertension is present.

For optimal management a multidisciplinary approach is essential and care should be in a facility with experience of high risk pregnancies, a neonatal intensive care unit, and the woman's care coordinated by an obstetrician and nephrologist from the outset.

Glomerular nephritis

This condition can follow a streptococcal infection and occurs in response to an abnormal antibody–antigen reaction.

Signs and symptoms
- Oedema
- Aching loins
- Dyspnoea
- Bradycardia
- Oliguria
- Haematuria.

Treatment
- Antibiotics
- Restricted protein diet
- Restricted fluids until diuresis begins
  Overall fetal loss is 21% with a preterm delivery rate of 19%.

Nephrotic syndrome

This can follow glomerular nephritis or be a result of diabetes or renal vein thrombosis.

Signs and symptoms
- Marked proteinuria
- Oedema

- Anaemia
- Decreased levels of plasma proteins
- Decreased osmotic pressure
- Decreased blood volume.

Treatment
- High protein, low sodium diet
- Carefully monitor electrolytes.
- Fetal loss is high.

Maintenance dialysis

Fertility generally decreases in women with end-stage renal disease but improved treatment can lead to a health improvement enough to restore fertility. There is however a low fetal survival rate, prematurity is a major problem and polyhydramnios is common.

Renal transplant recipients

There is a greater chance of a successful pregnancy with a gap of 2 years between transplant and conception. The incidence of preterm delivery is high as is IUGR. Fetal prognosis depends on how well the allograft continues to function and hypertension, proteinuria, and renal function must be closely monitored.

Recommended reading

Hnat M, Sibai B (2008). Renal disease and pregnancy. *Global Library of Women's Medicine* (ISSN: 1756-2228) 2008; DOI 10.3843/GLOWM.10157.

Part 2

Normal labour

Normal labour: first stage

Physiology of the first stage of labour

Definition of labour

The physiological process by which the fetus, placenta, and membranes are expelled through the birth canal. The first stage of labour is from the onset of regular uterine contractions until full dilatation of the cervix.

Normal labour

- Is spontaneous, occurs between 37 and 42 weeks' gestation.
- Culminates in the normal birth of a live, healthy infant.
- Is completed within 24h and there are no maternal complications.

The two main physiological changes that take place in the first stage are effacement and dilatation of the cervical os. These are initiated by the action of various hormones and prostaglandins, and the contraction and retraction of the uterine muscle. The mechanism by which labour is initiated is still not fully understood. Some theories suggest that it involves a very complex interaction between the mother, the fetus, and their environment.

Initiation of labour

Increasing levels of prostaglandins, oxytocin, and progesterone are thought to contribute to the initiation of the onset of labour. The levels then rise progressively, reaching highest levels at delivery of the head and after placental separation.

The myometrium

Individual cells within the myometrium are able to depolarize their cell membranes allowing the movement of ions, primarily calcium, which together with ATPase initiates the contraction of myosin fibres within the cell. The cells are able to communicate their activity via gap junctions. If this process occurs together, this results in a harmonized contraction, which can spread across the uterus. At term, muscle fibres are present in compact bundles, reducing the gap size, therefore the number of gap junctions increases and the potential to stimulate contractility is increased.

The cervix

The cervix consists of collagen fibres alternating with circular and longitudinal muscle fibres. Normally the cervix is firm and resistant to downward activity from the uterus and its contents. Towards term the percentage of water in the collagen fibres increases which decreases stability and therefore results in a softer, more compliant cervix.

Hormonal influences

Oestrogen enhances myometrial activity by increasing oxytocin and prostaglandin receptors, in turn this assists with the formation of gap junctions.

Prostaglandins are produced in the placenta, membranes, and decidua. PGE and PGF2a facilitate the production of calcium ions which increases their availability for binding to the myosin receptors. This enhances contractile action and results in harmonized contractions. The presence of prostaglandins in the cervix encourages the production of enzymes to reduce the amount of collagen, this leads to cervical ripening.

Oxytocin acts as a hormone and neurotransmitter and is produced by the hypothalamus, it is a powerful uterine tonic. An increase in oxytocin receptors, due to the action of oestrogen, dramatically increases uterine sensitivity to oxytocin at term. This facilitates the onset and maintenance of contractions by depolarization and stimulating the production of prostaglandins. Animal studies suggest that relaxin is instrumental in stimulating oxytocin-synthesizing neurons in the hypothalamus just before the onset of labour.

Physiological changes in the first stage

- The onset of labour is a process, not an event. Cervical ripening takes place from 36 weeks' gestation.
- *Contraction and retraction*: shortening of the uterine muscles occurs with every contraction, mainly in the upper segment. Progressive pull on the weaker lower segment results in effacement and dilatation of the cervix. The latent phase of the first stage is considered to be up to 3cm, whilst the active phase is from 3cm to 10cm.
- *Retraction ring*: a normal occurrence in all labours. Ridge formation occurs between the thick, retracted muscles of the upper segment and the thin, distended aspect of the lower segment. Only visible in obstructed labour, when a transverse ridge across the abdomen forms—known as Bandl's ring—indicates imminent rupture of the uterus.
- *Fundal dominance*: contractions commence from the cornua and pass in waves in an inwards and downwards direction. Intensity of uterine action is greater in the upper segment.
- *Upper active segment/lower passive segment*: shortening of the upper segment exerts pull on the passive lower segment. This initiates a reflex releasing oxytocin via the posterior pituitary, and assists with effacement and dilatation.
- *Polarity of the uterus*: coordination between upper and lower segments; a balanced, harmonious and rhythmical process. The upper segment contracts powerfully and the lower contracts slightly and dilates.
- *Resting tone*: during a contraction the blood flow to the placenta is impaired so that oxygen and carbon dioxide exchange in the intervillous spaces is reduced. The resting tone is the relaxation period between contractions which enables placental blood flow to resume normal levels, to ensure adequate fetal oxygenation. The uterus is never completely relaxed; the measurement of the resting tone is 4–10mmHg.
- *Intensity of contractions*: contractions cause a rise in intrauterine pressure (amplitude), which can be recorded. Contractions rise rapidly to a peak, then slowly diminish (resting tone).
  - Early labour, >20mmHg, 20–30s every 20min.
  - Established labour, >60mmHg, 45–60s every 2–3min.
- *Formation of forewaters and hindwaters*: the result of the descent of the fetal head on to the cervix, which separates a small bag of amniotic

fluid in front of the presenting part. The forewaters assist effacement of the cervix and early dilatation. The hindwaters fill the remainder of the uterine cavity; they help to equalize pressure in the uterus during contractions, thus providing protection to the fetus and placenta.

- *Rupture of the membranes*: is thought to occur as a result of increased production of PGE2 from the amnion during labour, together with the force of the contractions. In a normal labour without intervention, the membranes usually rupture between 2cm and 3cm,[1] around full dilatation or in the second stage.[2]
- *Show*: displacement of the operculum as a result of effacement and dilatation of the cervix. This can occur at any time during labour, but more commonly towards the end of the first stage or at full dilatation. Sometimes a show may occur before the onset of labour, however, this is not an indication that labour is apparent.
- *Fetal axis pressure*: this is the force transmitted by the uterine contractions down the fetal spine to its head.

Recommended reading

Fraser DM, Cooper MA (2009). *Myles Textbook for Midwives*, 15th edn. Edinburgh: Churchill Livingstone.

1 National Childbirth Trust (1989). *Rupture of the Membranes in Labour: Women's Views*. London: NCT.

2 Walsh D (2007). *Evidence Based Care for Normal Labour and Birth. A Guide for Midwives*. London: Routledge.

Diagnosis of onset of labour

Although the three cardinal signs listed below indicate the onset of labour, each woman will be individual in her response and adaptation to labour, dependent on her parity, expectations, and pain threshold. Therefore it is recommended that individualized care is undertaken at all times. The stages of labour should be loosely adhered to, to detract from rigid routine and impersonal care.

Pre-labour signs
- Nesting instinct and spurts of energy.
- Feeling generally unwell: flu-like symptoms or a cold.
- Diarrhoea or loose stools.
- Frequency of micturition.
- Heavy sensation/discomfort in the upper thighs and pelvic area.
- Lower backache as the fetus nestles deeply in the pelvis.
- Increase in Braxton Hicks contractions in the final few weeks.
- Feeling different, distant, and restless prior to going into labour.
- Mucoid loss or a show.
- Intermittent leakage of liquor.
- Pre-labour rupture of the membranes: most women will proceed into labour spontaneously within 24h.

Onset of labour
- *Show*. The mucoid, blood-stained loss that is passed per the vagina known as the operculum, seals the cervical canal. Dislodgement of this mucoid plug is an early sign of uterine activity, but not necessarily an indication of the onset of labour.
- *Contractions*. The most important sign, as cervical dilatation is not possible without regular contractions of the uterus. They may commence as tightenings, but become longer, stronger, and more regular as labour progresses. The contractions coincide with abdominal tightenings that can be felt on abdominal palpation. The contractions may commence at 20–30min intervals, lasting for 20–30s.
- *Rupture of the membranes*. This can occur at any time during or before labour. More commonly, in a normal spontaneous labour without intervention they will rupture at a cervical dilation of 9cm or more. Occasionally they do not rupture until the advanced second stage at delivery. The amount of amniotic fluid that is lost depends on the effectiveness of the fetal presentation to aid the formation of the forewaters. With a well-fitting head, that is sufficiently engaged in the pelvis, there will be little loss of fluid, with further small leaks. If the head is poorly engaged, then the loss of fluid may well be substantial.

Diagnosis
- *Uterine activity*: abdominal palpation, degree of discomfort or pain, observation of contractions—their regularity, strength, and length.
- *History so far*: when contractions started, evidence of a show, or ruptured membranes.
- Observation of vital signs, urinalysis, and general examination.
- Vaginal examination if clinically indicated.

- Observation of non-verbal behaviour, visual, and auditory signs.
- All observations, clinical findings and history of the labour so far should be clearly recorded in the maternal notes.
- The above information should form the basis for a plan of care to be discussed and agreed with the woman, which should be recorded in the maternity notes.

Differential diagnosis

Sometimes it may be difficult to ascertain the true onset of labour, due to compounding factors such as spurious labour and a long latent phase. The only way to manage this situation is to adopt a 'wait and see' policy, and it is only in retrospect that a definite diagnosis can be made.

Generally, regular contractions will cease after a few hours, with no dilatation of the cervical os, this is sometimes referred to as false labour. Obviously this can be very distressing for the woman, thinking that she has commenced labour.

In this case:

- Provide extra moral support and sound explanations to ease women through this difficult time.
- Some women may require pain relief.
- Promote coping tactics and utilize non-pharmacological means to relieve discomfort and anxiety.

Latent phase

Defining the start of labour can be arbitrary; many women may experience a long latent phase prior to the body going in to established labour. Therefore there is some debate as to how this should be managed.

- Labour should be seen as a dynamic event, not a mechanical process.
- Consider the individual needs and responses of the woman, as there is huge variation in experience.
- Established labour may not occur until the cervix is between 3cm and 5cm dilated.[1] The latent phase is the 'warming up' phase prior to established labour.
- Evidence suggests that labouring at home during early labour is preferable to early admission to the delivery suite.
- Admission for normal labour should be at home or in assessment areas sited away from the delivery suite.[2]
- The environment for assessment will affect progress, depending on certain inhibiting factors, such as medical procedures, clinical apparatus, bright lights, language, and being observed. Women tend to be subjected to more labour intervention as a result.[3]
- Provide psychological support, information, and clear explanations of the role of the latent phase. This will depend on the pain response and expectations of the individual.
- Utilize all your observational, clinical, and intuitive skills.
- A vaginal examination is not necessary if all observations, history, and findings are satisfactory.
- It may be advisable for the woman to return home to await the onset of established labour; that is, when the contractions are occurring every 5–6min and lasting for a longer period of time.

- Provide an efficient communication network so that the woman can phone and obtain advice regarding her progress and concerns during this phase.
- In some areas vaginal examination to assess progress may initially be undertaken at home by the community midwife, so that unnecessary visits to hospital are minimized and the woman remains in a non-threatening environment.
- Provide antenatal health promotion that focuses on clear explanations of the latent phase and spurious labour, so that women adopt a more realistic notion of what labour involves.

1 Gurewitsch E. Diament P, Fong J, et al. (2002). The labour curve of the grand multipara: Does progress of labour continue to improve with additional childbearing? *American Journal of Obstetrics and Gynaecology* **186**, 1331–8.

2 Lauzon L, Hodnett E (2006). Labour assessment programs to delay admission to labour wards (Cochrane Review), In: *Cochrane Library*, Issue 1. Chichester: John Wiley and Sons Ltd.

3 Rahnama P, Ziaei S, Faghihzadeh S (2006). Impact of early admission in labour on method of delivery. *International Journal of Gynaecology and Obstetrics* **92**(3), 217–20.

Support for women in labour

Research has shown that where women are supported through their birth experience by midwives in birth units or midwife-led areas there is:
- Less intervention—induction of labour, caesarean section, forceps, ventouse, and artificial rupture of the membranes[1]
- Less pharmacological analgesia
- Fewer episiotomies
- Less immobility during birthing and labour
- Less external fetal monitoring
- Fewer fetal heart abnormalities.
  In addition:
- There are more normal, spontaneous births
- Women experience greater satisfaction with their care
- Midwives express greater job satisfaction
- There is no difference in perinatal mortality or morbidity rates compared with births in other units.
  These outcomes rely on the following aspects relating to care.
- *Informational support*: full, accurate, and individualized information is provided about progress and procedures. There is a two-way process of information and communication between mother and partner and midwife.
- *Physical support*: physical activity is encouraged, tactile support is provided for some women, non-pharmacological means are provided to help women to cope better, e.g. warm baths, massage, freedom of movement, optimal positioning.[2] Reassurance is provided about physical changes and symptoms that occur during labour, e.g. show, rupture of membranes, feeling nauseated.
- *Emotional support*: it is important that the midwife appreciates the range of emotional feelings and behaviour that may be expressed during labour and birth:
  - Fear: of failure, pain, the unknown; perhaps influenced by a previous negative obstetric experience
  - Hostility: due to poor previous relationships with health professionals; a defence mechanism for unexpressed anxiety; unwanted pregnancy
  - Resentment: due to personal circumstances and difficult relationships
  - Positive emotions: excitement, confidence, fulfilment, etc.
  - Unrealistic expectations
  - Awareness of fears and anxieties of partner.
  Unrealistic expectations are addressed with sensitivity. Relaxation techniques, breathing awareness, and dialogue are encouraged to help allay fears.
- *Advocacy and empowerment*:
  - Birth and labour are viewed as a partnership within a social, cultural, and biophysical model of care.
  - The midwife acts as an intermediary for the woman when she may feel undermined by the environment of a hospital, experiences loss

of personal identity or loss of assertiveness to express her needs and anxieties.
- Empowerment is encouraged by assisting women with decision-making that reflects their needs and care plans.
- Facilitate choice and control for women.
- Respect is shown for women's ability to verbalize their wishes and requirements freely.
- *Environment*: known to have a huge impact on the release of endorphins, which will enhance the physiological process of labour.[3]
  - Women are encouraged to adopt upright/alternative positions and freedom of movement.
  - Appropriate props are provided: birthing balls, beanbags, easy chairs, stools, music, etc.
  - Low lights and low noise levels.
  - Creation of a home-from-home environment within a hospital setting: medical apparatus is removed or hidden, pleasant furnishings are provided, etc.
  - Complementary therapies are used, e.g. massage, aromatherapy.
  - Privacy is provided.
  - Key carers only are involved in care: continuous support from a midwife has been shown to be associated with less use of pharmacological analgesia and epidurals. Attendance of a birth supporter (partner, friend, sister, mother) has been shown to result in shorter labours and less intervention.[1,2]
- *Individualized care*: the ability to accommodate and appreciate the woman's personal needs, expectations, and views; to achieve a meaningful experience with respect to her social and cultural background, and her emotional, mental, and physical attributes. Providing the opportunity to discuss the woman's labour afterwards, to clear up any concerns or confusion.

1 Hodnett ED, Gates S, Hofmeyr GJ, Sakala C (2003). Continuous support for women during childbirth. *Cochrane Database of Systematic Reviews* **3**, CD003766.

2 Simkin P, O'Hara M (2002). Non-pharmacological relief of pain during labour: systematic review of five methods. *American Journal of Obstetrics and Gynaecology* **186**, S131–S59.

3 Walsh D (2006). Subverting assembly-line childbirth: childbirth in a free-standing birth centre. *Social Science and Medicine* **26**(6), 1330–40.

High- and low-risk labour

Determining whether a woman falls into a high- or low-risk category for labour is dependent on her previous medical and obstetric history. This will have been recorded in her notes at the booking visit, and recommendations made for her care in labour. For a list of these, 📖 see Screening for risk in pregnancy, p. 56.

Sometimes a woman may have had a theoretical risk factor during pregnancy which may have been resolved, e.g. a fetal abnormality which has been investigated and all is normal, or a woman with active herpes which has been treated and is not active when she presents in labour. Therefore, there may be overlapping situations where decisions are not verified until a woman commences labour.

Take a full and detailed account of the woman's current obstetric and medical health when she presents in labour.

In addition to the antenatal risk factors, circumstances may occur in the current pregnancy and early labour stage that will require high-risk care:

- Antepartum haemorrhage
- Breech presentation
- Malpresentation of the fetal head
- Preterm labour
- Premature rupture of the membranes
- Multiple pregnancy
- Placenta praevia
- Pre-eclampsia
- Pregnancy-induced hypertension
- Severe anaemia
- Renal conditions associated with pregnancy, such as pyelonephritis
- Abnormalities of the genital tract, such as bicornate uterus and female genital mutilation
- Intrauterine growth retardation
- Acute fetal distress
- Cord presentation or prolapse
- Maternal anxiety.

A low-risk labour may be viewed as one where the woman commences labour having experienced an uneventful pregnancy, is in good physical health, and has no known risk factors that would interfere with the normal physiological course of labour and birth.

Always discuss, and take into account, the woman's individual needs and choices before making decisions about care in labour.

Principles of care for low-risk women

Since the inception of medically managed care for labour and birth, there has been a steep rise in intervention and assisted birth, among a population of women who invariably have uncomplicated pregnancies. In view of the evidence to support midwives managing low-risk women in labour, it is important that the midwife is confident in all aspects of midwifery care to support women's choices and to enhance normal physiological principles.[1]

The midwife needs to assess suitability for low-risk care based on individual needs and predisposing conditions.

Assessment

- No predisposing medical or obstetric conditions.
- No antenatal pathology present.
- Maternal choice.
- Review of case notes, reports, ultrasound scan and birth plan.
- Discussion with the woman and her birthing partner/s.

Principles

- Ideally be cared for in separate midwife-led unit or section away from the high-risk area.
- Where possible provide a home environment with low lighting, privacy, birthing aids, hidden equipment.
- Consider home birth as an option.
- No CTG machines within immediate area.
- An admission CTG is not required if low risk.
- Auscultation of the fetal heart should be conducted with a fetal stethoscope (Pinard) or a Sonicaid for 60s at regular intervals. In well established first stage every 15–30min for 60s and every 5min in the second stage.
- If the woman is having a hospital birth, assessment at home in early labour is an option to avoid hospitalization too soon and the potential for unnecessary noise and distraction.
- Work towards the lower boundaries for interventions, e.g. 0.5cm per hour and a 4h action line to account for individual progress and avoidance of precipitate action.[2,3]
- Provide support and enhance confidence by encouraging relaxation and breathing techniques, mobility and change of position. Consider the possible use of complementary therapies to help with coping strategies.

1 Royal College of Midwives (2005). *Evidence-based Guidelines for Midwifery-led Care in Labour.* London: RCM.

2 Enkin M, Kierse M, Neilson J, *et al.* (2000). *A Guide to Effective Care in Pregnancy and Childbirth.* Oxford: Oxford University Press.

3 Lavender T, Alfrevic Z, Walkinshaw S (2006). Effects of different partogram action lines on birth outcomes: a randomized controlled trial. *Obstetrics and Gynaecology* **108**(2), 295–302.

Principles of care in the first stage of labour

The first stage of labour is primarily a stage of preparation, both physically and emotionally. The cervix has to undergo radical anatomical changes in order for birth to be possible, and the mother has to quickly adjust to the demands of labour. As it is the longest stage of labour, this may place a great deal of strain on the woman and therefore be challenging in terms of care. It is always important to give individualized care, based on the woman's choices and her progress in labour.

It is important when taking over care from a colleague, admitting a woman in labour, or visiting for a home birth that you familiarize yourself with all the necessary information about the woman.

- Be aware of previous medical or obstetric history that is relevant to the labour and birth.
- Be aware of any risk factors or possible problems that may necessitate potential referral to consultant care.
- Essential information that should be available:
  - Blood group and haemoglobin result
  - Allergies and drug reactions
  - The ultrasound report confirming the location of the placenta.
  Also double check the woman's gestation.
- Familiarize yourself with the birth plan and discuss any preferences the woman may have.
- Check any information about the history of the labour so far—whether membranes are intact, onset of contractions, loss per vagina, and so on.

Then carry out an assessment of the woman's physical condition, degree of comfort/pain, and how she is coping emotionally with the labour so far. This will involve observation, abdominal palpation, recording vital signs, direct questioning, and possibly a vaginal examination, only if indicated.

Discuss with the woman what her options of care are. You may need to raise questions such as:

- How far advanced in labour is the woman?
- Does she want to mobilize?
- Does she want a bath or analgesia?
- What about food and drink?
- Is the environment satisfactory?

Assess the woman's progress regularly, while also being flexible in responding to her individual needs.

- If the woman is not in established labour, give her a realistic and reassuring explanation of early labour, and that this could last for several hours and sometimes days before established labour begins in earnest.
- Encourage and assist with positions of comfort and hygiene. A shower or bath in early labour is often relaxing and refreshing.
- Encourage her to adopt upright positions and mobilization, to assist progress. These measures are known to result in shorter labours, less demand for analgesia and epidural anaesthesia, and less need for augmentation of labour.

- Encourage the woman to empty her bladder every 2h, to prevent trauma and delay in labour. Test the urine for protein, glucose, and ketones.
- Encourage the woman to maintain adequate fluid balance and nutrition during labour. For further information regarding food intake in labour, 📖 see Nutrition in labour, p. 226.
- Carry out regular observations of the woman's physical condition by monitoring the vital signs—2–4h in early labour, progressing to hourly, half hourly as appropriate, and record on the partogram.
- Observe for vaginal loss—a minimal blood-stained mucoid loss indicates a show. A copious show may coincide with full dilatation. When the membranes rupture, the amniotic fluid should be straw-coloured; a greenish appearance indicates the presence of meconium. A copious amount of thick meconium present in the liquor is associated with poor fetal outcome. Record the time of rupture of the membranes in the notes.
- Observe for signs of pretibial, finger, and facial oedema, which may be associated with a developing or worsening hypertensive state.
- Palpate uterine activity regularly—the timing, strength, regularity, and duration of contractions—to assess progress. Encourage the woman to relax between contractions.
- Carry out abdominal palpation prior to a vaginal examination and to assess position, progress, and descent of the fetal head.
- Monitor the effect of analgesia or other measures that may have been initiated, e.g. encouraging breathing, massage, complementary therapies such as aromatherapy.
- Carry out vaginal examination when appropriate and only if clinically necessary (📖 see Vaginal examination, p. 232).
- Reassure the mother regarding her progress and ability to cope. In their excitement, women, particularly primigravidae, often overestimate their progress. You will need to provide a realistic picture while acknowledging their excitement as well as their fears.
- Encourage the woman's coping skills by giving reassurance and emotional support. Encourage her to utilize breathing and relaxation techniques. Provide practical measures such as fans, birthing balls, back massage, positions of comfort, TENS, etc.
- Support the birthing partner and encourage involvement.
- Ensure that the woman's physical environment is private and conducive to her needs.
- Monitor the fetal heart regularly, either by auscultation via a Pinard stethoscope, Sonicaid, or CTG.

Home birth

When pregnancy is straightforward, there is no evidence to suggest any difference in mortality or morbidity between a hospital or home birth.[1] Studies have highlighted that, in low-risk women, there are: fewer caesarean births; fewer assisted births; fewer inductions; fewer episiotomies and severe tears; fewer low Apgar scores; less fetal distress; fewer neonatal respiratory problems; less birth trauma; and less PPH.[2] There was no difference in perinatal mortality rates, often cited as the reason for going into hospital to give birth.[3] Where women had given birth at home, they were very satisfied with their experience and care.

In order for women to make an informed choice as to where they would like to give birth, they require unbiased and realistic information about their choices. In some areas there may be the option for low-risk women to give birth in a midwife-led 'birth centre' or these women may feel more comfortable giving birth at home.

Planning and preparation

- During the first contact with the pregnant woman, discuss where she would like to give birth. Women should not feel pressurized to go into hospital.
- Discuss the risk factors thoroughly with the woman (see below) and, if she is deemed to be high-risk, advise her to consider giving birth in a consultant unit.
- The woman needs plenty of time to think over her options, therefore the decision to opt for a home birth can be taken at any time during pregnancy, or even delayed until the commencement of labour, provided this has been discussed and appropriate plans made for a home birth.
- Inform the supervisor of midwives when a home booking is made.
- Assess the home environment for suitability for a home birth. This includes:
  - The location of the home and ease of access in case an ambulance needs to be called
  - Heating and hot and cold water supply.
  - A hygienic environment for the birth, with adequate towels, blankets, and clothing for the baby
  - Adequate telephone communication.
- The woman's family and birth partner need to be supportive.
- Care of any other children should be considered, with preferably an adult to look after them.
- You (the named midwife) should ensure that your working colleagues are informed of a planned home birth and the relevant information, should they be on duty to assist or conduct the birth. Ideally colleagues who may be involved in the woman's care should be introduced to her in the antenatal period.
- A birth plan is advisable, outlining the woman's care options. Emphasize that if there are concerns antenatally or in labour regarding the welfare of the mother or the fetus, you will discuss the situation with your superiors and, if necessary, transfer to hospital care.

- Antenatal care should be based on the guidelines for low-risk women. If there is any deviation from the normal, you may wish to refer to consultant care with the agreement of the pregnant woman.

Labour

- Ensure that all equipment for the birth is delivered to the woman's home at 37 weeks, or as soon as possible after a decision is made, should it be later than this. Inhalational analgesia and oxygen should be stored at the home, adhering to health and safety regulations.
- Collect resuscitation equipment from the maternity unit as soon as possible, or make arrangements to transfer the equipment in readiness for the birth. Local policies vary.
- On receipt of a labour call, the named midwife, or midwife on call, will attend the woman. Other working colleagues and the labour ward must be informed.
- A second midwife will be required to attend for the birth.
- Follow the NMC and NICE guidelines for low-risk intrapartum care.
- Adhere to guidelines for the safe administration of drugs.
- The woman should have a bag or case packed in case urgent transfer to hospital is necessary.
- If transfer to hospital is necessary, an emergency call for a paramedic ambulance is made. The midwife must accompany the woman in the ambulance and provide details of the woman's labour so far to the attending hospital staff.
- If the woman does not agree with the decision to transfer, then the supervisor of midwives must be informed.

After delivery

- The woman's GP should be informed of the birth and asked to carry out the neonatal examination, unless the midwife has been trained to do this.
- Complete and maintain all records of the birth, according to the guidelines for records and record keeping.
- Dispose of clinical waste and sharps in a safe manner, with reference to the local trust policy. Return inhalational analgesia, oxygen, and drugs to the hospital.
- Undertake immediate postnatal care to ensure the well-being of both mother and baby before leaving their home.

Exclusion criteria for home birth

- *Parity*: primigravida over 37 years of age, parity of five or above. Trust policies may vary regarding parity and age.
- *Stature*: shorter than 152cm (5 feet).
- *BMI*: under 18 or above 31.
- *Previous medical history*:
  - Diabetes
  - Cardiac disease
  - Renal disease
  - Deep vein thrombosis
  - Pulmonary embolism
  - Hypertension

- IV drug abuse
- Hepatitis B antigen positive
- HIV positive
- Recent history of active genital herpes.
- *Previous obstetric history*:
  - Caesarean section—dependent on the reason for the previous LSCS
  - Hysterotomy
  - Rhesus antibodies
  - Severe pregnancy-induced hypertension
  - Eclampsia
  - Previous stillbirth or neonatal death
  - Shoulder dystocia
  - Retained placenta
  - Inverted uterus
  - Primary PPH.
- *Previous gynaecological history*:
  - Infertility
  - Major surgery
  - Myomectomy
  - Uterine anomaly (congenital or fibroids).
- *Current pregnancy*:
  - Twins
  - Malpresentation after 36 weeks
  - Preterm rupture of membranes
  - Antepartum haemorrhage
  - Intrauterine growth retardation
  - Sustained hypertension
  - Fetal anomaly
  - Poly- or oligohydramnios
  - Abnormal glucose tolerance test
  - Anaemia below 10g/dL
  - High head at term in primigravida
  - Previous anaesthetic problems
  - Post maturity.
- *Intrapartum*:
  - Malpresentation
  - Preterm labour
  - Poor progress in labour
  - Fetal heart rate abnormalities
  - Meconium-stained liquor
  - Maternal distress
  - Mother's request.

Basic equipment for planned home birth

- Delivery pack
- *Protection and safe disposal*:
  - Maternity pads
  - Inco pads
  - Non-sterile gloves

- Sterile gloves
- Plastic aprons
- Disposal bags
- Clinical waste disposal bags
- Venflon and intravenous therapy fluid (for cannulation in case of PPH)
- Sharps disposal container.
- *Supplementary equipment:*
  - Lubricating jelly
  - Amnihook
  - Pinard and fetal Doppler
  - Syringes and needles
  - Specimen bottles and request forms
  - Oxytocic drugs
  - Naloxone
  - Urinary catheter.
- *Equipment for mother's comfort:*
  - Bean bag
  - Birthing ball
  - Floor mattress
  - Hot water bottle.
- *Requirements for the baby:*
  - Tape measure
  - Cord clamp
  - Mucus extractor
  - Name bands (only if transfer is necessary)
  - Vitamin K
  - Scales.
- *For perineal repair:*
  - Lidocaine
  - Suture pack
  - Suture material
  - Torch.
- *Gases:*
  - Inhalational analgesia (Entonox), two full cylinders, plus mouth and mask attachments
  - Oxygen, together with adult and neonatal masks
  - Portable suction equipment.
- *Appropriate documentation* to include mother's notes, baby's notes, and birth notification.

1 Tew M (1998). *Safer Childbirth? A Critical History of Maternity Care*. London: Chapman and Hall.

2 Chamberlain G, Wraight A, Crowley P (1997). *Home Births: The Report of the 1994 Confidential Enquiry by The National Birthday Trust Fund*. Carnforth, Lancs: Parthenon Publishing Trust.

3 Olsen O, Jewell M (1998). Home versus hospital birth. *Cochrane Database of Systematic Reviews* **3**. 1998, issue 3. Art No: CD000352. DOI:10.1002/14651858. CD000352. Available from: ℘ http://www2.cochrane.org/reviews/en/ab000352.htm (accessed 22.2.11)

Hospital birth

A hospital is by far the most common place to give birth in the UK. This has been the result of government legislation arising from the 1970s (the Peel Report)[1] which advocated that all women should give birth in hospital where it was considered to be safer. This led to a radical change in the role of the midwife and maternity care, while increased intervention has brought a staggering rise in the of rate complications associated with pregnancy and labour and incidence of LSCS. Advanced technology and screening have contributed greatly towards better outcomes for high-risk women. However, in recent years there has been much opposition to these practices and interventions. The evidence for hospitalization of all women for birth is unfounded.[2] Women should be involved in deciding where to give birth following initial assessment in early pregnancy to identify any risk factors to be aware of their options and be able to make an informed choice.

Reasons for hospital birth
- Maternal illness or pre-existing medical condition.
- Obstetric history or present obstetric condition that warrants high-risk management.
- Maternal choice: feels safer in hospital, request for epidural analgesia.
- Unsupported mother: without partner, family, or friends who can provide immediate and ongoing care.
- Social circumstances: e.g. drug misuse, poor housing /living conditions.
- Emergency admission.
- Concealed pregnancy.
- Concerns over the well-being of the fetus.
  Invariably the length of stay in hospital is relatively short unless there are complications.
- 6h stay: the woman spends the latter part of labour and delivery in hospital, followed by a short 6h-recovery period prior to being discharged home to community care.
- 12–24h stay: this is most common for women who have had a normal birth and there are no complications.
- 24–48h stay: very often primiparous women, or women who have had a forceps or ventouse birth, may stay a little longer.
- 3–4 days: mainly women who have had an LSCS or where there are complications.

Admission
- Hospital environments tend to put labour and birth into the illness mode, which equates with disease or that something is wrong.
- The woman may be anxious about hospital admission for labour. She may not have been in hospital before and have pre-conceived ideas or had a previous bad experience.
- Build up of tension will produce stress hormones that interfere with the normal physiology of labour, and slows the process down. Consequently the chances of intervention are increased.
- The hospital environment may be very daunting and impersonal, care should be taken to make the woman feel comfortable and relaxed.

Provision of a home from home environment, with low lights, music facilities, and non-clinical furnishings should be standard.
• Hospital routines and unnecessary medical terminology should be kept to a minimum.
• Women should be encouraged to make a birth plan regardless of their parity, obstetric status, or mode of delivery, to ensure that their individual wishes are taken into account.
• Hospital birth may take place in a consultant-based unit, a midwifery-led birth suite, or a birth centre near to a hospital base.
• All maternity units should have a policy for the care of low-risk women within the hospital environment.

Recommended reading

National Institute for Health and Clinical Excellence (NICE) Guidelines (2007). *Intrapartum Care: Management and Delivery of Care to Women in Labour CG55*. London: NICE. Available from: ℘ http://guidance.nice.org.uk/CG55 (accessed 22.2.11).

1 Peel Report (1970). *Report of the Standing Maternity and Midwifery Advisory Committee (Chairman Sir John Peel)* Domiciliary Midwifery and Maternity Bed Needs. London: HMSO.

2 Tew M (1990). *Safer Childbirth—A Critical History of Maternity Care*. London: Chapman and Hall.

Water birth

Labouring in water is recognized as an appropriate method of assisting pain relief and relaxation, by the release of natural endorphins, raising oxytocin levels, and reducing catecholamine secretion. Water provides a secure, peaceful environment and aids buoyancy, which enables the woman to adopt positions of comfort and freedom more easily. There have, however, been several controversies regarding the use of water for giving birth such as: risk of fetal drowning; fetal hyperthermia; length of labour; genital tract trauma; use of analgesia; Apgar score; and blood loss. Birthing in water is associated with fewer third- and fourth-degree tears, however, labial tears, associated with naturally occurring trauma are more likely to occur.[1] Studies have found that there is no difference in the length of labour,[2] blood loss,[3] Apgar scores, or risk of infection[4,5] when using a birth pool.

Most maternity units have specific guidelines to ensure safe practice regarding water birth, while also considering the individual needs of the woman. Midwives should familiarize themselves with this mode of birth to ensure their competency when a woman chooses to labour or give birth in water.

Criteria

- Single cephalic presentation.
- Uncomplicated term pregnancy from 37 weeks until term +9–14 days, dependant on hospital policy.
- Woman's informed choice.
- Spontaneous rupture of the membranes of less than 24h.
- It may be appropriate for the mother to use the pool for the first stage only—maternal choice or anticipation of possible problems in the second stage, e.g. previous shoulder dystocia or previous PPH.

Exclusion

- Intrauterine growth retardation.
- Meconium-stained liquor.
- Following the administration of narcotics (pethidine, diamorphine), midwives need to use their discretion and professional judgement, and refer to their local guidelines, regarding re-entry to the pool. A minimum of 3–12h for diamorphine has been suggested.
- Intravenous infusion.
- Previous LSCS—not a universal exclusion, depends on the reasons for the LSCS, a risk assessment is advisable.
- Antepartum haemorrhage.
- Multiple pregnancy.
- Prolonged rupture of membranes of over 24h.
- Grand multiparity.
- Maternal pyrexia—37.5 or above.
- Epilepsy.
- Fetal heart rate abnormalities—bradycardia, tachycardia, decelerations.

- Any fetal or maternal finding during the course of labour and birth that deviates from normal, or where continuous CTG is required.
- Women should be able to enter and leave the pool independently—this may result in exclusion of some women with disabilities or poor physical mobility on safety grounds. A risk assessment is advisable.

Preparation for water birth

- There will be local policies in place for effective cleaning and preparation of the pool. Decontamination should involve the use of a chlorine-releasing agent which is effective against HIV, hepatitis B, and hepatitis C.
- If the pool has not been used for some time, leave the water to run for a minimum of 5min.
- Use a previously disinfected hose for each woman using the pool.
- Fill the pool to about two-thirds depth, approximately to the woman's breast level and sufficient to cover the uterus when in a sitting position.
- Maintain a temperature of between 35 and 37°C in the first stage of labour to avoid fetal hyperthermia, frequent observation of the pool temperature is therefore crucial. You may need to add hot water every 30min to achieve this.
- The following equipment should be available:
  - Thermometer to check the water temperature
  - Waterproof Sonicaid
  - Towels
  - Sieve for pool to remove debris
  - Patient hoist to be placed outside the pool room door
  - Sample bottles for microbiology checks on the pool water—refer to local guidelines
  - Portable Entonox or extended tubing for the woman to use while in the pool.
- Wear loose, comfortable clothing, and gauntlet gloves (or half a size smaller gloves) for the birth.
- Encourage involvement of the birth partner. If the partner wishes to enter the pool then suitable swimwear should be used.
- Adhere to health and safety principles while caring for a woman in the pool.

Care in the first stage of labour

- Allow the woman to enter and leave the pool as she wishes.
- The woman should be in established labour prior to entering the pool, i.e. 4–5cm dilated. Entering the pool too early is associated with slowing progress during labour.[5]
- Check the woman's temperature hourly, to help prevent fetal hyperthermia. A rise of 1°C above the baseline should indicate possible termination of pool use.[6]
- Check the pool water temperature half-hourly and top up to maintain pool temperature as appropriate. Record pool temperature on the partogram and in specified paperwork for pool use.

- Assist the woman in adopting a comfortable position.
- Avoid dehydration by encouraging the woman to drink freely. Diuresis is increased when immersed in water.
- Rehearse with the woman and her birth partner, the principles of vacating the pool in the event of an emergency, with regard to health and safety.
- Amniotomy and spontaneous rupture of the membranes (SROM) are not contraindicated if all other observations, progress, and criteria are satisfactory.
- It is possible to perform a vaginal examination while the woman is in the pool; however, this needs to be discussed with the woman and will depend on individual preferences.
- There are differences of opinion regarding the use of essential oils, generally they are not added to the pool—refer to local guidelines and information on administration of oils (📖 see Aromatherapy during labour, p. 248).
- Adhere to the guidelines for low-risk care during labour.

Care in the second stage of labour

- Continue with low-risk care as recommended.
- Adjust water temperature to 37°C and check pool temperature every 15min if birth in the pool is anticipated.
- Hands-off approach for the birth—touching the head is thought to stimulate the breathing response.
- A pool birth should be facilitated completely under water, to avoid premature cessation of the breathing response. No increase in perinatal morbidity or mortality has been found when comparing births in water and conventional vaginal births in low-risk women.[7]
- If at any time during birth the baby is exposed to air, then the baby must be born out of water.
- Once the head is delivered it is usually visible as a dark shadow under the water. Do not check for the cord routinely. If the baby is not delivered with the next contraction and the cord does require clamping and cutting, the woman should be eased out of the water on to the pool edge to undertake the procedure. The baby must then be born out of water.
- Allow the remainder of the body to deliver spontaneously; it may be appropriate to assist/encourage the woman to bring the baby to the surface herself, with the baby's face uppermost. Assistance to deliver the shoulders can be utilized in the same way as a birth out of water.
- If episiotomy is required, assist the mother to sit on the ledge or to get out of the pool for the procedure.
- Due to the more gentle birth, babies born in water often do not cry or appear to breathe instantaneously. The usual checks of the baby's colour, respiration, and heart rate should be observed. If there is any cause for concern, then the baby may be rubbed with a towel or lifted into the cooler air out of the water and this will usually result in a crying response.
- Cut and clamp the cord promptly (to avoid the risk of neonatal polycythaemia) before the mother leaves the pool. The vasoconstriction action of the cord may be delayed while in the water.

The third stage of labour

- Usually women like to vacate the pool for the third stage of labour. If active management of the third stage is chosen, then this should be undertaken out of the pool.
- If the woman chooses to stay in the pool, then a physiological third stage is the only option. Ensure that the woman is aware of this before she makes the decision to stay in the pool.
- Keep the mother and baby warm by submerging the baby's body under the water and draping a towel over the woman's shoulders.
- Blood loss may not be easy to assess. Normal amounts of bleeding associated with separation of the placenta will sink to the bottom of the pool. However, if the bleeding appears to be diffusing very quickly through the water, and there is any doubt, it is best to ask the woman to vacate the pool so that more accurate assessment of bleeding can be established.
- In the event of bleeding, administer an oxytocic drug when the mother has vacated the pool.
- Carry out examination of vaginal trauma as in normal labour.
- After use, empty the pool and decontaminate according to local policy. Thorough cleaning of the pool after use is essential.[4] Some units use a new pool liner for each woman.

Recommended reading

Cluett ER, Burns E (2009). Immersion in water in labour and birth (Cochrane review). In: *Cochrane Library*, Issue 2. Oxford: Update Software.

Da Silva FMB, de Oliveira SMJV, Nobre MRC (2009). A randomized controlled trial evaluating the effect of immersion bath on labour pain. *Midwifery* **25**(3), 286–94.

1 Garland D (2006). On the crest of a wave. Completion of a collaborative audit. *MIDIRS Midwifery Digest*: **16**(1), 81–5.

2 Andersen B, Gyhagen M, Neilson TF (1996). Warm tub bath during labour. Effects on labour duration and maternal infectious morbidity. *Journal of Obstetrics and Gynaecology* **16**, 326–30.

3 Lim SK (1994). *A Study to Compare Midwives Visual Estimation of Blood Loss in 'Water' and on 'Land'*. MSc Dissertation. Guildford: University of Surrey.

4 Forde C, Creighton S, Batty A, Hawdon J, Summers-Ma S, Ridgway G (1999). Labour and delivery in the birthing pool. *British Journal of Midwifery* **7**, 165–71.

5 Eriksson M, Mattson LA, Ladfors L (1997). Early or late bath during the first stage of labour: a randomized study of 200 women. *Midwifery* **13**, 146–8.

6 Charles C (1998). Fetal hyperthermia risk from warm water immersion. *British Journal of Midwifery* **6**, 152–6.

7 Gilbert RE, Tookey PA (1999). Perinatal mortality and morbidity among babies delivered in water: surveillance study and postal survey. *British Medical Journal* **319**, 183–7.

Mobility and positioning in labour

Women should be encouraged to adopt an upright position in labour.[1] This works with the laws of gravity to assist labour and facilitate birth, and has been shown to have the following physiological advantages:
- Shorter labour, bearing down easier[2]
- Reduced analgesia requirements
- Less need to speed up the labour with intravenous oxytocin
- Less intervention in labour
- Apgar scores higher at 1 and 5min.

Suggested positions
- Upright, walking freely—support during contraction from partner, wall, table, or other furniture.
- Sitting in a chair, either forward or astride, supported by pillows.
- Use of bean bags/wedges/pillows.
- Use of a birthing ball (pelvic rocking aids rotation).
- Left lateral position.

For the second stage of labour

Positions adopted in the second stage have the potential to maximize the pelvic outlet by up to 20–30% and to influence favourably stretching of the perineum.[3]
- The traditional semi-recumbent position: even when well supported with pillows, there is a tendency to slide down the bed leading to compression of the vena cava. The perineum is stretched adversely sideways when the legs are bent and the knees flopped open, thus substantially reducing the pelvic outlet. Therefore this position is not recommended in current midwifery practice.
- Left lateral position on a bed or mattress on the floor—particularly useful for when women require some temporary relief from an upright position or during a restful phase.
- Kneeling on the floor or a bed.
- Squatting (this is difficult to maintain without support).
- Supported squatting (partner, chair, parallel bars, furniture). Squatting positions open up the pelvic outlet, whereas the sacrum is fixed when lying flat.
- On all fours: the perineum is stretched favourably lengthways to form a continuation of the birth canal, maintaining flexion of the fetal head.
- Birthing chair or stool (linked to a higher incidence of haemorrhage).
- The laws of physics and gravity can improve the intravaginal pressures in upright and sitting positions. Sitting is 30% more effective than lateral or supine positions.[4]

The choice of analgesia, electronic fetal monitoring, and intravenous infusions will impair a woman's mobility. To make an informed choice, women need to be aware of these restrictions.

Recommended reading

Boyle M (2000). Childbirth in bed—the historical perspective. *Practising Midwife* **3**(11), 21–4.

Gupta J, Hofmeyr G (2006). Position for women during second stage of labour (Cochrane review). In: *Cochrane Library*, Issue 4. Chichester: John Wiley and Sons Ltd.

Walsh D (2007). *Evidence-based Care for Normal Labour and Birth*. London: Taylor and Francis Group.

1 Deakin BA (2001). Alternative positions in labour and childbirth. *British Journal of Midwifery* **9**(10), 620–5.

2 De Jonge A, Largo-Janssen ALM (2004). Birthing positions. A qualitative study into the views of women about various birthing positions. *Journal of Psychosomatic Obstetrics and Gynaecology* **25**, 47–55.

3 Downe S, Gerrett D, Renfrew MJ (2004). A prospective randomized trial on the effect of position in the passive second stage of labour on birth outcome in nulliparous women using epidural anaesthesia. *Midwifery* **20**(2), 157–68.

4 Walsh D (2000). Evidence-based care. Part five: Why we should reject the 'bed birth' myth. *British Journal of Midwifery* **8**(9), 556–8.

Nutrition in labour

Studies regarding nutrition in labour are sourced primarily from anaesthetics research into delayed gastric emptying.[1] Whenever a general anaesthetic is administered, there is a high risk of regurgitation and inhalation of stomach contents. The lower oesophageal sphincter is often impaired during pregnancy and intragastric pressure is raised due to the gravid uterus. There is some debate regarding the more common use of spinal anaesthesia for caesarean section and the reduced risk of regurgitation, however, the factors below should also be considered in the overall assessment and management of eating and drinking in labour.

- Delayed gastric emptying may be influenced by pain, anxiety, and, most significantly, the use of narcotics.
- Consequently, there is insufficient evidence to support fasting during labour. Nor is there support for increasing the calorie intake during labour. A recent study has highlighted that consumption of a light diet during labour did not appear to influence obstetric or neonatal outcomes.[2]
- The body stores fat during pregnancy, which can be used as fuel in labour if required.[3] The smooth muscle of the uterus metabolizes fatty acids/ketones as fuel. Therefore, mild acidosis is considered to be a normal, and probably beneficial, physiological state of labour.
- In normal labour there is little evidence to suggest that fluid balance needs correcting, however there has been recent caution regarding possible risk of fluid overload where women are over-zealous to drink copious amounts of water during labour.[4] The usual practice of sipping water between contractions should not pose a risk. IV infusions of glucose should be used sparingly, due to the risks of rebound hypoglycaemia in the newborn infant.

In order to achieve safety and comfort for women, and not to impose a strict, unreasonable regimen for the majority, it is important to consider the risk factors and to recognize those women who may need a caesarean section. As there is scant evidence of improved outcomes for the baby and mother regarding fasting in labour, women should be informed of the choices they have, taking into account their individual situation during labour. Management will therefore depend on the risk factors present and maternal choice.

Management

- Self regulation of food intake during normal labour has been recommended. Eating and drinking may help to make a woman feel healthy and normal.
- No restrictions of food intake after induction, prior to the onset of labour and beyond if the labour proceeds normally.
- Drinks and light diet during early labour; established normal labour without narcotics; uncomplicated labour with an epidural.
- Alcohol and fatty foods should be avoided at all times.

- Small amounts of clear fluids only, if labour is established with one or more of the following factors:
  - Narcotics used for pain relief
  - Suspicious CTG recording
  - Trial of labour, breech, twins, etc.
  - Severe pre-eclampsia
  - Antepartum haemorrhage.
- No food or drink is permitted if an operation is likely, to ensure the woman's safety due to the increased risk of regurgitation and delayed gastric emptying.

Recommended reading

Campion P, McCormick C (2002). *Eating and Drinking in Labour*. Cheshire: Books for Midwives Press.

Young D (2007). Eating in labour: The issue deserves revisiting…. *Birth* **34**(4), 279–81.

1 Sleutal M, Golden S (1999). Fasting in labour: relic or requirement. *Journal of Obstetric, Gynaecology and Neonatal Nursing* **28**(5), 507–12.

2 O'Sullivan G, Liu b, Hart D, Seed P, Shennan A (2009). Effect of food intake during labour on obstetric outcome: randomized controlled trail. *British Medical Journal* **338**, b784.

3 Odent M (1998). Labouring women are not marathon runners. *Practising Midwife* **1**(9), 16–18.

4 Ophir E, Solt I, Odeh M, Bornstein J (2007). Water intoxication—a dangerous condition in labour and delivery rooms. *Obstetrical and Gynaecological Survey* **62**(11), 731–8.

Assessing progress of labour

The means by which the midwife evaluates and assesses the progress being made, will influence the care and responses she gives based on the individual needs and choices of women in her care.

Assessing progress during labour should not just involve monitoring the vital signs, assessing cervical dilatation, and intensity of uterine contractions.[1] The midwife should also use her hands on skills such as abdominal palpation, observation of the mother's changing physical and emotional behaviour, vocalizations, and positioning.[2] Assessment of progress does not rely on just one set of parameters, consideration of all of the previous pointers makes for holistic assessment.

First stage

- Verbal and observational history from the woman at onset and throughout labour.
- General examination and vital signs.
- Abdominal palpation and inspection (initially to give a baseline for future care), uterine activity, establish position and descent.
- Vaginal examination: the midwife should ensure that sound clinical reasons are indicated prior to the procedure to safeguard against unnecessary intervention, exposure, and distress for the mother.
- Psychological and emotional aspects, coping strategies, and support from birth attendants.
- Loss per vagina: show, colour of amniotic fluid, rupture of membranes, meconium.
- Record all ongoing assessments, examinations and overview of care on a partogram.

Assessment in labour is based on a medical environment and perspective, therefore the commonly used baselines, such as length of labour/latent phase of first stage/action curves, etc., may not reflect the normal physiology of labour. Some would suggest that this has led to increased intervention and ultimately a rise in LSCS rates.

Latent phase

- Definition of onset of the first stage varies considerably; it is a dynamic process, therefore individualized care is important.
- A prolonged latent phase may mean that the onset could be up to 3/4/5cm dilatation.
- There is evidence to support: minimizing early admission to a labour ward, maximizing assessment at home or in assessment areas, encouraging women to stay at home during the early stages.[3,4]

Active phase

- No differences in outcome or LSCS rate have been reported with an action line, this describes the timing of intervention/augmentation that is considered during labour of 2 or 4h. Reduced intervention has been reported with a 4h action line.[5]
- Assuming a baseline rate of 0.5cm/h as opposed to 1cm/h reduces unnecessary interventions and accounts for the slower labours of primigravidas.[6]

- Other means of assessing progress: pattern of contractions; women's behaviour; auditory/visual cues; intuitive skills.

Second stage

- Close observation of the woman's subtle behaviour, vocalizations, and emotional responses provide the midwife with key information about her progress, for instance: a quiet restful time prior to strong pushing urges; changing position; pelvic rocking; renewed strength; grunting during a contraction etc.
- Observation of the physical signs of descent of the presenting part (📖 see also Mechanism of labour, p. 270). If all observations are satisfactory and progress of the vertex is not apparent after a reasonable period of time, then review or possibly augmentation/intervention may need to be considered.
- Progress should be reflected by maternal and fetal condition.
- Women's choice for care should be taken into consideration, regarding position; care of the perineum; and monitoring the fetal heart
- Time restrictions for the second stage should be reconsidered, and an holistic approach taken, based upon individual progress.
- Clear evidence of the presenting part is apparent, such as pouting of the anal sphincter.
- Encourage the woman to adopt a comfortable position to aid progress, upright postures tend to shorten the duration of the second stage.[7]
- Encourage the woman to push spontaneously with the surges of her contractions to help her assist with descent and progress of the presenting part.

1 Warren C (1999). Why should I do vaginal examinations? *Practising Midwife* **2**(6), 12–13.

2 Baker A, Kenner A (1993). Communication of pain: vocalization as an indicator of the stages of labour. *Australian and New Zealand Journal of Obstetrics and Gynaecology* **33**(4), 384–5.

3 Holmes P, Lawrence W, Oppenheimer W, Wu Wen S (2001). The relationship between cervical dilatation at initial presentation in labour and subsequent intervention. *British Journal of Obstetrics and Gynaecology* **108**, 1120–4.

4 McNiven P, Williams J, Hodnett E, Kaufman K, Hannah M (1998). An early labour assessment program: A randomised controlled trial. *Birth* **25**(1), 5–10.

5 Lavender T, Wallymahmed A, Walkinshaw S (1999). Managing labour using partograms with different action lines: a prospective study of women's views. *Birth* **26**(2), 89–96.

6 Enkin M, Kierse M, Neilson J, Crowther C, Duley L, Hodnett E (2000). *A Guide to Effective care in Pregnancy and Childbirth*. Oxford: Oxford University Press.

7 Simkin P, Ancheta R (2000). *The Labour Progress Handbook*. Oxford: Blackwell Science.

Abdominal examination

Abdominal palpation in labour is one of the key clinical skills that the midwife uses to assess progress and determine the position of the fetus. At the first contact with the woman in labour the midwife will carry out a detailed abdominal examination to establish the progress and individual status of the woman's labour so far. This information will enable the midwife to plan care, discuss care with the mother and her partner. The examination should be carried out between contractions avoiding any discomfort to the woman. The midwife will then need to palpate the fundus during a contraction if they are present to determine their strength and length.

In normal labour the findings should be:

- Lie: longitudinal, an oblique or transverse lie should be detected early and the woman referred.
- Presentation: should be cephalic, any other presentation should be reported immediately.
- Position should be established (Fig. 11.1).
- Engagement of the fetal head should be determined in fifths above the brim of the pelvis. In primiparous women this is usually engaged prior to labour. When the head is engaged the occipital protuberance is barely felt from above.
- Auscultation of the fetal heart should be between 110 and 160 beats per minute (bpm).
- For information on how to perform an abdominal palpation, 🕮 see Abdominal examination, p. 74.

During labour an abdominal palpation is repeated at regular intervals as above to assess position, lie, and descent of the fetal head. In addition palpation of uterine contractions throughout labour is important:

- Palpation of the fundus of the uterus with the palm of the hand during contractions provides valuable information on the progress of labour.
- The frequency of contractions—if they are occurring very close together and strong, this may indicate fetal hypoxia; therefore careful monitoring of the fetal heart is advised. Hyperstimulation with oxytocics may be one of the reasons for this, in which case the infusion should be stopped and a review of progress should be made. Contractions may be weaker and less often, which will indicate slow progress or fatigue of the mother. Encouraging ambulation and/or repositioning may re-establish uterine activity.
- The strength and length of the contractions—assessing the strength of contractions may be subjective as the midwife cannot relate to the intensity of the pain the woman may be experiencing in relation to what is felt abdominally. This will depend on the individual's pain threshold and perception.
- Contractions are described and recorded in three ways:
  - Mild—the fundus feels tense throughout the contraction, but can be easily indented with the fingertips.
  - Moderate—the fundus feels more tense throughout the contraction and it is difficult to indent it with the fingertips.
  - Strong—the fundus feels tense, hard and rigid during the contraction.

- The uterus should return to feeling soft between contractions.
- Contractions may last from 30s up to 90s. The midwife notes the time of the start of the contraction and how long it lasts.
- Uterine contractions are not felt by the woman at the beginning and the end. However the midwife can detect the start of the contraction by palpation before the woman. This may well be useful for using pain relief such as inhalational analgesia or for encouraging coping mechanisms in labour such as breathing and relaxation techniques.

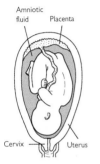

(a) Left occipito-anterior

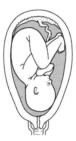

(b) Right occipito-lateral

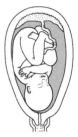

(c) Right occipito-posterior

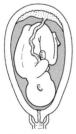

(d) Right occipito-anterior

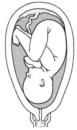

(e) Left occipito-lateral

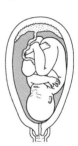

(f) Left occipito-posterior

Fig. 11.1 Cephalic presentations prior to labour.

Reproduced from *Acupuncture in Pregnancy and Childbirth*. Zita West (2001) Copyright © Elsevier Limited 2001, reprinted by permission of the publisher.

Vaginal examination

In normal labour, vaginal examination is performed at the discretion of the midwife, dependent on the individual needs of the woman, consent, and her progress through labour. Sensitivity should be employed at all times, as many women find vaginal examinations uncomfortable and traumatic. Where possible, examinations should be kept to a minimum (only when clinically indicated) and ideally should be performed by the same person.

Indications

Vaginal examination may be undertaken to:
• Confirm the establishment of labour
• Provide a baseline for subsequent progress
• Assess progress in labour and detect abnormal indices
• Assess the presenting part/position if in doubt (Fig. 11.2)

Occipito-posterior position

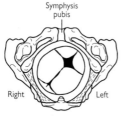

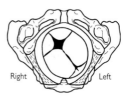

Sacrum
right occipito-posterior

Sacrum
left occipito-posterior

Occipito-anterior position

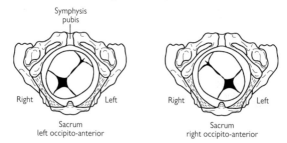

Sacrum
left occipito-anterior

Sacrum
right occipito-anterior

Fig. 11.2 Occipito-anterior and occipito-posterior positions.

Reproduced from *Acupuncture in Pregnancy and Childbirth*. Zita West (2001) Copyright © Elsevier Limited 2001, reprinted by permission of the publisher.

- Confirm progress to the second stage of labour
- Determine the position and station of the presenting part
- Determine the cause of delay/lack of progress in the second stage
- Rupture membranes if indicated
- Apply a fetal electrode
- Exclude cord prolapse following rupture of the membranes when ill-fitting or non-engagement of the presenting part or polyhydramnios is encountered.

Method

Discussion with the woman is essential before examination, to explain the procedure, reassure, and gain consent.

- Encourage the woman to empty her bladder.
- Assist in making her comfortable.
- Carry out an abdominal examination and auscultation of the fetal heart prior to examination.
- Clean the surrounding labial area/apply gloves (dependent on local policy).
- Assess the external genitalia (lesions, scars, varicose veins, discharge).
- Assess the cervix: consistency, position, effacement and dilatation.
- Assess the membranes: absent or intact, observation of liquor.
- Auscultate the fetal heart after the procedure.
- Explain your findings to the woman.

The partogram

The partogram is a graphical overview of the physical elements and events that take place in an individual woman's labour. This has proved to be an invaluable, at a glance, visual aid and reference for midwives during their care of women in labour. It is especially useful when handing over the woman's care to a colleague, as it provides an instant summary of the woman's progress to date. The partogram is usually commenced when the woman is in established labour. Details recorded on the partogram are:

- Hospital number, name of woman, age, parity, date of birth, and expected date of confinement
- The fetal heart rate, plotted at regular intervals (see 📖 Electronic fetal monitoring, p. 238, for NICE guidelines on frequency of auscultation of the fetal heart rate)
- Observation of the liquor, and what time the membranes ruptured
- Cervical dilatation and descent of the presenting part, plotted diagrammatically
- Oxytocic agents if used during labour
- Uterine activity: the length and strength of the contractions per 10min
- Drugs, inhalational analgesia, and non-pharmacological interventions used
- Urinalysis
- Blood pressure and pulse.

Legally the partogram provides a complete and comprehensive record of care and should include the following information:

- Time of birth, gender of baby, and weight
- Any abnormalities noted at birth
- Mode of birth
- Apgar score and any resuscitation/intervention/drugs given to the baby
- Length of the first, second, and third stages of labour
- Blood loss
- Perineal repair or status of perineum
- Whether meconium or urine passed during or post birth
- Feeding intention and summary of feeding/skin to skin contact.

  Originally, it was noted that use of the partogram would easily recognize cases of prolonged labour, so that appropriate action/intervention could be taken. However, this also tends to create a structured and rigid approach to care, which some midwives find restrictive, while not addressing the woman's individual needs.

- Most research on the first stage of labour is based on a medical model of care, where interventions are commonplace, and may not reflect normal labour and physiology.
- The length of labour may well be much longer than originally anticipated, particularly in primigravid women.

- Provided progress in labour is steady and the fetus is uncompromised, more flexibility in care and less rigid action lines result in less intervention and the promotion of more spontaneous births.
- A 4h action line, as opposed to a 2h action line, is associated with fewer caesarean sections and less use of oxytocin.
- More recently, it has been suggested that a cervical dilatation rate of 0.5cm/h is more realistic than 1cm/h. This again resulted in fewer interventions in labour, with equally favourable outcomes for the mother and fetus. (See Assessing progress of labour, p. 228.)
- Debate about the effectiveness and use of the partogram for normal, uncomplicated labour should not detract from the keeping of contemporaneous records during labour and delivery.

Cardiotocograph monitoring

Documentation
When continuous monitoring is commenced it is important to maintain a satisfactory tracing of fetal heart activity and contraction of frequency and strength. Maintain the CTG machine in good working order to ensure a satisfactory and accurate recording. Record the following information on the CTG paper:
- Date and time of commencing the CTG
- Name of the woman
- The woman's hospital number
- The woman's pulse rate—to establish that the tracing is the fetal heart rate
- Significant events, such as vaginal examination, siting of an epidural and epidural top-ups, augmentation with oxytocin, rupture of the membranes, and fetal blood sampling
- The CTG should be signed, dated, and the time noted
- When the birth is complete, the date, time, and mode of birth should be recorded, and the end of the trace marked clearly to verify that the whole of the trace has been retained.

Fetal heart rate patterns
- **Baseline rate**: the normal baseline rate is between 110 and 160bpm. This is defined as the mean level of the fetal heart rate (FHR) when it is stable, which excludes periods of accelerations and decelerations.
- **Baseline variability**: is the variation in the baseline rate over 1min, excluding accelerations and decelerations. Normal baseline variability is greater than or equal to a minimum of 5bpm between contractions. Good variability is an important sign of fetal well-being.
- **Reactivity**: is the presence or absence of accelerations. In labour an acceleration is interpreted as a rise in the FHR of at least 15 beats for a minimum of 15s.
- **Decelerations**: a transient fall in the baseline rate of at least 15 beats for at least 15s. Decelerations are defined depending on their depth, shape duration, and time lag.
  - Early: these are usually a repetitive and consistent pattern. There is a slowing of the FHR with the onset of the contraction, returning to the baseline at the end of the contraction.
  - Variable: these are intermittent and variable in their timing, frequency and shape. The FHR slows down rapidly at the onset and are of short duration. May not occur with contraction cycle.
  - Late: a uniform and repetitive slowing of the FHR which commences at the mid to end of the contraction. The lowest point of the deceleration may be more than 20s past the peak of the contraction and finishing after the contraction.
  - Isolated prolonged: an abrupt decrease in FHR to levels below baseline that last at least 60–90s.

The most common abnormalities of the FHR pattern during labour are decelerations, baseline tachycardia, and loss of baseline variability.

Of these, the most worrying is loss of baseline variability together with shallow decelerations occurring after the peak of contractions.

- *Tachycardia*: the baseline fetal heart rate exceeds 160bpm. A baseline rate between 160 and 180bpm is regarded as within normal limits, provided there are no other abnormal indices.
- *Bradycardia*: the baseline fetal heart rate falls below 110bpm. A baseline rate between 100 and 110bpm is regarded as normal, provided no other abnormal indices are present. A baseline rate below 100 suggests fetal hypoxia. Care should be taken to ensure that the maternal pulse rate is not being monitored instead of the fetal heart rate.

A useful pneumonic to use for interpretation of the CTG trace is shown in Table 11.1.

Table 11.1 DR C BRAVADO to indicate:

DR	=	document risks
C	=	contractions
BR	=	baseline rate
A	=	accelerations
VA	=	variability
D	=	decelerations
O	=	overall plan—this will involve some kind of decision making, for example: maintain observation, discontinue monitoring, or stop an oxytocin infusion.

Monitoring fetal well-being

The fetal response to coping with the stress of labour can be assessed by the observational skills of the midwife and by clinical means, as follows:

- Fetal movements are always an indication of fetal well being, particularly during a contraction. Fetal activity may be felt abdominally or the woman questioned about the movements she is feeling.
- Auscultation of the fetal heart using a Pinard® fetal stethoscope, Sonicaid®, or electronic fetal monitor.
- Intrapartum events, such as augmentation with oxytocin, epidural anaesthesia, bleeding, etc. Electronic fetal monitoring needs to be commenced if the woman develops risk factors during labour.
- Condition of the amniotic fluid: meconium present in the amniotic fluid is of some value, but not always predictive of fetal distress. However, thick, fresh meconium may be indicative of fetal compromise and it is recommended that continuous electronic monitoring is commenced to establish any changes in the normal pattern of the fetal heart. Potential morbidity due to inhalation of meconium at birth must be prepared for. However, morbid inhalation of meconium is more likely to occur in utero when severe hypoxia causes agonal respirations prior to terminal apnoea.
- Because of the very close relationship between a mother and her fetus, a mother's overanxiety regarding fetal well-being should be taken as a cue to start continuous monitoring.

Electronic fetal monitoring

Electronic fetal monitoring (EFM) was introduced initially to reduce perinatal mortality and cerebral palsy. While a fall in the incidence of these conditions has not been demonstrated clinically, there has been a steep rise in interventions during labour. This has led to much debate about the value of continuous EFM in normal, low-risk labours.[1]

- The NICE guidelines[2] recommend that in normal labour the admission trace should be abandoned and auscultation of the fetal heart should be carried out intermittently, with a Pinard® stethoscope or Sonicaid®, for up to 60s after a contraction, every 15min in the first stage of labour and every 5min in the second stage of labour unless the woman develops any risk factors. However the timings selected are not based on sound research evidence. Certainly during the early stages of normal labour, women are encouraged to remain at home and this amount of monitoring could be regarded as extremely intrusive.
- On admission, the maternal pulse should be recorded at the same time as the fetal heart, to differentiate between the two.
- EFM is poor at detecting normality, due to its high false-positive rate.[3]
- Intrapartum hypoxia is a relatively rare occurrence. Therefore the risk of acidaemia is negligible if the pattern of the fetal heart rate falls into the reassuring classification.
- EFM affects the birth environment, changes relationships, and increases anxiety for the woman, birth supporters, and clinicians.[4]
- With intermittent auscultation, the fetus is protected from recurrent, transient, and mild hypoxic episodes during labour. Therefore

individual variations in the fetal response to cope with labour is unmeasurable.[5] Due to high levels of stress hormones the fetus is able to cope with prolonged periods of hypoxia and lowering of the heart rate during contractions.

- Intermittent auscultation provides more flexible, one-to-one care, which is more personalized.
- Ideally, low-risk women should be cared for in separate areas to high-risk women.
- Ideally, no EFM machines should be housed in normal birth areas.[7]
- Several randomized controlled trials have been carried out indicating that EFM results in a negative labour and birth experience for many low-risk women, due to restriction of movement and concern centred on the monitoring procedure rather than the standard of care given.[6,7] However, informed consent about EFM is important and some women may not share these views.
- Important to weigh up the risks/benefits of using technology in low-risk labours before using them. Establishing the boundaries of normal labour is key.[8–10]

Recommended reading

National Collaborating Centre for Womens's and Children's Health (2007). *NICE Guidelines for Intrapartum Care—Care of Healthy Women and Their Babies During Childbirth.* London, RCOG Press.

1 Thacker S, Stroup D, Peterson H (2003). Continuous electronic fetal monitoring during labour. (Cochrane review). In: *Cochrane Library*, Issue **1**. Oxford: Update Software.

2 National Institute of Clinical Excellence (2001). *The Use of Electronic Fetal Monitoring.* London: NICE. Available at: ℘ www.nice.org.uk.

3 Hillan E (1991). Electronic fetal monitoring—more problems than benefits? *MIDIRS Midwifery Digest:***1**(3), 249–51.

4 Walsh D (2001). Midwives and birth technology: the debate that's overdue. *MIDIRS Midwifery Digest:***11**(3), S3–S6.

5 Harrison J (1999). Fetal perspectives on labour. *British Journal of Midwifery* **7**(10), 643–7.

6 Alfrevic Z, Devane D, Gyte G (2006). Continuous cardiotocography (CTG) as a form of electronic fetal monitoring (EFM) for fetal assessment during labour. *Cochrane Database of Systematic Reviews*, 2011 Issue 2. The Cochrane Collection. London: John Wiley and Sons Ltd.

7 Walsh D (2007). *Evidence-based Care for Normal Labour and Birth.* London: Routledge.

8 Thacker S (1997). Lessons in technology diffusion: The electronic fetal monitoring experience. *Birth* **24**(1), 58–60.

9 Hindley C (2001). Intrapartum electronic fetal monitoring in low risk women: a literature review. *Journal of Clinical Excellence* **3**, 91–9.

10 Walsh D (2001). Midwives and birth technology: the debate that's long overdue. *MIDIRS Midwifery Digest:* **11**(3)Supp 2, S3–S6.

Chapter 12

Pain relief: non-pharmacological

Massage

The basis of massage is touch, which many midwives incorporate into their care of the labouring woman. Regular massage from 36 weeks and during labour has been shown to reduce levels of stress hormones in women.[1] Professional massage involves the use of vegetable oils, using basic remedial techniques. The three basic strokes are:

• *Effleurage*: long, smooth strokes used at the beginning and end of a treatment.
• *Kneading*: both hands work together, alternately picking up and squeezing the muscle, resulting in a kneading movement.
• *Frictions*: using the thumbs, fingers, or heels of the hand; these strokes are used to penetrate deep muscle tissue.

Essential oils may be added to enhance the therapeutic effect. Care should be taken to ensure that the use of essential oils are not contraindicated, that the midwife is trained in their use and is familiar with safety precautions (🕮 see Aromatherapy, pp. 122–6, and Aromatherapy during labour, p. 248).

Physiological and psychological benefits

• Improves the circulation.
• Relaxes the muscular system.
• Stimulates diuresis and reduces oedema.
• Stimulates the lymphatic system.
• Speeds up the elimination of waste products.
• Encourages the production of endorphins.
• Aids digestion.
• Aids sleep.
• Enhances mental and physical relaxation.
• Encourages release of emotional tension.
• Encourages communication.

However, precautions do need to be taken prior to a massage session, to address general and pregnancy-specific contraindications. Awareness of the woman's medical and obstetric history should always be considered and consent needs to be obtained beforehand.

General contraindications

Massage should not be given, or caution should be taken, under the following circumstances:

• After a meal or alcohol; allow at least 1–2h before massage
• If there is infection, pyrexia, or inflammation
• If there has been recent injury or surgery
• Varicose veins: work very gently over these areas
• Thrombophlebitis
• Carcinoma: exert no direct pressure over the diseased site
• Sciatica: take extreme caution in the affected area
• Burns, bruising, and open wounds
• Sensitive skin: take care with these patients.

Pregnancy-specific contraindications

Avoid:

- Suprapubic or sacral massage during first trimester
- Deep massage to the calves if the woman has a history of thrombosis
- Vigorous massage around the heel: this relates to the pelvic zone in reflexology
- Shiatsu points that are contraindicated in pregnancy
- Massage of women with hypotension or a tendency to faint; monitor blood pressure
- Abdominal massage if the woman has history of antepartum haemorrhage
- In cases where the midwife or practitioner expresses any uncertainty. For further information see ✆ www.childbirth-massage.co.uk.

1 McNabb MT, Kimber L, Haines H, McCourt C (2006). Does regular massage from late pregnancy to birth decrease pain perception during labour and birth? – A feasibility to investigate a programme of massage, controlled breathing and visualization, from 36 of pregnancy until birth. *Complementary Therapies in Clinical Practice* **12**(3), 222–31.

Homoeopathic remedies for labour and birth

Homoeopathic remedies can contribute a great deal to supporting women physically and emotionally throughout labour and birth. It enables a woman to be empowered to progress through this physiological event without resort to chemical drugs and unnecessary interventions. It provides another option for care that is not harmful to the mother or the fetus. An informed woman may wish to self-medicate (comprehensive birth kits are available), or a woman may choose to be attended by a homoeopath who has gained permission prior to labour, or the midwife may be qualified in homoeopathy. For general principles of homoeopathy, 📖 see Homoeopathy, p. 120.

Arnica

The most commonly used remedy for childbirth is arnica. This remedy is used extensively for emotional and physical trauma, so therefore is an invaluable remedy for labour and the early postnatal period. It can be taken during labour and immediately following birth (preferably before the cord is cut) to minimize the general effects of trauma and to assist with pain relief. Taken for a few days after the birth, arnica will aid healing and help with after pains.

Other common remedies

- **Aconite**: for anxiety and fearfulness at any time during labour, but especially before labour and afterwards where there has been a sudden or traumatic birth.
- **Belladonna**: for severe, distressing, and spasmodic pains. The woman feels like she wants to escape. The face is hot, red, and flushed, often accompanied by a headache.
- **Caulophyllum**: for exhaustion and slow progress in labour. Helps to establish regular and effective contractions.
  ❶ This should not be taken during pregnancy as it is a powerful uterine tonic and may initiate premature labour.
- **Chamomilla**: for unbearable pain and extreme irritability.
- **Cimicifuga**: for sharp, shooting pains in all directions and failure to progress. A feeling of wanting to give up accompanied by anxiety and possibly hysteria.
- **Gelsemium**: the uterus feels heavy, sore, and squeezed, with pains radiating to the back. There may be fear, trembling, and weakness, especially in the transition stage.
- **Pulsatilla**: for an erratic, changeable, and tearful emotional state. The pains tend to be cutting and tearing, and move around. The remedy helps to establish regular contractions and restores emotional balance.
- **Sepia**: a sensation of the uterus being dragged down and heavy. Experienced by women in the second stage of labour at the crowning of the head. The overwhelming urge to bear down feels like the muscles of the pelvic floor are stretched beyond their limits. The woman is usually irritable, indifferent, and self-absorbed.
- **Nux vomica**: for irritability, chilliness, and finding fault with carers.

Recommended reading

Geraghty B (1997). *Homoeopathy for Midwives*. London: Churchill Livingstone.

Lockie A, Geddes N (1992). *The Women's Guide to Homoeopathy*. London: Hamish Hamilton.

Moskowitz R (1992). *Homoeopathic Medicines for Pregnancy and Childbirth*. Berkeley, California: North Atlantic Books.

Breathing awareness

Women are encouraged to become aware of their own breathing patterns and how adjustments can be made during labour and birth to help relieve tension and aid coping skills. A non-directive approach to breathing awareness ensures that the mother follows instinctual cues for working with her contractions. This prevents hyperventilation and enables more efficient exchange of oxygen and carbon dioxide.

- SOS breathing—Sigh Out Slowly. The outgoing breath is a naturally relaxing part of respiration; extending the outgoing breath will help to counteract hyperventilation. Inhalation naturally follows exhalation and therefore there is no need to emphasize breathing in.
- Pant Pant Blow or Puff Puff Blow breathing is a modification of panting, for the end of the first stage and transition, where there may be a premature urge to push.
- Panting—breathing out short/light breaths to help at crowning, allowing the baby's head to be born slowly and to help minimize perineal trauma. Care should be taken not to breathe in this way for long periods as this can lead to hyperventilation and lightheadedness.

Valsalva's manoeuvre: continued use of this technique is no longer recommended. Involves fixed diaphragm, closed epiglottis and breath holding, usually commenced at the beginning of contraction. Leads to increased intrathoracic pressure; decreased venous blood return to the heart; reduced cardiac output;[1] less O_2 from lungs; lowered arterial pressure and reduced O_2 to placenta.[2]

Disadvantages

- Prolonged decrease of O_2 to fetus.
- Lower cord pH.
- Fetal heart rate abnormalities.
- Lower Apgar score.
- More vaginal wall damage.
- Oedema of maternal face.
- Burst blood vessels.
- Headache.
- Maternal hypoxia.
- Maternal exhaustion.
- Undermines women's own natural birthing instincts.
- Ignores the optimum timings for pushing within a contraction—the extra surges that occur up to 3–4 times during a contraction.

1 Thompson A (1995). Maternal behaviour during spontaneous and directed pushing in the second stage of labour. *Journal of Advanced Nursing* **22**, 1027–34.

2 Bosomworth A, Bettany-Saltikov J (2006). Just take a deep breath. *MIDIRS Midwifery Digest* **16**(2), 157–65.

Hypnosis and visualization

Hypnosis is a naturally induced state of relaxed concentration—a state of union between the mind and body that communicates suggestions to the subconscious mind. The subconscious mind governs what we think and feel, while influencing the choices that we make. In essence, it can control pain. The aim of hypnosis and visualization is to equip the woman with supportive techniques that will help her prepare and cope with labour and birth. These techniques consist of self-hypnosis, guided visualization, and breathing methods. The philosophy of hypnosis maintains that when fear, stress, and tension are absent, then the woman can utilize her natural instincts more effectively, resulting in a more calm and fulfilling birth experience.[1]

Women using hypnosis have been compared with controls using traditional breathing and relaxation techniques. It was found that those in the hypnotically prepared group experienced:

• Reduced pain
• Shorter first-stage labours
• Less medication
• Higher Apgar scores
• Higher incidence of spontaneous deliveries.[2]

Pregnant women can access courses and classes to learn self-hypnosis and visualization. The techniques do not involve deep, trance-like states, rather a state more like redirected focus is involved, similar to daydreaming or being absorbed in a book. The mind and body are relaxed while also being in control and conversant with the surrounding environment.

Benefits

In addition to the above indications, hypnosis purports to have many benefits:

• Inspires confidence and optimism
• Promotes relaxation and inner peace
• Eliminates the fear–tension–pain cycle during labour
• Enhances a calm, peaceful birth environment
• Reduces fatigue during labour
• Enhances production of natural endorphins
• Eliminates the risk of hyperventilation from shallow breathing
• Enhances natural birthing instincts and behaviours
• Fewer complications during labour and birth
• A fulfilling and meaningful experience of childbirth
• A dedicated role for the birth partner
• Promotes mother, baby, and partner relationships
• Quicker postnatal recovery.

1 Melh Madrona LE (2004). Hypnosis to facilitate uncomplicated birth. *American Journal of Clinical Hypnosis* **46**(4), 299–312.

2 Cyna AM, Andrew MI, McAucliffe GL (2006). Antenatal self-hypnosis for labour and childbirth: A pilot study. *Anaesthesia and Intensive Care* **34**(4), 464–9.

Aromatherapy during labour

The use of essential oils in labour can enhance the woman's coping strategies when used alone or in conjunction with other complementary therapies, other coping mechanisms, such as breathing and relaxation techniques or conventional methods of pain relief.

The main contributions of essential oils during labour and childbirth are to:
• Assist with pain relief
• Relieve stress and anxiety
• Assist with efficient functioning of the uterus
• Prevent fatigue.

For details of the safe administration and therapeutic properties of essential oils, 📖 see Aromatherapy, pp. 122–126.

The following oils are some of the most commonly used essential oils for labour and delivery. Some aromatherapy practitioners/midwives may wish to use other oils not listed here.

• *Lavender*: is a very versatile oil, with relaxing, antispasmodic and pain-relieving properties. It is therefore useful to help ease the pain of contractions, and as a general, all-round, helpful oil throughout labour. It is best avoided by people with hay fever and asthma. Take care with vaporizing the oil, as some women find the aroma unpleasant and overpowering; it may also cause headaches in some people.
  ❶ *Do not* use lavender in conjunction with epidurals because it has hypotensive properties. It may also possibly interact with narcotics, so care should be taken in conjunction with pethidine or diamorphine.

• *Chamomile*: is calming and relaxing during labour. It has significant anti-inflammatory and antispasmodic properties. Chamomile should not be used until late pregnancy because it has emmenagogic properties, which theoretically may induce menstruation, and therefore bleeding.

• *Clary sage*: a uterine tonic and euphoric oil, it is useful for stimulating contractions and pain relief. Clary sage has emmenagogic properties, so should not be used in pregnancy until near term and if overused may cause drowsiness and headaches.
  ❶ Driving is not recommended if exposed to Clary sage for lengthy periods, and it should not be combined with alcoholic drinks.

• *Frankincense*: is a very useful oil for calming anxiety and panic, especially where this is associated with hyperventilation. May not be suitable for asthmatic people due to its strong aroma and conflicting reports regarding its benefits for asthma.

• *Jasmine*: is a uterine tonic that has been used traditionally as an aid to childbirth. It helps to strengthen contractions, while also having pain-relieving and antispasmodic properties. It is reputed to be useful as a compress, placed on the lower abdomen, to help expel a retained placenta. Emotionally it has energizing and antidepressant qualities.
  ❶ *Do not* use jasmine until the onset of labour.

• *Lemon*: is an antiseptic and astringent, also reputed to be a circulatory tonic. A gentle, uplifting oil with a pleasant, fresh aroma. Often mixed with other oils to minimize pungent aromas, this makes it a versatile oil to use at any time during labour and birth. Lemon has phototoxic properties, therefore after use care should be taken to reduce exposure to sunlight, as with most citrus oils.

- *Mandarin*: a refreshing and gently uplifting oil, with a delicate aroma. Helpful for nausea and anxiety. Has antispasmodic properties and helps to balance the metabolic rate. This makes mandarin a safe, all-round oil for use in labour. Slightly phototoxic.
- *Rose*: aids uterine action due to its homone-like action. It stimulates the pituitary gland and releases dopamine. It also possesses antispasmodic properties and is a general circulatory tonic. Rose is said to have a strong affinity to the female reproductive system, making it a special oil for labour and childbirth.
- *Petitgrain*: a useful oil for the transition phase, as it helps to soothe emotions especially where there is panic and loss of control.
- Other oils that are beneficial during labour and birth include grapefruit, lime, sweet orange, neroli, sandalwood, geranium, eucalyptus, and ylang ylang.

Recommended reading

Burns E, Blamey C, Ersser S (2000). The use of aromatherapy in intrapartum midwifery practice: an observational study. *Complementary Therapies in Nursing and Midwifery* **6**, 33–4.

Lawless J (1992). *The Encyclopaedia of Essential Oils*. Shaftesbury, Dorset: Element Books Limited.

Price S, Price L (1995). *Aromatherapy for Health Professionals*. London: Churchill Livingstone.

Tiran D (2000). *Clinical Aromatherapy for Pregnancy and Childbirth*, 2nd edn. London: Churchill Livingstone.

Reflexology during labour

Reflexology is one of many complementary therapies that can assist with the mother's coping abilities during labour. The woman may be attended by a midwife/reflexologist or have arranged for an independent reflexology practitioner to attend her during labour. It is important that all practitioners are fully conversant with the physiology of labour and the potential problems. Reflexology is a powerful tool and can have a dynamic therapeutic effect when used wisely. The overall care of the woman rests with the midwife or doctor in charge and, in the event of complications, complementary therapy may not always be appropriate. Midwives may have received in-house training to perform specific techniques in reflexology relating to labour care—untrained personnel should never dabble.

- Encourage the woman to adopt a comfortable, well-supported position appropriate to labour, to prevent postural hypotension while maintaining good eye contact and communication. Adjust your posture to accommodate the mother's varying positions throughout labour.
- Familiarize yourself with the woman's relevant medical and obstetric history and present labour circumstances.
- Obtain consent from the woman.
- Adhere to the local policy for treatment using complementary therapies.

Uses in labour

- General relaxation.
- Relief of stress and anxiety.
- Helps to relieve the pain of contractions and backache.
- Minimizes nausea and vomiting.
- Relief of cold feet in labour.
- Encourages strong rhythmic contractions—may assist with augmentation. It is important to work within local policy and liaise with medical staff if used as a measure to augment labour.
- Induction of labour should not be undertaken by a midwife or practitioner unless there is a local policy clearly stating the conditions when complementary therapies can be used for induction of labour, or with the agreement of the woman's consultant.
- For the third stage of labour, reflexology may be used in uncomplicated retained placenta.
- Treatments may consist of general reflexology massage for relaxation or shorter, more specific treatments focusing on a particular area, e.g., the ankles pertaining to the pelvic area or the pad of the thumb pertaining to the pituitary gland.
- Treatments should be recorded in the woman's notes.
- Reflexology is also very useful in the postnatal stage. Some of the conditions that respond to treatment are:
  - Retention of urine
  - Painful perineum
  - Breast engorgement
  - Constipation
  - Inadequate lactation
  - Oedema.

Recommended reading

Mackereth PA, Tiran D (2002). *Clinical Reflexology—A Guide for Health Care Professionals.* London: Elsevier.

Tiran D (2004). Midwives enthusiasm for complementary therapies: a cause for concern? *Complementary Therapies in Nursing and Midwifery* **10**(2), 77–9.

Tiran D (2006). Midwives responsibilities when caring for women using complementary therapies during labour. *MIDIRS Midwifery Digest* **16**(1), 77–80.

Tiran D (2009). *Reflexology for Pregnancy—A Definitive Guide for Healthcare Professionals.* London: Elsevier.

Acupuncture in labour and childbirth

Some midwives may be qualified acupuncturists, or an acupuncturist practitioner may attend a woman; however, it is important that the practitioner has in-depth knowledge of the appropriate points to use in labour and how to needle them effectively. Insight into a woman's behavioural patterns and emotional needs will also influence the choice of points used to maximize effective treatment for the individual.

Four patterns of disharmony that may be manifested in labour have been identified:[1]

- **Deficiency of Qi and blood**: this may be due to premature rupture of membranes to labour or it can be the result of heavy periods or blood loss following previous deliveries.
- **Kidney deficiency**: this may be due to multiple pregnancies or *in vitro* fertilization (IVF) pregnancies; short gaps between pregnancies deplete the kidney energy.
- **Spleen and stomach deficiency**: this may be due to a lack of proper nourishment prior to labour.
- **Ki and blood stagnation** (*liver Qi stagnation*): this is due to emotional problems or bad premenstrual tension prior to pregnancy.

Acupuncture offers many benefits to the labouring woman, it helps to release endorphins, which will enhance relaxation, aid pain relief, and assist with coping mechanisms. A variety of techniques may be used, from traditional needling of the points, moxibustion, electro acupuncture, and ear acupuncture; shiatsu techniques may also be utilized.

First stage of labour

- In early labour the points used are to facilitate uterine action and help with general pain relief.
- As labour progresses acupuncture may be used to augment weak or irregular contractions.
- Specific pain relief, as in posterior position and backache.
- Helps to boost and maintain energy levels.
- Helps to dispel fear and anxiety at any stage.
- Helps with the difficulties associated with the transition stage.

Second stage of labour

- Helps to alleviate exhaustion.
- Helps to dispel fear and anxiety, which blocks the mother's energy network.
- Augments contractions if they are becoming too far apart.
- Many of the points forbidden in pregnancy will be used during labour as they generally have a strong downwards movement of energy in the body, which greatly enhances the birthing process.

Third stage of labour

- Chinese philosophy dictates that vessels are depleted of blood following birth and therefore are vulnerable to attack from external pathogens. Very often tonifying treatment to build up the blood is commenced soon after birth.
- Retained placenta: points that have a strong downwards movement will be used to initiate uterine action.
- Others points may be used help to regulate uterine action and stimulate the movement of blood.

The main disadvantage of acupuncture treatment in labour is that it cannot be used in conjunction with water birth. Some women may find needling a little bit painful, and some points may not be accessible due to the variety of positions and restlessness of the woman at times.

Shiatsu

Shiatsu helps the woman to tune into the powerful and changeable energy patterns associated with labour, which makes it an ideal therapy to complement normal midwifery practice and provide individual and woman-centred care. The main focus is to help the woman's energies to flow freely from the onset of labour, rather than waiting until the energies become blocked. Various techniques may be used to move or balance energy, such as strong pressure and holding of key points along the meridian lines, knuckling, hooking, stroking and massage to selected areas or acupoints. Shiatsu can be used throughout the whole of labour if the woman wishes, and will certainly be extremely beneficial if used in this way.

Benefits in labour

Shiatsu shares the same benefits as previously mentioned in the acupuncture section as it is a manual form of acupuncture, accessing the key meridian lines and points without needles. This makes it less invasive and easily combined with normal midwifery care given by the midwife. In addition Shiatsu has the following benefits:

• Emotionally releasing—tension and emotional stasis may block the process of birth
• Relieves headaches and assists concentration
• Helps to calm the baby. Helps the woman to connect and focus her energy on her baby rather than on the pain
• Provides a supportive role for the midwife.

Working on the meridians located in the back is key. The Governing Vessel (GV) is the main source of Yang energy, which is required for labour to proceed effectively. By working on the GV the therapist can tap into and balance all of the energy sources in the body. The Bladder (BL) meridian located in the back is important to work on in the first stage of labour to relieve fear and anxiety. Sacral work is effective to relieve pain and tension, particularly on the sacral grooves, which helps to release energy to the uterus, perineum, and vagina.

If the woman feels comfortable for the therapist to work in the abdominal area, this has a direct link with the uterus and represents earth energy, which helps the woman ground herself. Kidney One is located on the underside of the foot, being the lowest point of the body; this point links to earth energy and is very grounding and calming.

Encouraging the birth partner to assist with some of the techniques enables the midwife to attend to other care commitments for the woman and provides a key role for involvement of the partner.

Recommended reading

Yates S (2003). *Shiatsu for Midwives*. London: Elsevier.

1 West Z (2001). *Acupuncture in Pregnancy and Childbirth*. London: Churchill Livingstone.

Transcutaneous electrical nerve stimulation

Transcutaneous nerve stimulation (TENS) is a self-administered form of non-pharmacological pain relief that can be used throughout all stages of labour. The equipment can be hired or loaned by the pregnant woman for use at home before transfer to the labour ward.

Pain relief is thought to be activated by the passage of a mild electrical stimulus across the nerves of the spine at the level which transmits pain impulses from the uterus and cervix. This works in two ways by influencing the pain gate mechanism and stimulation of naturally occurring endorphins.

Electrodes in the form of adhesive pads are placed on either side of the spine and these are attached to a small control device by coated wires. Hand control buttons allows the user to select the power level required; as labour progresses a more intense level of stimulation can be selected as the contractions become longer, stronger, and more frequent. The device has a booster feature which can be operated throughout a contraction to obtain more pain relief and then a return to the selected programme once the contraction has subsided.

Effectiveness varies and is thought to be enhanced if the device is used from the earliest contractions onwards, before the labour becomes established. This enables the initial build up of endorphins to take effect e.g. 40min, thus allowing the mother to gain benefit before strong contractions commence.

Instruction needs to be given to the woman and her birth partner regarding the placement of electrodes:
• One on either side of the spine just below the bra line, vertebral level T10–L1 and placed 3cm apart.
• One on either side of the spine, over the sacral dimples, vertebral level S2–S4 and placed 3cm apart.

Advantages
• TENS is safe to use alongside other methods of pain relief such as nitrous oxide and oxygen, opiates and complementary therapies.
• Mother is in control.
• Non-invasive.
• No adverse effect on fetus.
• May reduce need for pharmacological analgesia.

Disadvantages
• TENS cannot be used submerged in water or alongside epidural analgesia.
• There have been occasional reports of TENS possibly disrupting CTG tracings which midwives ought to be aware of.

Recommended reading

Johnson MI (1997). Transcutaneous electrical nerve stimulation in pain management. *British Journal of Midwifery* **5**(7), 400–5.

Mainstone A (2004). Transcutaneous electrical nerve stimulus (TENS). *British Journal of Midwifery* **12**(9), 578–80.

Rodriguez MA (2005). Transcutaneous nerve stimulation during birth. *British Journal of Midwifery* **13**(8), 8–9.

Trout KK (2004). The neuromatrix theory of pain: implications for selected non-pharmacological methods of pain relief for labor. *Journal of Midwifery and Women's Health* **49**(6), 482–8. Reprinted in: *MIDIRS Midwifery Digest* **15**(1), 73–8.

Bach flower remedies during labour

Childbirth presents an enormous physical and emotional challenge, consequently emotional reserves of strength and staying power may well be put to the test. The Bach flower remedies may help by assisting the mother to stay calm and work with her body, resulting in the release of endorphins and encephalins which greatly assist in the process of labour.

Rescue Remedy is the most useful remedy for labour and can be sipped from a glass of water between contractions for the duration of labour. For dosages and administration, 📖 see Bach flower remedies, pp. 128–130.

Other remedies that may prove useful at this time are:

- **Olive**: may be useful when the woman is emotionally and physically exhausted, perhaps due to a long labour.
- **Gorse**: may help when there is a feeling of wanting to give up, cannot go on any longer.
- **Beech**: may help when there are feelings of intolerance towards birth partners and carers.
- **Red chestnut**: may be useful for overanxiety for the baby during labour and birth.
- **Cherry plum**: may help when there is fear of losing control, or behaving in an irrational way.
- **Aspen**: may help when apprehension or fear of the unknown is experienced.
- **Clematis**: for when there is too much detachment and distance from the process of birthing, possibly causing delay/disruption to progress.
- **Impatiens**: for feeling impatient and irritable with those around her or with the slow pace/progress of labour.
- **White chestnut**: may assist to relieve constant anxiety and worrying.
- **Mimulus**: for fear of pain, procedures, or the hospital environment.
- **Walnut**: may help in adjusting to the changes occurring during labour and birth, and extra protection to be able to cope better.
- **Gentian**: may help when there are feelings of despondency, perhaps because of slow progress or setbacks during labour.
- **Willow**: for feelings of self-pity and resentment.

If the mother uses up less energy on anxiety and stress related to labour, she can then retain more energy to cope physically with labour.

During labour, the calming effect of the remedies may also impact on the fetus in adjusting and coping with the stress of birth.

Chapter 13

Pain relief: pharmacological

Nitrous oxide and oxygen administration

This is a very good method to use in practice as:
- It is easily available to all midwives
- The woman controls it herself
- It works quickly, usually within three to four contractions
- It wears off quickly when administration stops
- It is safe to use in conjunction with other methods of pain relief
- It is useful as an aid to enhance coping strategies over 'a rough patch', or while waiting for other forms of pain relief to be effective.

Method

A mixture of N_2O 50% and O_2 50% is delivered from a cylinder via Entonox® apparatus.

How to use it

- Start use as soon as a contraction begins—to achieve maximum relief at the height of the contraction.
- You will need to palpate contractions and warn the woman to start breathing through the mask or mouthpiece (ask her preference!). A mask should cover the nose and mouth with a good seal. Listen to ensure that the valve is delivering the gas mixture correctly.
- The gas mixture should be inhaled throughout the contraction.
- It may take up to three contractions before good pain relief is experienced.
- Once started, onset of relief is usually within 20s.
- Recovery takes place between contractions. If the woman is too drowsy to operate the apparatus effectively, then no gas will be delivered and she will quickly recover. It is very unlikely to cause sleep or loss of consciousness.
- You may need to remind the woman that she does not need to inhale the gas mixture when there is no contraction.

Disadvantages

- It may cause drowsiness, dizziness, and nausea.
- Some women do not like the odour.
- Use over more than 6h is not recommended.
- Some concern regarding the possibility of cross-infection and staff safety has arisen – however, is still considered a safe and simple method of pain relief for women.[1]

The *Midwives Rules and Standards*[2] outline the midwife's responsibilities in the administration of pain relief.

---

1 Rosen MA (2002). Nitrous oxide for relief of labor pain: a systematic review. *American Journal of Obstetrics and Gynecology* **186**(5), S110–S26.

2 Nursing and Midwifery Council (2004). *Midwives Rules and Standards*, Rule 7. London: NMC, p. 19.

Opiates

Considerations for the use of opiates during labour

The use of opiates for the relief of pain during labour has been somewhat superseded by the growing popularity of epidural analgesia. There does remain a place for an alternative to epidurals, and midwives do need to be able to advise mothers about a range of choices.

In discussion, clients need to be made aware of the following issues:

- The efficacy of analgesic effect[1,2]
- The effect upon the fetal heart rate and features of the CTG trace if this is in progress
- The effect on labour
- The potential depressant effects on the neonate following birth with respect to the initiation of respiration and establishment of breast feeding.[3,4]

The commonly used opiates are pethidine and morphine derivatives, for example diamorphine. Meptazinol, a drug introduced in the 1980s is less commonly offered, probably due to its cost.

Pethidine

- Usual dosage 50–100mg via intramuscular injection.
- Narcotic—respiratory depressant.
- Antispasmodic.
- Can cause nausea and vomiting.
- Reduces gastrointestinal motility.
- Crosses the placenta.
- Action reversed by naloxone 100micrograms/kg body weight.

Diamorphine

- Usual dosage 10mg via intramuscular injection.
- Strongly narcotic—respiratory depressant.
- Can cause nausea and vomiting.
- Reduces gastrointestinal motility.
- Crosses the placenta.
- Many standing orders only allow a single dose to be administered.

1 Tsui MHY, Kee WDN, Ng FF (2004). A double blinded randomized placebo-controlled study of intra-muscular pethidine for pain relief in the first stage of labour. *BJOG International Journal of Obstetrics and Gynaecology* **111**(7), 648–55.

2 Wood C, Soltani H (2005). Does pethidine relieve pain? *Practising Midwife* **8**(7), 16, 18–20, 22–5.

3 Hunt S (2002). Pethidine: love it or hate it? *MIDIRS Midwifery Digest* **12**(3), 363–5.

4 Sosa CG, Buekens P, Hughes JM, *et al.* (2006). Effect of pethidine administered during the first stage of labor on the acid-base status at birth. *European Journal of Obstetrics and Gynecology and Reproductive Biology* **129**, 135–9.

Lumbar epidural analgesia

This is a very effective method of pain relief which has gained in popularity since its use in obstetrics became more widespread in the 1970s.

A senior anaesthetist must be present or readily available during administration of lumbar epidural anaesthesia. This limits the use of this technique in units or centres that cannot provide 24h anaesthetic cover. However, recently ODAs and nurses have begun to insert epidurals for labouring women.

What is an epidural?

- A local anaesthetic, usually bupivacaine hydrochloride (Marcain®) injected into the epidural space between the second and third lumbar vertebrae.
- This drug acts on the spinal nerves at this level to produce a sensory and partial motor block.
- The sensory block produces excellent pain relief, as it affects the uterine and cervical nerve plexuses, which are the main transmitters of pain sensation during uterine contractions.
- The partial motor block leaves the woman unable to walk around, so she is cared for in bed.
- There is a reflex relaxation of the blood vessels in the lower body, leading to increased warmth and a feeling of heaviness in the lower limbs.
- This haemodynamic shift results in rebound hypotension, improved circulation in the lower body, and relaxation of the pelvic floor.
- As labour advances, contraction pain is centred on the rectum and pelvic floor, and the sacral nerve plexus is then involved in the transmission of pain. A stronger dose of bupivacaine can be administered with the woman in a more upright position to give effective pain relief at this time (referred to as a second-stage top-up).

Types of epidural

An epidural anaesthetic can be administered in several ways.

Standard: 10mL of bupivacaine 0.25–0.5% via an epidural cannula. Each dose lasts 1–2h, therefore the drug is readministered as required (epidural top-up).

Combined epi-spinal: a combination of low-dose bupivacaine (0.15%) into the epidural space, with a small dose of opiate (3micrograms fentanyl) into the subarachnoid space, is used to produce a less-dense motor block, allowing the woman more mobility. This is sometimes referred to as a mobile epidural, but it does not mean the woman can walk about! She will have improved motor control so she will be able to move around in bed more easily. Regular injections every 1–2h of bupivacaine into the epidural space will still be required.

Continuous lumbar epidural infusion: once the epidural block is established, 10–15mg/h of a 0.1 or 0.125% solution of bupivacaine (with or without opiate) is administered via an infusion pump attached to the epidural cannula. This can be combined with a patient-controlled device that allows the woman to top up the dose, within a strict limit (a very popular option with mothers and midwives!).

Choice between the above methods depends on availability (midwives to administer the top-ups), unit protocol, and the mother's preference.

Before asking for consent, explain the risks and benefits of the procedure to the woman who is considering epidural analgesia.

Indications

- If *instrumental or operative delivery is necessary* epidural analgesia provides excellent pain control during operative procedures, avoiding the risks of general anaesthesia.
- *Malpresentations or malpositions* (e.g., breech, occipito-posterior), where there is a higher risk of slow progress and intervention. The advantages of epidural analgesia have to be balanced against the loss of pushing sensations and failure of the presenting part to rotate and descend, which are crucial to achieve a vaginal delivery.
- *Multiple pregnancy*, where there is a higher than normal risk of delivery problems with the second twin.
- Women with *breech presentations* or *multiple pregnancy* who aim to give birth vaginally may refuse an epidural and their wishes should be respected.
- *Pregnancy-induced hypertension*. Lowered blood pressure induced by an epidural anaesthetic offsets the increased blood pressure due to the response to painful contractions, making the blood pressure easier to control during labour.
- *Induction of labour*. The drugs used to induce labour create artificially high levels of uterine contraction for a longer period of time. The length of labour is often extended, so adequate pain relief becomes more problematic.
- *Maternal request*: This is not a good option for low-risk deliveries in normal spontaneous labour, as the side-effects often outweigh the benefits. Women need good preparation, midwifery support, and encouragement to try other pain-relief options first. However, if a woman has understood and given careful consideration to the information given, then her choice should be respected.

Contraindications

- Abnormalities of the spine: refer to an anaesthetist during pregnancy if the woman is keen to have epidural analgesia during labour.
- Systemic infection, because of the added risk of spread into the epidural site.
- Bleeding/clotting disorders, because of the risk of haematoma formation in the epidural space.
- Maternal reluctance: if the woman is not keen, she has not given proper consent!
- Absence of adequate levels of midwifery staff/anaesthetic staff to ensure safe care.

Complications

- Impaired descent and rotation of the presenting part. This can sometimes be countered by use of IV oxytocin during the second stage. This is the main cause of the increase in instrumental delivery associated with epidural analgesia.
- Sudden profound hypotension can be prevented by adequate loading of the maternal circulation throughout. Emergency resuscitation drugs should be available in the room at all times.
- Dural tap: the spinal needle or cannula pierces the dura mater, allowing cerebrospinal fluid (CSF) to escape and causing severe headache. Pushing efforts may need to be restricted. Following delivery, the mother must be nursed flat for 24h. A blood patch may be performed to seal the dura mater.
- Infection at the site of introduction.
- Fetal hyperthermia due to the increased warming effect in the woman's lower body. This increases as the length of labour increases. Continuous electronic monitoring of the fetal heart is required throughout. This can be offset by delaying the commencement of epidural analgesia by using other methods, such as an opiate or inhalational analgesia, during early labour; and then by using the lowest doses possible to achieve maternal comfort.
- Neurological problems: injury/trauma to the spinal cord caused by drug or operator errors.

Care of the woman during epidural analgesia

How is the lumbar epidural commenced?

- Before inserting the epidural, 500mL of IV normal saline (or equivalent) is used to pre-load the maternal circulation, to offset the hypotensive effects of the epidural. This infusion must be maintained throughout labour until the epidural analgesic is no longer required (approximately 1h following delivery).
- A senior anaesthetist, appropriately trained nurse, or operating department assistant (ODA) sites the epidural cannula, and the first dose is administered at this time.
- The cannula is inserted through a spinal needle, which is used to locate the epidural space. The woman's position during insertion is critical: she must sit up with her legs over the edge of the bed, feet supported, or lie flat, on her left side with her spine curved outwards and legs flexed, and lie completely still until the cannula is in place.
- This position is very difficult to achieve and maintain during frequent painful contractions. The midwife must assist the woman and remain with her until the procedure is completed.
- If the anaesthetist needs assistance, a second midwife should be present.
- During insertion it is very important to have a clear record of the fetal heart, and the midwife may need to use a hand-held ultrasound transducer to achieve this.
- The cannula is secured firmly with adhesive dressings and the filter on the distal end is left easily accessible.

- The anaesthetist ensures that the woman has an adequate block before leaving her in the care of the midwife. The anaesthetist also leaves precise instructions about dosage and frequency of any top-ups, and dosage during the second stage of labour and for instrumental vaginal delivery.

Care as labour progresses

- After the initial and subsequent doses, measure maternal blood pressure, pulse, and the fetal heart every 5min for 15min. Medical staff should be alerted if the readings give any cause for concern, e.g. if the fetal heart rate is below 110bpm or the maternal systolic blood pressure below 100mmHg.
- Thereafter, measure pulse, blood pressure, and contractions half-hourly, and monitor the fetal heart continuously.
- Help the woman to change position frequently, to avoid pressure sores.
- Absence of sensation in the bladder is a feature of this method of pain relief and the woman will not be aware of the need to pass urine. Help her to empty her bladder every 2h, by urinary catheter if necessary. This prevents injury to the urinary tract and obstruction of labour due to a full bladder.
- Do not allow the woman to lie supine unless the midwife is in attendance. This may reduce blood flow to the placental site leading to fetal bradycardia. Avoid aorto-caval compression by positioning the woman on her side, or with a small wedge/pillow under her side, to tilt her abdomen.
- The fetus-ejection or pushing reflex is often lost as a result of epidural analgesia. Therefore, during the second stage of labour, direct care towards ensuring an adequate but safe maternal effort during pushing, as the mother will not know when to push and will often become discouraged by, what seems to her, a lack of progress. Ideally the presenting part should be either visible or below the ischial spines before you encourage the woman to push.

Chapter 14

Normal labour: second stage

Recognition of the second stage

The sometimes difficult transition between the first and second stages of labour is usually an indicator of the changes and readjustments that are made physically and emotionally, in order for labour to continue successfully. Changes in the woman's behaviour and physical demeanour provide the midwife with visual and auditory clues, which are characteristic of the end of the first stage of labour and the onset of the second stage. During this time the stress hormones associated with labour are at their peak, suggesting a favourable physiological response to labour.

Visual, auditory, and physical signs

Women may:
- Experience contractions that come very close together, feeling more intense and painful (due to the action of stretch receptors and the effect of oxytocin).
- Feel a sensation of wanting to bear down, although the cervix is not quite fully dilated—there is no rationale for preventing women from bearing down if they so desire.
- Rest or sleep for periods, sometimes women enter a sleepy phase, where contractions are weaker and less frequent.
- Appear to be in trance-like state; distant and withdrawn from carers and difficulty in concentrating, the focus is mainly on giving birth.

This is thought to be the result of the maternal release of β-endorphins during labour, which peak at birth. In a drug-free and non-interventionist labour the woman (and the baby) will be impregnated with opiates which also contribute to the early dependency (attachment) of mother and baby following birth. Women may:
- Lose control or feel unable to cope
- Strongly vocalize their needs by:
  - Distressed statements such as 'Get me an epidural, I am going home. Get this baby out!'
  - Swearing or using language that is uncharacteristic
  - Shouting and groaning
- Feel strange, shaky, trembling
- Feel nauseated or vomit
- Experience extremes of hot and cold
- Express body language of restlessness and irritability; often women curl their toes during contractions.

Latent phase: physiology

The anatomical recognition of the second stage is full dilatation of the cervix, but this does not necessarily coincide with expulsive contractions.
- The contractions may subside for a period of 10–12min, or up to 2h, women often take this opportunity to sleep or doze. Often referred to as the 'rest and be thankful' phase.
- Contractions and the urge to push may be absent or weak.
- Once the presenting part has passed through the cervical walls, some adjustment due to decreased volume may be needed. This requires the muscle fibres of the upper segment of the uterus to shorten and

thicken further; only when the slack has been taken up can progress be made to expulsive contractions and descent down the birth canal.
- Stretch receptors in the vagina, rectum and perineum communicate changes in volume, tension, and tone, possibly accounting for the complexity of symptoms experienced at the transition stage.
- Passive descent should be allowed until the fetal head becomes visible.
There is scant evidence to suggest that active pushing in the latent phase of the second stage achieves much other than exhausting and discouraging the mother.

Early physical and auditory signs of the active second stage
- If the membranes are intact, they will commonly rupture at full dilatation.
- The woman has a sensation of wanting to have her bowels open during a contraction.
- A bright red loss may be observed.
- The woman shows renewed strength and excitement, and ability to work with her contractions.
- A purple line may appear, extending from the anus to the nape of the buttocks. It is not recognizable in all women, due to obesity or upright positions.[1]
- The woman may grunt at the height of a contraction and show facial congestion during pushing efforts.

Advanced signs of the second stage
- Vulval and perineal areas bulge and gape.
- The anus pouts and then flattens. The woman may empty her bowels during a contraction.

Active phase: physiology
- The urge to push allows the presenting part to descend to compress the tissues of the pelvic floor.
- Approximately 1cm above the ischial spines, pressure from the fetal presentation stimulates nerve receptors in the pelvic floor (Ferguson's reflex) and an uncontrollable urge to bear down is experienced.
- During expulsive contractions, muscle fibres of the vagina and uterus draw up and tighten the lining of the birth canal, providing a taut surface against which the presenting part can slide down.
- Beynon's (coat/sleeve) analogy. When an arm is quickly put in a coat sleeve, the lining is dragged out with hand; if the lining is held at the top everything stays in place. In childbirth, when told to push immediately at the beginning of a contraction, the pulling up mechanism may be diminished or prevented, leading to delay or damage.
- Odent[2] identifies the 'fetal ejection reflex' when there is a steep rise in the release of catecholamines during the last few contractions before birth. This is recognized by the woman suddenly becoming more alert and energized. She may need to drink a glass of water and perhaps hold on to someone. This ensures that the woman is alert and therefore protective for when the baby is born. The fetus also releases its own catecholamines at this time and is observed in the wide eyed, alert baby who gazes at its mother directly after birth.

Contractions of the second stage

$$\text{Contraction alone} = 70\text{–}80\text{mmHg}$$
$$+$$
$$\text{Extra surges at peak of contraction} = 70\text{–}80\text{mmHg}$$
$$\text{Therefore total effort} = 140\text{–}160\text{mmHg}$$

Stretch receptors and pushing

Stretch receptors are activated in the wall of the vagina, rectum, and perineum, especially during the surges of the contractions:

Uterine surges + abdominal pressure + receptors = overwhelming desire to push

Recommended reading

Downe S (2009). Transition and the second stage of labour. In: Fraser D, Cooper A (eds) *Myles Textbook for Midwives*, 15th edn. Edinburgh: Churchill Livingstone.

1 Hobbs L (1998). Assessing cervical dilatation without VEs. *Practising Midwife* **1**(11), 34–5.

2 Odent M (2001). New reasons and new ways to study birth physiology. *International Journal of Gynecology and Obstetrics* **75** Suppl 1, S39–S45.

Mechanism of labour

During labour the fetus makes a series of passive movements, collectively known as the mechanism of labour (Fig.14.1). These enable the fetus to adapt to the changes of the pelvis and birth canal, making use of the best space available. It is important to have a sound understanding of this mechanism, so that the normal manoeuvres of the fetus at delivery are anticipated and situations when assist- ance may be necessary recognized. This is best depicted diagrammatically.

- Descent commences before labour begins in the primigravidae; in multigravidae this may not occur until labour is established. Further descent is facilitated during labour, particularly during the second stage, when auxiliary muscles (diaphragm and abdominals) are employed to aid expulsion.
- Flexion is the natural attitude of the fetal head at commencement of labour. Flexion becomes more marked as labour progresses. Resistance of the birth canal exerts pressure through the occiput.

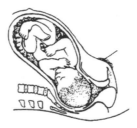

Fig. 14.1a First stage of labour. The cervix dilates. After full dilatation the head flexes further and descends further into the pelvis.

- Internal rotation occurs when the occiput (or whichever denominator meets the pelvic floor first) meets the resistance of the pelvic floor, rotating through one-eighth of a circle. The contour of the pelvic floor assists by presenting the longest diameter of the pelvic outlet (antero-posterior diameter). The occiput is then able to escape under the pubic arch and crowning takes place.
- Crowning of the head occurs when it has emerged under the pubic arch and does not recede between contractions. The widest diameter of the head (biparietal) is apparent.
- Extension of the head takes place to facilitate the bregma, forehead, face, and chin to sweep the perineum and accommodate the changed contour of the pelvis.
- Following birth of the head, restitution (untwisting of the fetal head) takes place to enable realignment of the head and shoulders, in preparation for delivery of the shoulders and body.
- The shoulders then undergo internal rotation, lying in the antero-posterior diameter of the outlet, to follow the direction of restitution.

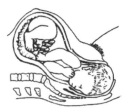

Fig. 14.1b During the early second stage the head rotates at the levels of the ischial spine so the occiput lies in the anterior part of pelvis. In late second stage the head broaches the vulval ring (crowning) and the perineum stretches over the head.

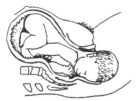

Fig. 14.1c The head is born. The shoulders still lie transversely in the midpelvis.

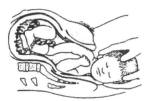

Fig. 14.1d Birth of the anterior shoulder. The shoulders rotate to lie in the antero-posterior diameter of the pelvic outlet. The head rotates externally, 'restitutes', to its direction at onset of labour.

- The anterior shoulder is then born by applying gentle downward
  traction. The posterior shoulder and trunk are then born by lateral
  flexion. If traction is not applied, it is not uncommon for the posterior
  shoulder to be born first.

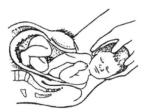

Fig. 14.1e Birth of the posterior shoulder.

Principles of care in the second stage of labour

The second stage of labour places extra emotional and physical demands on the woman. Extra vigilance is required in terms of midwifery care and support.

- *Vital signs*. In normal labour unnecessary recordings of the blood pressure (BP) and pulse will hinder the woman's concentration and focus. She may be affected by pain, anxiety, fear, and contractions, therefore taking the BP is of minimal value when the woman is actively pushing. Auscultate the fetal heart every 5min and between contractions in the latter part of the second stage.
- *Contractions*. Note frequency, strength, and length. Identify the different phases of the second stage—strong expulsive contractions for the active phase.
- *Vaginal loss*. Observe amniotic fluid or blood loss. Be aware of any abnormalities.
- *Bladder*. Encourage the woman to empty her bladder at commencement of the second stage. Failure to do this can lead to delay and trauma to the bladder at delivery.
- *Cleanliness and comfort*. Due to the woman's extra physical efforts and emotional strain, it may help to:
  - Sponge her face, or use a fine water spray/mister
  - Sponge her hands, neck, and arms
  - Give her sips of iced water or mouthwash between contractions
  - Have a fan in room if it is hot
  - Give her simple massage, particularly if she is prone to cramp
  - Give her physical support during contractions
  - Clean/swab her vulval area and provide a clean pad as frequently as required
  - Use complementary therapies if she wishes
  - Explore positions for comfort and to assist with the birth—an upright position will aid descent of the fetus and give the woman more control over the process
  - Play music if she wishes
  - Encourage her to use breathing awareness
  - Encourage the involvement of her birth partner.
- *Emotional support*
  - Give verbal and non-verbal encouragement.
  - Appreciate the woman's individuality and needs.
  - Be informative and gain consent for procedures.
  - Be aware of birth plan choices.
  - Communicate and give reassurance.
  - Understand, appreciate, and be tolerant of her vocalizations, behaviour, and expressions during the second stage.
  - Prepare her to welcome the baby into the world.

Directed sustained versus spontaneous physiological pushing

Breath holding, closed glottis, and fixed diaphragm—commonly known as the Valsalva's manoeuvre—is no longer recommended due to its negative effects (☐ see Breathing awareness, p. 246)[1,2]. At the peak of a contraction the utero-placental blood flow ceases—a physiological factor that the fetus can cope with for short periods.

This technique is said to reduce the length of the second stage, however, a technique for pushing infers that something needs to be done in place of the body's own efforts, which undermines the mother's ability and instincts.[1,2,3]

Spontaneous physiological pushing

This allows the woman's body to tell her what to do. If she is left to push spontaneously, she will do so three to five times within a contraction, to coincide with extra surges. The length of pushing may be significantly reduced, but it is more intense and productive if the woman tunes into this natural pattern.[4]

Disadvantages

• It is challenging for the woman to work with her own body and its intense sensations.

Advantages

• All fetal and maternal complications are minimized.
• Spiritual and psychological fulfilment/empowerment.
• Breathing awareness will automatically become easier and therefore assist with coping abilities.
• The woman can save her strength for the active/perineal phase.

1 Bosomworth A, Bettany-Saltikov J (2006). Just take a deep breath... A review to compare the effects of spontaneous versus directed Valsalva pushing in the second stage of labour on maternal and fetal welbeing. *MIDIRS Midwifery Digest* **16**(2), 157–65.

2 Byrom A, Downe S (2005). Second stage of labour: challenging the use of directed pushing. *Midwives* **8**(4), 168–9.

3 Davies L (2006). Maternal pushing: to coach or not to coach. *Practising Midwife* **9**(5), 38–40.

4 Perez-Botella M, Downe S (2006). Stories as evidence: why do midwives still use directed pushing. *British Journal of Midwifery* **14**(10), 596–9.

Care of the perineum

Care of the perineum is an important part of the birthing process, both for the midwife and the mother. Perineal trauma can have far-reaching effects, influencing the woman's physical, emotional, and sexual relationships for the rest of her life. Perineal trauma is associated with:

• Urinary incontinence
• Faecal/flatus incontinence
• Dyspareunia
• Psychosocial factors as a result of the above
• A negative experience of motherhood.

Much of the routine care of the perineum is based on custom and practice; however, recent studies have shown how changes in management can help to enhance perineal integrity and minimize trauma.

Management

• Keeping the perineal area clean and free from faecal contamination is universally recognized.
• Conduct of the second stage of labour and perineal management should be discussed with the woman, to ensure informed choice and consideration of her birth plan.
• There is no evidence to suggest that applying hot flannels and pads to the perineum is beneficial; however, it may provide some temporary comfort for the woman if there are no objections to this practice.
• Antenatal massage of the perineum appears to be advantageous, however, there is no evidence to support massage of the perineum in the second stage of labour.
• Upright positions for birth generally enhance perineal integrity.
• There is no evidence to suggest that guarding the perineum is beneficial as opposed to hands-free management. There is a correlation between hands-free management and fewer episiotomies and third-degree tears.
• Women's participation and confidence to breathe or pant the baby's head out slowly, to gradually stretch the perineum, is beneficial.
• The midwife's rapport and relationship with the woman and her birthing partner during labour is crucial, leading to less intervention in management of the perineum.
• Episiotomy should be reserved for fetal reasons only.

There has been much debate about whether applying pressure on the fetal head to maintain flexion, and the Ritgen manoeuvre to assist extension, are of value. Review of the key physiological principles would suggest that intervention using these techniques interferes with normal birthing mechanisms, by increasing the diameter of the fetal skull, thus inevitably leading to potential perineal trauma rather than preventing it. This is best highlighted diagrammatically: see Fig. 14.2.

Flexion technique

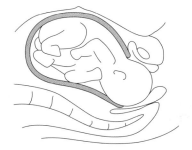

Fig. 14.2a The smallest diameter of the fetal head is maintained by an attitude of flexion. Further flexion applied by the birth attendant changes the position of the head to a larger diameter. This puts unnecessary pressure on the perineum, instead of its important role as a pivotal mechanism. Flexibility of the neck ensures the smallest diameter is maintained throughout the whole of the birth process.

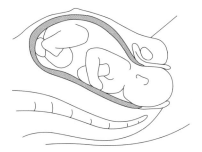

Fig. 14.2b The presenting part is halfway through the 90% curve of the birth canal. Partial extension occurs to maintain the smallest diameter (suboccipito-bregmatic). Extension of the head already occurs before it is visible therefore flexion at this point only maintains a larger diameter. As the birth canal is not straight there is no rationale for this technique.

Ritgen manoeuvre

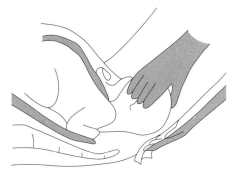

Fig. 14.2c The Ritgen manoeuvre. As the fetal head emerges from the introitus, if over-extension is applied this results in the occipito-frontal diameter presenting – a considerably larger diameter. In an unassisted mechanism the head increasingly extends through the 90% angle so that it is able to utilize the resistance and pivotal force of the perineum and the pubic bone. This maintains the smallest diameter at the vaginal orifice.

Performing an episiotomy

In 1996 the World Health Organization (WHO) recommended an episiotomy rate of less than 10% for normal deliveries. The only real indication for an episiotomy should be if the fetus is compromised in the second stage of labour and birth needs to be facilitated quickly. In rare cases a rigid perineum that is unquestionably obstructing the process of delivery may require episiotomy. Evidence suggests that:[1]

- Protection against sphincter damage is unfounded
- Episiotomy may predispose to third-degree tears
- There is no difference between tears and episiotomies as far as pain and dyspareunia are concerned
- Episiotomy is more likely to cause unnecessary perineal trauma
- There is a risk of healing complications
- Episiotomy is contraindicated for third-degree tears, except in the event of shoulder dystocia, to prevent extensive perineal damage when undertaking internal manoeuvres to release the impacted fetal shoulder.

Awareness of anatomical structures is important, especially the location of the external sphincter muscle, which extends 2.5cm around the anus (see Fig. 14.3). A medio-lateral incision is used, as opposed to the midline incision, which is associated with increased incidence of third-degree tears.

Performing an episiotomy

- Obtain consent after explaining the rationale determining the procedure.
- Prepare the necessary equipment:
  - Sterile swabs
  - Lidocaine 0.5% (10mL) or 1% (5mL)
  - 10mL syringe
  - Gauge 21 needle.
- Clean the skin with antiseptic using aseptic technique.
- Insert the first and second fingers of your gloved hand into the vagina to protect the fetal skull from injury and anaesthetic.
- Episiotomy is usually performed on the right side. Insert the needle via the fourchette and direct it at a 45% angle from the midline for 4–5cm, to ensure a medio-lateral incision (Fig. 14.3).
- Withdraw the piston before infiltrating anaesthetic, to check that the needle is not in a blood vessel. If so, the needle must be withdrawn and repositioned.
- Lidocaine can be injected slowly as the needle is withdrawn. However, it is considered to be more effective if 3–4mL are injected initially and then, before removing the needle, the remaining lidocaine is injected either side of the initial injection, in a fan shape.
- At least 4–5min must be given for the analgesic to be effective prior to incision (Fig. 14.3).
- Use blunt-ended scissors.
- Insert two fingers into the vagina, as before.

- Open the blades of the scissors; insert the blade accessing the vagina flat over the fingers, and then rotate into the cutting position with the outer blade.
- Make a cut of approximately 4cm within the anaesthetized area.
- Cut concisely and deliberately at the height of a contraction, when the perineum is maximally stretched, to minimize bleeding and pain.
- A medio-lateral incision is commonly used or sometimes a 'J' shaped incision. Both methods help to prevent extension of the incision to the anal sphincter.
- Preparation for an imminent delivery is important. It is vital to deliver the head carefully and prevent the shoulders being expelled before restitution has occurred.
- If the delivery is delayed, control bleeding by applying pressure to the episiotomy.

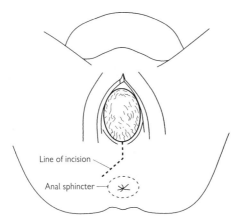

Fig. 14.3 Episiotomy.

1 Carroli G, Belizan J (2006). Episiotomy for vaginal birth (Cochrane review). In: *Cochrane Library*, Issue 3. Chichester: John Wiley and Sons.

Female genital mutilation

Female genital mutilation (FGM), also known as female circumcision, is deeply rooted in the traditions and religion of about 30 countries. In the UK it is most commonly seen amongst immigrants from Somalia, Eritrea, Mali, Sudan, Ethiopia, Sierra Leone, and Nigeria. The practice has been outlawed in the UK, and parents found to be carrying out this practice, or returning to their country of origin for this to be undertaken, are at risk of severe penalties.

Definition

FGM involves a variety of invasive procedures that result in partial or total removal of the external female genitalia and/or other injury to the female genital organs, for cultural or any other non-therapeutic reason.

Classification

- Type 1: excision of the prepuce, with or without excision of part or all of the clitoris.
- Type 2: excision of the prepuce and clitoris, together with partial or total excision of the labia minora.
- Type 3: excision of part or all of the external genitalia and stitching/ narrowing of the vaginal opening (infibulation).
- Type 4: unclassified: includes pricking, piercing, or incision of the clitoris and/or labia; stretching of the clitoris and or labia; cauterization by burning the clitoris and surrounding tissues; scraping of the vaginal orifice or cutting the vagina; introduction of corrosive substances to the vagina to cause bleeding, or herbs placed in the vagina to cause tightening or narrowing of the vagina; any other procedure that falls under the above definition.

Cultural and historical background

- Most parents believe they are doing their best for their daughters and that they are adhering to sound cultural practices.
- A circumcised woman is regarded as spiritually pure and clean. An uncircumcised woman is regarded as shameful and unnatural by society and therefore not fit to marry or have children.
- It is believed she must undergo this procedure in order for her to identify with the everyday hardships of being a woman.
- Religious reasons—some women see it as a religious obligation. There are no references in the Bible or the Koran referring to FGM.
- It is claimed to promote chastity and virginity.
- It negates sexual pleasure.
- It is advocated as improving fertility and preventing maternal and infant mortality. The opposite is true, FGM puts the health of the woman and the baby at great risk during pregnancy and childbirth.
- It is claimed to ensure that a woman is faithful to her husband, thereby preventing promiscuity.
- It is believed to promote cleanliness.
- Parents believe that FGM ensures a good marriage for their daughters.

Prevalence

FGM is commonly performed on girls between the ages of 4 and 10 years, but may also be performed soon after birth, at adolescence, at the time of marriage, or during the first pregnancy. The procedure is usually carried out by a traditional midwife or a woman within the local community. FGM is practised widely on the African continent, with countries such as Somalia and Sudan performing infibulation on 90–98% of girls. The WHO estimates that over 120 million women from 30 different countries have undergone FGM.

Complications

Following FGM, immediate complications are haemorrhage, pain, shock, infection, urine retention, injury to surrounding tissue, ulceration of genital area, and death. Long-term complications include:

- Delayed wound healing, keloid formation, and severe scarring
- Pelvic infection, recurrent urinary tract infection
- Formation of epidermoid cysts and abscess
- Neuromata
- Haematocolpos—vaginal closure leading to scarring can impair the flow of menstrual blood and exacerbate dysmenorrhoea
- Trauma and fears during childbirth
- Painful coitus
- Infertility
- Psychological trauma.

Complications during labour and birth

- Prolonged obstructed labour, due to tough scar tissue formation commonly found in type 3 FGM. Clitoridectomy does not cause obstructed labour.
- Perineal laceration.
- Uterine inertia, due to prolonged labour.
- Fetal distress caused by obstructed labour; may lead to fetal death (a common occurrence in Africa).
- Postpartum wound infections.
- Re-infibulation is commonly practised in Africa but is outlawed in the UK. Where possible, it is important to identify women who may have been subjected to FGM early in pregnancy, by asking sensitive but leading questions. In an area with a high ratio of African residents there may well be a specialist midwife. Reversal of infibulation can be carried out at about 20 weeks to allow for complete healing prior to labour. This will also provide access to the urethra and vaginal orifice during labour. However, some women prefer to have reversal performed during labour, so that the pain of de-infibulation is combined with the pain of labour. Adequate pain relief is crucial so that the woman is not further traumatized by the procedure. With the woman's consent, an anterior midline incision that exposes the urethra and clitoris (which is often buried under scar tissue) is performed during labour. Prompt assessment of suturing requirements following birth should be attended to, and sensitive follow-up care of the woman's physical and psychological welfare should be ongoing.

Recommended reading

Momoh C (ed.) (2005). *Female Genital Mutilation*. Abingdon: Radcliffe Publishing Ltd.

Conduct of normal vaginal delivery

If a woman and her birthing partner have established a good rapport with their midwife, the environment is peaceful and unhurried, there is low lighting and privacy, with good communication and information, then the woman is likely to have a positive and empowering experience of birth.

The woman should be enabled to adopt a position for birth that she feels comfortable with, and should be relaxed enough to verbalize (shouting, grunting, etc.) to relieve tension and anxiety and to prevent breath-holding.

Preparation

- When birth is anticipated, put on protective glasses (in case of blood spillages).
- Wash your hands thoroughly, put on protective wear and gloves, and prepare the necessary equipment. A sterile area for equipment will need to be organized and accessible.
- The immediate birthing area should be prepared, e.g. mattress, birthing chair, etc.
- Prior to the birth, wash the vulva with water/lotion, drape sterile towels around the immediate area, and place a sterile pad over the anus to prevent faecal contamination.
- If the woman is in an upright position, the anal area will need to be kept free from faecal material.

Delivery

- Encourage the woman to work with her contractions as before.
- At crowning, encourage her to breathe gently and/or to pant her baby's head out in a slow and controlled way. This helps to minimize perineal trauma, empowers the mother's experience, and prevents the need for too much hands-on intervention.
- Be ready to prevent sudden delivery of the head. There is no physiological rationale for the application of firm pressure and resistance to maintain flexion, which serves only to increase the diameters of the fetal skull (see Flexion technique, p. 277).
- Encourage the mother, both verbally and by non-verbal communication. This is crucial in helping to maintain her efforts and confidence. Make plenty of eye contact and give her praise, using a quietly spoken and supportive tone throughout.
- The Ritgen manoeuvre is generally not required if the birth is proceeding normally. Grasping the parietal eminences to overextend the head serves only to increase the diameters of the fetal skull (see Care of the perineum, pp. 276–8).
- Checking for the cord around the neck of the baby can cause considerable discomfort for the woman, and opinions are mixed as to whether this procedure is routinely necessary.
  - If the cord is around the neck, it can usually be untangled following delivery.
  - If the cord is very tight, some suggest cutting the cord: two pairs of artery forceps are applied 2.5cm apart and the cord cut between

them, using cord scissors, and then unwound. However, this can often be a difficult procedure and may result in lower Apgar scores.
  • Others suggest that cutting the cord is unnecessary, as the baby will be born through the loops of cord.
• If necessary, remove mucus gently from the baby's nose and mouth.
• The mother may wish to touch or watch the baby's head as it delivers; she may wish to assist with the birth of the trunk.
• Following restitution (after the head is born it realigns itself with the shoulders) observe for external rotation of the head, assist in delivery of the shoulders by placing your hands on either side of the baby's head and applying downwards traction with the next contraction to free the anterior shoulder, and then upwards traction to deliver the posterior shoulder and trunk by lateral flexion.
• If the mother is in an upright position, it may be difficult to see the baby, but be ready to receive the baby's head and body and assist if necessary. Upright positions maximize the diameters of the pelvic outlet and therefore the need for manoeuvres is less likely.
• Place the baby directly on to the mother's abdomen/chest/arms to encourage immediate bonding. Cover the baby and keep him/her warm by maintaining skin-to-skin contact with the mother.
• Note the time of birth.
• Cut the cord after pulsation has ceased, unless there are specific reasons not to.
• Keep contemporaneous records of the labour and birth.

Normal labour: third stage

Care during the third stage of labour

The third stage of labour is potentially hazardous for the woman due to the increased risk of haemorrhage, particularly immediately following delivery of the placenta. Life-threatening haemorrhage occurs in approximately 1 per 1000 births. However, estimates of PPH vary widely—from 4% to 18%.[1]

Definition of primary postpartum haemorrhage

Primary PPH is traditionally defined as the loss of >500mL of blood from the genital tract within the first 24h after the birth. If haemodynamic changes manifest in the newly delivered woman with loss <500mL, this may also be regarded as a primary PPH. Recently a blood loss of 1000mL has been considered as a more realistic definition of primary PPH.

Causes and risk factors associated with primary PPH

History
- Previous PPH or previous retained placenta
- Previous precipitate, prolonged, or traumatic labour
- Previous APH
- Uterine scar
- HIV/AIDS
- Uterine fibroids or other anomalies.

Pregnancy
- High parity
- Multiple pregnancy
- Polyhydramnios
- Coagulation disorders
- Anaemia
- Placenta praevia
- APH
- Pre-eclampsia.

Labour
- Precipitate labour
- Prolonged labour
- Induction of labour or augmentation of labour
- Large doses of narcotics and/or epidural analgesia
- General anaesthesia
- Tocolytic drugs (used to suppress uterine activity in preterm labour)
- Infection—chorioamnionitis
- Ketoacidosis.

Third stage
- Incomplete separation of the placenta
- Full bladder
- Retained cotyledon, placental tissue, or membranes
- Mismanagement of the third stage, disrupting the rhythm of myometrial activity
- Inversion of the uterus.

There are two ways in which the third stage may be managed: either by active management (see Active management of the third stage, p. 292) or by physiological management (see Physiological management of the third stage, p. 290). However, it has been suggested that the third stage should not be managed at all, and that attention to creating the right environment to enhance physiological efficiency is far more important; therefore preventing intervention that is likely to lead to complications.[2]

General care

- You should be proficient with the proposed management of the third stage.
- Note the latest haemoglobin results and blood pressure recordings in pregnancy. Review blood pressure recordings and any complications arising in labour before third stage management is determined.
- Ensure that the woman is fully conversant with, and understands, the process of the third stage and her involvement.
- Maintain positions of comfort and dignity throughout.
- Careful observation of blood loss, and arrange for assistance to be available should abnormal bleeding occur.
- Blood loss >500mL is considered to be significant. Generally, blood loss tends to be underestimated, especially the greater the blood loss.
- Some schools of thought suggest that healthy women can cope with a blood loss of up to 1000mL.[3] However, accurate estimation of blood loss is crucial for both active and physiological management.
- If blood loss is significant, watch the woman's condition carefully, looking for symptoms of shock and observing the lochia and vital signs regularly following or during the third stage.
- Check the placenta and membranes thoroughly following delivery, to ensure there are no abnormalities and that they are complete. Retained products can result in sepsis and secondary PPH. Any suspicion of ragged membranes or missing placental tissue should be recorded in the notes and the information passed on to the receiving midwife taking over the woman's care.
- The woman should be alerted to monitor her lochia and report any abnormally heavy bleeding or clots.

1 Harrison K (1998). Management of postpartum haemorrhage. *Prescriber Update* **16**, 4–9.

2 Odent M (1998). Don't manage the third stage of labour! *Practising Midwife* **1**(9), 31–3.

3 Bose P, Regan F, Paterson-Brown S (2006). Improving the accuracy of estimated blood loss at obstetric haemorrhage using clinical reconstructions. *BJOG International Journal of Obstetrics and Gynaecology* **113**, 919–24.

Physiological management of the third stage

A physiological third stage of labour may be the choice for women who prefer to avoid intervention during childbirth. Placental separation occurs physiologically without resorting to oxytocic drugs, and expulsion of the placenta is achieved by maternal effort The average length of the third stage is 15–60min, although in some cases, provided there are no abnormal signs, it may occasionally last up to 120min. The Bristol trial indicated that there is a higher incidence of PPH with a physiological third stage.[1] However, criticisms of the trial suggest that inexperience in managing the third stage of labour was a serious flaw. More recent studies have found no difference in the incidence of PPH between active and physiological management of the third stage.

Physiology of the third stage

- Detachment of the placenta commences with contractions that deliver the baby's trunk.
- Once the baby is born, the uterus is greatly reduced in size due to the powerful contraction and retraction of the uterine muscles.
- Consequently, the placental site is also greatly reduced. When the placental site is reduced by one-half it becomes puckered and starts to peel away from the uterine wall.
- This is assisted by the tightly compressed and contracted uterus. As a result, fetal blood is pumped into the baby's circulation. Maternal blood is driven back into the spongy layer of the decidua.
- The congested veins are then forced to rupture. The effused blood from the congested veins results in detachment of the placenta. The veins are caused to rupture as the blood in these veins cannot return to the maternal circulation.
- Bleeding is controlled by the presence of 'living ligatures'. Plain muscle fibres of the uterus entangle around the exposed bleeding blood vessel site, preventing further blood loss.
- When separation of the placenta is complete (usually 3–5min), the upper segment of the uterus contracts strongly, forcing the placenta into the lower segment and then the vagina.
- Detachment of the membranes commences in the first stage of labour, when the membranes rupture they are shorn from the internal os. This is then completed in the third stage when the weight of the descending placenta allows them to peel away from the wall of the uterus.

Methods of detachment

Schultze method: approximately 80% of cases detach by this method. The placenta starts to detach from the centre and leads its descent down the vagina. The fetal surface of the placenta therefore appears first at the vulva, with the membranes trailing behind. The retroplacental clot is situated inside the membrane sac. Minimal visible blood loss is the result.

Matthews Duncan method: separation of the placenta commences at the lower edge, which allows the placenta to slide down sideways, exposing the maternal surface. This usually results in increased bleeding due to the slower rate of separation and no retroplacental clot being formed.

Expectant or physiological management of the third stage

It is important that midwives familiarize themselves with the principles and practice of the physiological third stage (as opposed to active management, with which they may have more experience). It is equally important to ensure that consent from the woman has been obtained, and that she understands her role. A physiological third stage is not recommended when the preceding stages have not been conducted physiologically.

Management

- Do not give oxytocic prophylaxis.
- Leave the cord unclamped until completion of the third stage. This practice allows the physiological action of contraction and retraction of the uterus to proceed naturally, and is thought to minimize any delay in separation and to prevent excessive bleeding. Delayed clamping of the cord will cause fetal-maternal transfusion and is therefore not advised for Rh-negative women. Some schools of thought suggest that early clamping of the cord shortens the length of the third stage.
- Ideally, the baby should be put to the breast to suckle, as this ensures the continued release of oxytocin to assist separation and expulsion of the placenta.
- Ensure that the bladder is empty; failure to do this may cause delay in the third stage and possibly predispose to bleeding.
- A 'hands off the abdomen' approach is crucial, as any manipulation of the uterus disturbs the rhythmical coordination of the uterine muscles, and will negate the physiological process.
- Observe vaginal loss to ensure that bleeding is not excessive. A gush of blood indicates the beginning of separation.
- A squatting position is most beneficial to aid expulsion of the placenta as this works with gravity and gives increased intra-abdominal pressure.
- Await the onset of expulsive contractions—this is usually an indication that the placenta has separated and descended into the lower segment. The weight of the placenta causes stimulation and pressure in the vagina, which triggers off expulsive contractions. Often the woman will involuntarily bear down and push the placenta out.
- Advise the woman that expulsive contractions are similar, but often not as strong as the contractions experienced in the second stage, and may easily be missed.
- As the uterus descends, it becomes rounder and smaller, the fundus rises and becomes harder and more mobile.
- The cord lengthens—this is another indication that the placenta has descended into the lower segment and is ready to be expelled.
- If you are sure that the placenta has separated and the woman does not experience contractions, encourage the woman to push down in a similar way to the second stage of labour to expel the placenta.
- Once the placenta is delivered, assist with easing the membranes out of the vagina. Either attach artery forceps or hold the placenta in both hands, rotating it so that the membranes form a rope-like appearance, then use very gentle traction to avoid tearing and retention of membranous material.

Recommended reading

Walsh D (2007). *Evidence-based Care for Normal Labour and Birth*. London: Routledge.

1 Prendiville W, Harding J, Elbourne D, Stirrat G (1988). The Bristol third stage trial: active versus physiological management of third stage of labour. *British Medical Journal* **297**, 1295–300.

Active management of the third stage

The third stage of labour, if managed actively, will usually be a short, passive stage for the woman, lasting no more than 10min, while she will be focused on her baby. However, this is also the most dangerous stage of labour as the risk of haemorrhage is at its greatest. Therefore sound physiological knowledge and the expertise of the midwife is essential to ensure a safe outcome for the woman.

Active management for the third stage has been the routine for many decades; however, in recent years women and midwives have increasingly been returning to a physiological managed third stage. In order for women to be fully informed about their care in the third stage, discuss the options prior to labour, so that they can make an informed, unhurried choice.

Active management is associated with less blood loss, shorter duration, fewer blood transfusions, and less need for therapeutic oxytocics. However, there is some debate that when the effect of oxytocic drugs wears off, women may experience heavier postnatal blood loss than those who had a physiological third stage.[1,2]

Management

- Ensure that the woman is comfortable, whether in the dorsal or an upright position.
- Based on an earlier explanation of the third stage, reinforce what the procedure involves, to encourage the woman's cooperation.
- Maintain a high standard of hygiene and aseptic technique throughout, to prevent contamination and infection.
- An oxytocic drug will have been administered at the birth of the anterior shoulder, intramuscularly into the upper lateral aspect of the thigh. This is usually one ampoule of Syntometrine®, which contains 5IU oxytocin and 0.5mg ergometrine. Oxytocin acts within 2–3min, whereas ergometrine acts within 6–8min, the effects lasting up to 2h.
- Ergometrine is not recommended for women with the following conditions:
  • Hypertension
  • Cardiac disease
  • Following β-agonist infusion, such as salbutamol or ritodrine
  • Raynaud's disease
  • Severe asthma.
In these situations oxytocin 10IU, given intramuscularly, is usually used. Check the local guidelines relating to management of the third stage.
- Ergometrine can cause nausea, vomiting, and hypertension.
- Wait for the signs of separation and descent of the placenta, i.e. the cord lengthening at the vulva, minimal fresh blood loss, and contraction of the uterus. The uterus will change from feeling broad to firm, central, and rounded at the level of the umbilicus.
- Do not manipulate the uterus in any way, in order to avoid overstimulation or incoordinate activity.

- Once you are happy that the uterus is contracted and separation has occurred, deliver the placenta and membranes by controlled cord traction.
- Cover the woman's abdomen with a sterile towel. Place one hand (usually the left) above the level of the symphysis pubis, with the palm facing towards the umbilicus. Apply firm upwards pressure to achieve counter traction and to guard the uterus.
- With the other hand, grasp the cord firmly and wrap it around your index and middle finger. Maintain firm, steady, and consistent traction in a downwards and backwards direction in line with the birth canal to guide the placenta and membranes into the vagina.
- If strong resistance is felt, or you feel that the membranes are breaking, then cease traction and use maternal effort instead.
- The object is to deliver the placenta in one continuous, controlled movement; however, there may need to be pauses in the process until the placenta is visible. Always reinstate your guarding hand before attempting traction after such a pause.
- Once the bulk of placenta is visible, the direction of the traction becomes horizontal and upwards, to follow the contour of the birth canal.
- Once the whole of the placenta has become visible, cup it in both hands to gently ease it out of the vagina without causing damage to the delicate membranes.
- In order to prevent tearing of the membranes, with two hands holding the placenta, help to coax the membranes out of the vagina with an upwards and downwards movement or a twisting action, forming a rope. This action is repeated until the membranes are completely free.
- Collect the placenta and membranes in a sterile receiver placed near the perineum.
- Assess the blood loss as accurately as possible.
- Inspect the perineum for trauma.
- Ensure the comfort and hygiene of the woman by cleaning the immediate perineal area, applying clean sanitary towels, etc.
- Check the placenta and membranes to ensure they are complete. Report any abnormalities to a senior doctor and to the receiving midwife on the postnatal ward.

1 Wickham S (1999). Further thoughts on the third stage. *Practising Midwife* **2**(10), 14–15.

2 Harris T (2001). Changing the focus for the third stage of labour. *British Journal of Midwifery* **9**(1), 7–12.

Assessing and repairing the perineum

Women who require suturing to the perineum following childbirth may well experience confused and turbulent emotions, from exhilaration to tiredness and anxiety. The prospect of the repair may well prove to be daunting and stressful for her. Midwives are increasingly trained and fully supervised to carry out perineal repair as this is now covered in midwifery training. Not only is it important for the midwife to carry out the procedure in a skilful and competent manner, but it is also important to ensure that the woman's experience is not a lonely, undignified, and threatening ordeal. This can be achieved by considering the following:

- The environment
- The comfort and position of the woman
- Presence of supportive carers
- Information and explanation about the procedure
- Consideration of the woman's birth experience
- Thorough assessment of the perineal damage, and referral to obstetrician if necessary
- Satisfactory pain relief.

Midwives involved in perineal repair should be aware of their limitations in suturing more complex trauma. It is not the midwife's responsibility to repair the following, and these should be referred to an obstetrician:

- Third/fourth degree tears
- Extended episiotomy
- Vulval varicosities
- Severe haemorrhoids
- Severe bruising of the perineum or a haematoma
- Labial lacerations
- Vulval warts
- Following previous third degree tear or extensive scar tissue.

Assessing perineal trauma

- Anterior labial tears: there is some debate about the merits of leaving these unsutured. This depends very much on the degree of bleeding. Oozing immediately following childbirth may resolve itself after a short period if a sanitary towel is placed securely between the legs, however, sometimes just one suture may be required to stabilize haemostasis.
- Posterior perineal trauma: spontaneous tears are classified by degrees of trauma relating to the anatomical structures involved.
  - First degree tears: this involves the skin of the fourchette only. This may be left to heal spontaneously or a single suture inserted—discussion with the woman about her options may determine the management.
  - Second degree tear and episiotomy: this involves the skin of the fourchette, the perineum, and perineal body. The superficial muscles affected are the bulbocavernosus and the transverse perineal muscles. Deeper muscle layer trauma may involve the pubococcygeus.

- Third degree tear: in addition to second degree trauma, there is damage to the anal sphincter.
- Fourth degree tear: this describes trauma that involves all of the above structures which extends into the rectal mucosa.

Preparation for perineal repair
- Ensure the woman is in a comfortable position. To minimize the risk of deep vein thrombosis, do not put the woman into the lithotomy position for suturing until all preparations are in hand to commence the procedure.
- Make the environment as comfortable as possible. The mother may like to cuddle and hold her baby throughout the procedure or even breastfeed. Ensure that she is not alone—ideally she should have her partner close by to comfort and distract her.
- Give a full explanation of the trauma, what her options may be and what the procedure involves. Reassure and relieve any anxieties she may have.
- Assess the woman's general and obstetric condition. Ensure that the uterus is well contracted, her lochia is not excessive, and her vital signs are stable.
- Gather requirements for the procedure—a perineal sterile pack, local anaesthesia, suture materials, syringes and needles, sanitary towel, incontinence pad, and sterile gloves.

Procedure
- Ideally the wound should be sutured as soon as possible following birth. A good directional light over the perineum is essential, but dimmed lights otherwise may help to create a more relaxed environment.
- Assist the woman into the lithotomy position to ensure a clear view of the perineum. Other positions of comfort may need to be explored if the woman finds this uncomfortable.
- Prepare the trolley and sterile field.
- The midwife then scrubs to prepare for aseptic technique.
- The wound is cleaned with warm antiseptic solution.
- The woman is draped with sterile towels to ensure a clean sterile field.
- Inspect the perineum to assess damage and whether you can carry out the repair. If there is any doubt an obstetrician or doctor experienced in perineal repair should be called for.
- Analgesia: prior to the procedure adequate analgesia is crucial:
  - Infiltration of the wound with 1% lidocaine—up to 20mL maximum dose within an hour and inclusive of the amount used for infiltration prior to episiotomy.
  - Epidural if *in situ* can be topped up to provide analgesia for the procedure.
  - Additionally the woman may like to use inhalational analgesia to assist if she is anxious.
- Infiltration: the whole of the area to be sutured should be infiltrated.
  - The needle should be inserted into the wound at the fourchette, passing superficially up the vagina; withdraw the plunger to ensure

the needle is not in a blood vessel, then infiltrate as the needle is slowly withdrawn.
- Using the same site of entry pass the needle into the perineal body and infiltrate. The perineal skin is then infiltrated in the same way.
- While waiting for the anaesthesia to take effect, you can check that you have everything ready for the repair and ensure the woman is comfortable and warm.
- Suturing: repair is usually undertaken in three layers, this ensures that the repair is performed in a logical way and nothing is missed (Fig. 15.1). The layers are the vaginal epithelium, the perineal muscle, and the perineal skin. Care should be taken to align the edges of the tissues as accurately as possible throughout the repair, to ensure a neat symmetrical result. Sutures should not be pulled too tight as oedema and bruising to the site will cause pain and slow healing.
  - A taped vaginal tampon should be inserted into the vault of the vagina prior to the procedure to prevent blood oozing from the uterus obscuring the operator's view. The tape of the tampon should be secured to the draped towels with a pair of forceps, so that it is removed following the procedure. On no account should loose cotton wool or gauze be used.
  - Absorbable suture material usually recommended is polyglycolic acid (Dexon), polyglactin 910 (Vicryl) or Vicryl Rapide, dependent on local provision.
  - Vaginal epithelium: identify the apex of the tear/episiotomy and secure the first suture, not going too deep as the rectum is in close proximity. Proceed using a continuous locking stitch, becoming a little deeper nearing the fourchette. Ensure good approximation of the edges and secure with a knot at the fourchette.
  - Perineal muscle: interrupted sutures (Fig. 15.1b) are used to achieve haemostasis and reduce dead space, thus helping to prevent haematoma formation. Identify the torn edges of the muscles and feel with the fingertips to judge the depth of suturing required. The first sutures are put into the deep tissues to bring the perineal body together, more sutures may be placed more superficially to bring the skin edges together (Fig. 15.1c).
  - Perineal skin: the perineal skin edges should be almost together at this stage. Various techniques may be used to aid healing; interrupted transcutaneous sutures, apposing the superficial edges and allowing natural healing and more commonly the use of continuous subcuticular sutures (Fig. 15.1d).
  - There is some debate regarding non-suturing of perineal skin—a large trial found no significant differences between sutured and non-sutured groups of women with regard to short-term pain.[1]
  - Alternatively, a continuous method of suturing may be used for all layers (Fig. 15.1a).
  - On completion of the suturing the tampon should be removed and the vagina inspected to ensure there are no bleeding points. The vagina and introitus should admit two fingers.

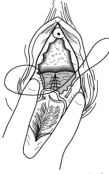
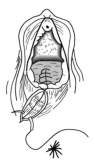

(a) Continuous suture to vaginal wall

(b) 3-4 interrupted sutures to fascia and muscle of perineum

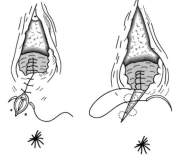

(c) Interrupted sutures to the skin

(d) Subcuticular skin suture

Fig. 15.1 Repairing an episiotomy.

- Cleanse and dry the perineal area. A rectal examination should be performed to exclude the presence of sutures. If sutures are found, medical aid should be sought as the sutures will need to be removed and re-suturing performed as soon as possible.
- Place a sanitary towel over the area, remove the drapes and assist the woman into a more comfortable position.
- Offer analgesia.
- Make sure that all needles and swabs are accounted for.
- Explain to the woman that the sutures will dissolve and not require removal. She may find pieces of suture coming from the vagina.
- Record and sign the perineal repair section in the patient notes.

1 Gordon B, Mackrodt C, Fern E, *et al.* (1998). The Ipswich Childbirth Study: 1. A randomized evaluation of two stage postpartum perineal repair leaving the skin unsutured. *British Journal of Obstetrics and Gynaecology* **105**, 435–40.

Examining the placenta and membranes

Appearance of full-term placenta

The placenta is approximately 18–20cm in diameter, about 2.5cm thick in the centre and progressively thinner towards the outer edges. It is round or oval in shape and weighs approximately one-sixth of the weight of the fetus. It has two surfaces—the fetal and the maternal.

The maternal surface is deep red in colour and attached to the uterine decidua, it is indented with deep grooves, or sulci, into 15–20 lobes, known as cotyledons. The fetal surface lies to one side of the fetus and is attached by the umbilical cord. From the insertion of the cord at the placental site, blood vessels radiate to the periphery, forming subdivisions of the blood vessels that burrow into the substance of the placenta. Each cotyledon has its own branch of the umbilical artery and vein. The surface is covered with the amnion.

Examination

- Examine the placenta and membranes as soon as possible after birth to detect any abnormalities that may have a direct influence on the neonate or provide information about intrapartum events.
- Wear protective clothing and gloves.
- Wash the placenta in running water to remove any clots. Retain the clots to estimate maternal blood loss.
- Hold the placenta firmly by the cord to check that the membranes are complete—there should just be one hole through which the fetus has passed.
- Separate the amnion from the chorion to ensure that both membranes are present.
- Turn the placenta over with the fetal surface resting on the hand, and with the membranes hanging down. Carefully examine the maternal surface to see whether all the lobes are complete, there should be no spaces or ragged areas.
- Note any areas of infarction on the lobes, recognized as firm, fibrous whitish patches. Gritty areas may also be seen.
- Check the edge of the placenta for signs of the blood vessels permeating the membranes, which may be indicative of a succenturiate lobe.
- Occasionally one vessel is seen that tracks its way back into the placenta—this is known as an erratic vessel.
- Examine the umbilical cord carefully, noting its insertion into the placenta; the length, the number of vessels, and any abnormalities.
- Usually the cord is inserted centrally into the placenta and is about 50cm long and 2cm thick, covered in a jelly-like substance known as Wharton's jelly. There should be one large umbilical vein and two umbilical arteries. Occasionally only one artery may be detected, this may be indicative of fetal abnormality and the baby should be examined thoroughly by a paediatrician.

- Measure blood loss as accurately as possible, including the loss that may have soaked into bed linen and pads.
- Record all findings in the maternal notes.

Abnormalities of the placenta and umbilical cord

- *Succenturiate lobe*: a small accessory placenta that has developed away from the main body of the placenta and is attached by blood vessels permeating the membranes. If blood vessels are detected leading to a tear in the membranes at the distal end, this would indicate that the missing cotyledon has been retained in the uterus. Consequently, cautions regarding blood loss and the passage of the products of conception need to be recorded in the woman's notes and explained to the mother. A doctor also needs to be informed of these findings.
- *Bipartite placenta*: the placenta is divided into two distinct lobes.
- *Circumvallate placenta*: the chorion, instead of being attached to the edge of the placenta, forms on the fetal surface, some distance from the edge of the placenta.
- *Placenta accreta*: the placenta is abnormally adherent to the uterine muscle surface, either partially or totally. Although extremely rare, there appears to be increased risk associated with repeated surgical procedures involving the uterus, such as myomectomy, caesarean section, and termination of pregnancy.
- *Infarctions*: these are red, or more commonly white, patches detected on the maternal surface, due to localized death of placental tissue. They may be seen occasionally in most placenta, but when found in substantial amounts they are often associated with pre-eclampsia.
- *Calcification*: small, whitish-grey areas that have a gritty feeling are lime salt deposits. They may be more noticeable in the postmature placenta.
- The umbilical cord may be either too short (causing delay in delivery) or too long, predisposing to prolapse of the cord. Occasionally it may be excessively thin or thick, in either case extra vigilance is required when clamping the cord and observing for haemorrhage.
- Knots in the umbilical cord are caused by fetal movements prior to birth, whereby the fetus is able to slip through a loop of cord. These 'true' knots may cause tightening of the cord during labour, depending on the location of the knot along the length of the cord. 'False' knots are formed by the blood vessels being longer than the cord itself, thus doubling back in the Wharton's jelly, or a similar appearance may occur due to the formation of irregularities and nodes.
- The cord may be inserted into the placenta in an irregular manner instead of centrally:
  - *Eccentric insertion*: the cord is attached to one side of the placenta
  - *Battledore insertion*: the cord is attached to the placental margin
  - *Velamentous insertion*: the vessels of the cord divide and run through the membranes prior to reaching the placenta. This is particularly dangerous if the vulnerable blood vessels lie over the internal os. This condition is known as *vasa praevia* and is extremely rare, but can be a cause of severe fetal hypoxia or fetal death should one of the blood vessels rupture.

Chapter 16

Immediate care of the newborn

Apgar score

Failure of the baby to establish respiration at birth may be due to:
- Obstruction due to mucus, blood, liquor, or meconium
- Analgesics given during labour—pethidine, diamorphine, and general anaesthesia
- Tentorial tears, which cause pressure on the fetal cerebellum and medulla, where the respiratory centre is sited
- Congenital abnormalities, such as choanal atresia, hypoplastic lung, diaphragmatic hernia, and anencephaly
- Prematurity—lack of surfactant, intrauterine hypoxia, immature respiratory centre, and associated muscle structures
- Severe intrauterine infections, such as pneumonia
- A method of observing the baby's responses at birth and 5min later, the Apgar score (Table 16.1), uses five vital signs to indicate the necessity for resuscitation: respiratory effort; heart rate; colour; muscle tone, and response to stimuli.
- Each sign is given a score of 2, 1, or 0 and then totalled.

Table 16.1 Calculating the Apgar score

Respiratory effort	Absent/no attempt to breathe (0)	Slow/weak attempts to breathe (1)	Spontaneous breathing/crying (2)
Heart rate	Absent/weak (0)	Slow <100 (1)	>100 (2)
Colour	Blue/pale/grey (0)	Body pink, extremities blue (1)	Completely pink (2)
Muscle tone	Limp/pupils dilated (0)	Partial flexion of extremities (1)	Active/good tone (2)
Reflex irritability	No response (0)	Grimace (1)	Crying/cough (2)

- A score of 8–10 indicates a baby in good condition, a score of 4–7 represents mild/moderate asphyxia, modest resuscitative measures are usually all that is required. Although initially there may be substantial cyanosis, often babies will recover spontaneously or only require tactile stimulation and light oxygen around the face and mouth via a face mask. Care should be taken not to be over-zealous with intervention in this middle group as this may worsen the situation rather than resolve it. A score of 1–3 represents severe asphyxia, requiring urgent resuscitation. 📖 See Neonatal resuscitation, p. 454.

Examination of the newborn

Shortly after birth, examine the baby carefully to check for obvious external abnormalities. Follow a logical sequence from head to toe and perform the examination in front of the parents, so you can provide explanations as you proceed.

Throughout the examination the baby should be naked, in warm surroundings with a good light, so that you can clearly see the baby.

Procedure

- Wash hands thoroughly prior to examination to prevent infection.
- Note any skin blemishes or abrasions, whether any vernix caseosa (white greasy substance) is present on the skin or lanugo (fine downy hair), normally only found abundantly in premature babies.
- Throughout the examination, observe and note the baby's overall muscle tone, movements, and symmetry.
- Colour and respirations: the term baby should be pink with slightly less colour in the hands and feet, which may not pink up for several hours following birth. If one or both nostrils are blocked with mucus, this may result in cyanosis and difficulties with breathing. The term baby should be breathing regularly, with no gasping or chest recession.
- Head: note the size, shape, and symmetry. Sometimes the head may be distorted by moulding or trauma caused during birth:
  - *Caput succedaneum*—this a soft, spongy oedema caused by pressure, which is present at birth and usually disappears within 24h.
  - *Cephalhaematoma*—this is caused by trauma and tends to appear and to get larger following birth. Occasionally there may be a double haematoma on either side of the head. This may take 4–6 weeks to resolve; no treatment is necessary. Examine the formation, width, and tension of the sutures and fontanelles on the skull. A wide anterior fontanelle may be indicative of hydrocephalus or immaturity. An extra fontanelle between the anterior and posterior fontanelles may indicate Down's syndrome.
- Check the face and neck for the following:
  - Eyes: symmetry, that both eyeballs are present with a clear lens. Oedema or bruising that may have occurred during birth, and haemorrhage under the conjunctiva can look alarming, but disappear quickly and are not significant. The spacing between the eyes is usually up to 3cm. The presence of wide, slanting epicanthic folds and white spots on the iris may be associated with Down's syndrome.
  - Ears: symmetry, low-set ears may be associated with various syndromes. Accessory skin tags in front of the ears may be present and should be noted.
  - Mouth: the mouth should be opened and the palate inspected with a finger. The hard palate should be arched, intact, and the uvula in a central position. At the junction of the hard and soft palate there may be small white spots known as Epstein's pearls. Occasionally teeth may be present, which are usually loose, normally these are extracted to prevent inhalation. Tongue-tie may be observed where

the frenulum seems to anchor the tongue to the floor of the mouth. This rarely causes major problems, but may cause difficulties with latching onto the breast for feeding.

- Capillary naevi: small, pink marks may be observed on the upper eyelids, midline of the forehead, the upper lip, and the nape of the neck. These are common and fade over a period of months. Capillary naevi found elsewhere may be extensive, such as port wine stain.
- Neck: observation and inspection of the neck area is important to exclude webbing, a short neck, a large fold of skin at the back of the neck, and any swellings.

- Chest: observe breathing and symmetry of the chest wall. Spacing and positioning of the nipples and any accessory nipples present.
- Abdomen: the shape of the abdomen should be rounded, any obvious variations should be noted such as: a scaphoid or boat-shaped abdomen or swelling. The state of the cord should be observed, ensuring that it securely clamped. The cord should have three vessels and there should be no swelling or protrusions at the base. Absence of a vessel should be brought to the paediatrician's notice immediately, as this may indicate cardiac or renal abnormalities.
- Limbs and digits: count carefully and open the hands fully to expose any accessory digits, webbing, or trauma. The axillae, elbows, groins, and popliteal spaces also need to be inspected. The limbs should be inspected for equal length and observed for normal movement. The feet and ankles should be inspected for talipes.
- External genitalia: in boys, observe the position of the urethral orifice, both testes should be situated in the scrotum. The foreskin should not be retracted as this is still adherent to the glans. Any obvious swelling in the inguinal area should be noted. In girls, gently inspect the labia— the urethral and vaginal orifices should be evident and a thick, white discharge may be present. Refer any discrepancy about the sex of the baby to the paediatrician promptly.
- Back and spine: turning the baby over into the prone position, palpate and observe the back for any unevenness, swellings, dimples, or hairy patches that may be associated with an occult spinal abnormality. A baby from Asian or African ancestry may have a bruised appearance over the sacral area, this is normal and is referred to as the Mongolian blue spot. The presence and position of the anus can be observed. It is also important to record in the notes whether the baby passes meconium at birth or shortly after, to confirm patency of the anus.
- Hips: Ortolani or Barlow's test, or possibly a modification of the two, is performed routinely to check for dysplasia of the hips. Depending on local policy, this will be carried out by the midwife or the paediatrician. Reference to local guidelines and any additional training required should be done prior to undertaking this procedure. If the paediatrician performs the test within the first day of birth, there is no reason to do it at the initial examination.
- Measurements: the head circumference and length may be recorded. However, different units may have differing policies. Unless calibrated equipment is available, measuring the crown to heel length is grossly

inaccurate. If a calibrated device is used, it is essential that the baby's legs are fully extended; this may require two people to assist to ensure accuracy. Measurement of the head circumference may be deferred to the third day, by which time any swelling will have subsided. A measuring tape is used to encircle the head at the occipital protuberance and the supra-orbital ridges.

- Record the baby's temperature.
- Record your findings in the baby's notes. Communicate any abnormalities to the paediatrician or GP, and pass the information on to the midwife taking over the mother's care on the postnatal ward. Inform the parents if a paediatrician needs to be notified and give the reasons why.

Immediate care of the newborn

The midwife should be familiar with the transitional requirements of adaptation to external uterine life, so that she can make appropriate preparations for the newborn's arrival.

• The birthing room, whether at home or hospital, should be warm, ideally 21–25°C. Switch off fans and draw curtains to reduce heat loss within the environment.
• As the baby's head is born, wipe excess mucus from his/her mouth.
• Touching the nasal nares may stimulate reflex inhalation of mucus and debris into the trachea and is not recommended.
• Following the birth of the trunk, lift the baby on to the mother's abdomen or chest, unless this has been declined by the mother.
• Most babies will start to breathe and maintain a clear airway without intervention.
• Aggressive and deep suction is not recommended. When suction is required, use a mucus extractor or a soft suction catheter. It is important to aspirate the oropharynx first before aspirating the nasopharynx, to prevent mucus being drawn down the trachea when the baby gasps due to suction stimulation of the nasal passages.
• Cut the cord approximately 2–8cm from the baby's umbilicus, between two cord clamps. Once the cord is clamped securely to prevent blood loss, cut the cord between the two clamps. Placing a gauze swab over the cord while cutting it will prevent blood spray over the delivery area.

Identification of the newborn is important if the baby is born within a maternity unit; however, a home birth does not require labelling, unless the baby is a twin. Individual units will have their own policy on this; however, basic principles apply:

• Apply name bands immediately following birth, in some units this may be before the cord is cut
• Usually two bands are applied—most commonly to both ankles
• Write the name bands legibly, clearly identifying the family surname, the time and date of birth, and the baby's gender. If gender is in any doubt, explain to the parents that you need to seek further help on this matter
• The mother or father should confirm that the information is correct before applying the name bands
• Ensure that both bands are not too tight nor too loose, but fixed securely and not causing trauma to the baby's skin
• Check the bands daily and replace them if they become loose or fall off while the baby is in the hospital.

Preventing heat loss in the time immediately following birth is crucial. The baby has an immature heat regulatory system, therefore provide a warm environment, as above.

• Reduce heat loss by drying the baby at delivery. Wet towels need to be replaced with warm, pre-heated towels to prevent further heat loss.
• Skin-to-skin contact with the mother helps to reduce heat loss if the remaining exposed skin of the baby is covered.
• Cover the baby's head, as substantial heat is lost through the head.

- Loose clothing and comfortable swaddling with blankets will help to conserve body heat.
- Some units may be provided with overhead heaters in the labour rooms. Care with overheating should be acknowledged. Hot water bottles used to pre-warm the cot at a home birth should be used with caution.
- Routine bathing of the baby following birth is not necessary unless the baby is overly soiled from the birth process or there is risk of contamination. Deferring non-urgent procedures such as bathing helps to maintain thermoregulation.
- Observe the baby regularly for colour and skin temperature, to ensure that hypothermia is not present. Record the body temperature following birth.

The baby may require a dose of vitamin K, given as prophylaxis against bleeding disorders. This should have been discussed thoroughly with the woman prior to birth, so that she could make an informed choice regarding the risks/benefits. Depending on local policy, this may be given orally or by intramuscular injection.

The period immediately following birth should allow some time for the parents and the baby to communicate and develop the important relationship and rapport necessary for the baby's well-being. Very often the baby is very alert following birth (unless drugs used in labour have blurred this response), resulting in an active three-way process of communication between the mother, father, and baby.

Skin-to-skin

All mothers should be encouraged to hold their naked baby against their skin in a calm and unhurried environment immediately following birth, regardless of their feeding intention. Mothers should be given the opportunity prior to birth to discuss how this can be acceptably achieved. Cultural influences need to be considered within this discussion, as they may make implementation of skin-to-skin unacceptable.

Newborn babies find their mother's breast partly by smell, and this instinctive process can be interfered with by clothing, wrapping in hospital towels, and separation, therefore these should be avoided whenever possible, 🕮 see Management of breastfeeding, p 662.

Benefits of skin-to-skin contact

- Babies gradually become more active, begin to root, and are at least three times more likely to suckle successfully.
- Babies demonstrate less distressed behaviour and cry less than those separated from their mothers, for example during suturing.
- Increased nurturing behaviour has been seen in mothers whose babies have touched their nipples and areolae within the first half hour of birth. Mothers planning to bottle feed could still enjoy and benefit from this instinctive interaction.
- The likelihood of PPH could be reduced as early contact and suckling stimulates the uterus to contract.
- Babies are much more likely to be breastfed for longer when uninterrupted skin-to-skin contact has occurred at birth.
- Mothers will feel higher levels of satisfaction with motherhood and have more positive feelings overall if they have been able to enjoy the first hour after birth without interruption.

Physiological effects on the baby

- Skin-to-skin contact is an effective measure against hypothermia and hypoglycaemia.
- The blood chemistry of babies who have been acidotic or had a period of 'fetal distress' rectifies itself more quickly when skin-to-skin contact has occurred.
- Skin-to-skin contact is particularly important for babies who have had a traumatic birth, required resuscitation, and who need to be warmed. It should be initiated as soon as possible.

Routine care practices which interfere with this process should be reconsidered and abandoned unless proven to be of benefit to the infant or mother in the circumstances in which they are initiated.

❶ Hospital routine should not take priority over the needs of the mother and child.

Part 3

Complicated labour

Management of malpositions and malpresentations

Occipito-posterior position

These are cephalic presentations where the occiput is directed towards the right or left sacro-iliac joint—right occipito-posterior (ROP) and left occipito-posterior (LOP). These positions are the most common of all causes of mechanical difficulty in labour.

Causes
- No definite cause has been established but on occasion it may be linked to abnormal shape of the maternal pelvis.
- There is a belief that maternal posture and lack of physical activity during pregnancy may be a predisposing factor, but this is not evidence based.
- Frequently the fetus has an attitude of deficient flexion of the head and spine.
- The occipito-posterior positions are the most common reason for non-engagement of the fetal head at term in the primigravida.
- Ultrasound scan may reveal an anteriorly placed placenta.

Diagnosis

Abdominal examination
- On inspection the abdomen is flattened below the level of the umbilicus.
- On palpation of the abdomen, the head is high and deflexed, limbs are felt on both sides of the midline. The back may be felt with difficulty laterally or may not be palpable.
- On auscultation of the fetal heart sounds are audible in the flank, over the fetal back; they are also easily heard in the midline because of the proximity of the fetal chest to the maternal abdominal wall.

Clinical features during labour
- Continuous backache.
- Slow progress.
- Irregularly spaced contractions which tend to couple together.
- More frequent incidence of non-reassuring FHR patterns in labour.
- Early spontaneous rupture of the membranes.
- Slow descent of the fetal head.
- Increased rectal pressure towards the end of the first stage of labour resulting in an urge to push prior to full dilatation of the os uteri.

Vaginal examination
- The degree of flexion of the head can be assessed during labour.
- The anterior fontanelle lies centrally or anteriorly.
- The posterior fontanelle may be out of reach.
- Caput and moulding are common
- When the head is deflexed the occipito-frontal diameter of 11.5cm presents.
- The presenting part is poorly applied to the cervix.
- The cervix may become oedematous as labour progresses.
- The head does not engage or descend easily, with risk of the following consequences.

Consequences
- Prolonged labour
- Delay in the second stage of labour

- Greater risk of instrumental delivery
- Difficult or traumatic delivery
- Infection
- Possible fetal hypoxia
- Intracranial haemorrhage.

Outcomes

Long rotation of the occiput

- In two-thirds of cases, following engagement the head flexes.
- When the occiput meets the resistance of the pelvic floor it makes a long rotation forwards through three-eighths of a circle.
- The fetus is then born in the occcipito-anterior position.

Deflexed head

In one-third of cases, flexion of the head remains deficient and the mechanism of internal rotation is affected by the following:

- *Deep transverse arrest*: an attempt at long rotation fails, the head being arrested with its long diameter between the ischial spines. Instrumental rotation with forceps or ventouse is required to complete the delivery. Alternatively an LSCS may be performed.
- *Persistent occipito-posterior*: the sinciput lying lower than the occiput is rotated one-eighth of a circle towards the symphysis pubis and the occiput turns to the hollow of the sacrum. Delay in the second stage occurs, but with good contractions the head advances, the root of the nose escapes under the pubic arch and the head is born in the face-to-pubes position. When contractions are less effective, no advance occurs and instrumental delivery is required.

Midwifery care and management

- The first stage is long and tedious, and often accompanied by severe backache. Give continuous explanation, empathy, and support.
- Mobility and an upright position encourage rotation and descent.
- All fours or squatting may assist rotation of the head.
- Maternal comfort, hydration, and prevention of infection are important.
- Encourage the woman to empty the bladder regularly, as a full bladder may add to discomfort and delay progress.
- Deal promptly once delay and fetal and/or maternal distress are recognized. Avoid language which may demoralize the woman, e.g. 'failure to progress'.
- Pain relief requirements may be increased.
- Consider the use of epidural analgesia carefully, as its effects may contribute to poor flexion of the fetus, lack of descent, and failure of the rotational mechanism.
- However, if an instrumental delivery is anticipated then epidural analgesia is the preferred method of pain relief.
- The second stage is characterized by considerable dilation of the anus, while the fetal head may not be visible.
- The squatting position may increase the sagittal diameter of the pelvic outlet, which may aid delivery.
- Perineal trauma is common. Look for signs of central rupture.
- Occasionally episiotomy may be needed to expedite the delivery.

Face presentation

When the attitude of the head is one of complete extension, the occiput of the fetus will be in contact with its spine and the face will present. Most cases develop in labour from occipito-posterior positions (secondary face presentation). Rarely, face presentation is apparent before labour and may be associated with congenital abnormality (primary face presentation).

Causes
- The uterus is tilted sideways (anterior obliquity)
- Contracted pelvis
- Tight or entangled cord
- Polyhydramnios
- Congenital abnormality (e.g. anencephaly)
- Multiple pregnancy.

Diagnosis
- Antenatal diagnosis is unlikely as the presentation usually develops in labour.
- On palpation: if the mentum is anterior, the presentation may not be detected. If the mentum is posterior, a deep groove may be felt between the occiput and the fetal back.
- On vaginal examination:
  - The presenting part is high and irregular
  - The orbital ridges, eyes, nose, and mouth are palpable
  - There may be confusion between the mouth and anus; differential signs are: open, hard gums, ridged palate, and the fetus may suck the examining finger
  - To determine the position, the mentum is located
  - Vaginal examinations should be undertaken with care so as not to injure or infect the eyes.

Course and outcomes of labour
- Prolonged labour
- With a mentoanterior position: spontaneous delivery.
- With a mentoposterior position: following rotation of the mentum to the anterior, a spontaneous delivery is possible.
- Persistent mentoposterior: the chin is in the hollow of the sacrum, so no further mechanism takes place. Instrumental assisted birth or LSCS is the outcome.

Management of labour and delivery
- Labour is often prolonged, the presenting part is ill fitting, so there is slow progress.
- Maternal comfort and support are important.
- Communicate and empathize, as the woman may become discouraged and anxious about her abilities.
- Prior to delivery explain the possible facial bruising to the parents
- Recognize delay or complications at an early stage.
- Avoid the use of a scalp electrode.
- Avoid the use of IV oxytocin.

- Birth may be facilitated by supporting the extended fetal position and applying gentle pressure on the sinciput until the mentum escapes.
- An episiotomy may be indicated, before the occiput sweeps the perineum.

Complications

- Obstructed labour, as the face is resistant to moulding
- Early rupture of the membranes
- Cord prolapse
- Facial bruising and oedema
- Cerebral haemorrhage
- Perineal lacerations and perineal trauma.

Brow presentation

When the attitude of the head is one of partial extension, the frontal bone presents. Brow presentation is less common than face presentation, occurring once in about 1000 births. The causes are the same as those for face presentation.

Diagnosis
- On abdominal palpation the presenting part is high and appears unduly large. A groove may be felt between the occiput and the back.
- On vaginal examination there may be difficulty in reaching the presenting part.
- If the brow is detected, the anterior fontanelle may be felt to one side with the orbital ridges or root of the nose felt on the other side.
- The presenting diameter is the mentovertical—13.5cm.

Management
- The midwife should call the obstetrician.
- Vaginal birth is rare.
- Usually LSCS for obstructed labour.
- Occasionally may convert to a face presentation.
- Complications are the same as those of face presentation.

Shoulder presentation

A non-longitudinal lie may be transverse or oblique, both can result in a shoulder presentation if not corrected.

Causes
- Laxity of uterine and abdominal muscles
- Placenta praevia
- Multiple pregnancy
- Polyhydramnios
- Uterine abnormality
- Contracted pelvis
- Uterine fibroid.

Diagnosis
- A transverse lie is usually detected in pregnancy by the appearance of the shape of the abdomen: there is a bulge on each side of the abdomen and the fundus appears very low.
- On palpation the head and the breech lie in opposite iliac fossae.
- There is no presenting part descending into the pelvis.
- Ultrasound may be used to confirm the condition and detect any fetal abnormality.

Management
- External version may be attempted, followed by induction of labour if successful.
- Monitor labour closely by EFM and diligent observation of the maternal condition.
- Providing normal progress in labour continues, the membranes may be ruptured once the fetal head enters the pelvis.
- Detect shoulder presentation by abdominal palpation and report this immediately to a doctor.
- Carry out vaginal examination (if placenta praevia has been previously excluded).
- LSCS may be the mode of delivery if the lie is persistently oblique or transverse, if there are any complications, or if there is a poor obstetric history.
- In the case of a second twin in the transverse position, correct the lie immediately by external version, while rupturing the membranes to hasten the birth and maintain the longitudinal lie.

Chapter 18

High-risk labour

Principles of care for high-risk labour

Definition

A 'high-risk' pregnancy is one in which the mother, fetus, or newborn is, or will be, at an increased risk of morbidity or mortality before, during, or after delivery.

On admission to the labour ward each antenatal patient will have been assessed to determine any risk factors. A high-risk or complicated pregnancy usually falls into one or more of the following categories:[1]

- Antepartum, intrapartum, or postpartum complication arising in a previous pregnancy, for example:
  - Stillbirth or neonatal death, subfertility
  - Caesarean section, any uterine scar, i.e. myomectomy, hysterotomy
  - Shoulder dystocia
  - PPH
  - Severe hypertension or eclampsia
  - Thromboembolism
  - Bowel or bladder surgery.
- Antepartum, intrapartum, or postpartum complication arising in the current pregnancy, for example:

Antepartum:

- Suspected small for gestational age fetus
- Woman suspected of being at risk of cephalopelvic disproportion
- Oligohydramnios, polyhydramnios
- APH
- Placenta praevia
- Multiple pregnancy
- Rh or other red cell antibodies
- Pregnancy-induced hypertension/pre-eclampsia
- Anaemia—haemoglobin less than 9g/dL
- Liver disease, e.g. cholestasis of pregnancy.

Intrapartum:

- Preterm labour (<37 completed weeks)
- Preterm rupture of membranes (<37 completed weeks)
- Post-term labour (>42 completed weeks)
- Malpresentation, e.g. breech presentation or transverse lie.
- Maternal pyrexia (greater than 38°C)
- Known GBS positive
- Intrapartum haemorrhage
- Meconium-stained liquor
- Induced labour
- Administration of oxytocin infusion to augment labour
- Regional analgesia (epidural or combined spinal-epidural)
- Slow progress in first or second stages of labour
- Suspicious FHR on auscultation
- Abnormal fetal heart pattern
- Planned home delivery admitted to hospital
- Unbooked women or transfers from other hospitals.

Always inform the consultant on call if any of the following are anticipated:
- Emergency ceasarean section
- Instrumental delivery in obstetric theatre
- Multiple birth
- Vaginal breech delivery.

Postpartum:
- PPH
- Third- and fourth-degree tear
- Postpartum severe pre-eclampsia.

The woman has a chronic medical disorder; for example any of the following:
- Diabetes
- Neurological, e.g. epilepsy, multiple sclerosis, myasthenia gravis
- Connective tissue disorder, e.g. systemic lupus erythematosus
- Cardiac disease
- Renal disease
- Thyroid, parathyroid, pituitary, or adrenal disease
- Respiratory disease (other than mild asthma)
- Coagulation disorder/thrombophilia
- Inflammatory bowel disease.

Ensure that all patients defined as high risk:
- Are treated sensitively, recognizing that women experiencing complications in labour may be extremely stressed and anxious, or have a different interpretation of their pregnancy than the clinically defined view. Give these patients:
  - Full, unbiased explanations
  - The chance to ask questions
  - Adequate support
  - Freedom to make choices in care
- Receive consultant-led care on admission to the labour ward or are transferred from midwifery-led care to consultant care when the problem arises.
- Are seen by a registrar as soon as they attend the hospital or the complication arises.
- Have a birth plan, devised in the antenatal clinic in consultation with a senior doctor, documented in the case notes. Review the notes to find plans for labour and delivery. Discuss the plan with the woman to ensure that it is up to date.
- Are monitored continuously for electronic FHR in labour (unless defined as high risk due to a previous postnatal complication, e.g. third-degree tear). Some instances of referral for high-risk care may require the midwife to inform the hospital clinical risk manager.

1 The Practice Development Team (2010). *Jessop Wing Labour Ward Guidelines 2009–2010.* Sheffield: Sheffield Teaching Hospitals NHS Trust.

Trial of labour for vaginal birth following previous caesarean (or other uterine scar)

A woman may request VBAC because:

- She wishes to avoid the stress of abdominal surgery and a longer hospital stay and recovery
- Vaginal deliveries have less risk of infection or haemorrhage
- She would like a satisfying experience of birth.

It is the responsibility of the obstetrician to ensure that a plan for delivery is made antenatally. However, the midwife should be aware of the risks and benefits of VBAC so that she/he can support the family in their choice of care.

- Most women who opt for VBAC do deliver vaginally.[1,2]
- Rare complications can occur—uterine rupture is increased with VBAC: 1:10 000 (repeat caesarean), 50:10 000 (VBAC).[1]
- Intrapartum fetal death is rare, about the same risk for a primigravida, but increased compared to planned repeat caesarean (1:10 000).[1]
- If the trial of labour includes induction there is a further increased risk of uterine rupture, especially if prostaglandins are used.

Because of these risks precautions are recommended:

- Admission to a regional unit with access to emergency caesarean and blood transfusion should this be required
- Continuous EFM during labour
- Careful use of prostaglandins for induction.

  However, a woman has the right to choose home birth or water birth after caesarean section and needs accurate information to make a choice appropriate for her needs. During the antenatal period the supervisor of midwives should be involved: discussion, planning, and documentation are paramount.

  When admitting a woman anticipating VBAC to the delivery suite:

- Recognize the psychological distress that may have been caused by a previous long labour and emergency caesarean. Give clear explanations, positive support, and discuss in detail the plans for the birth.
- Admit as for 'high risk' care:
  - Inform the woman's consultant obstetrician
  - Have a management plan documented in the hospital notes
  - Be aware of signs of uterine rupture (□ see Uterine rupture, p. 398).
- Obtain consent from the woman to monitor the fetal heart continuously in established labour, ensuring the woman's comfort and being flexible about maternal position. Review for variable and late decelerations and bradycardia.
- Site IV access, take and dispatch blood samples from the mother for group and save (G&S) and FBC.
- Monitor maternal blood pressure and pulse half hourly in established labour.
- In consultation with the anaesthetist and the woman, discuss what food and drink would be acceptable in labour. Total fasting is not

now recommended under normal circumstances. It can lead to poor progress.[3]

- Support the woman in her choice of pain relief. Epidural anaesthesia is recommended by some obstetricians in case caesarean is required, but it could mask severe pain or may have side-effects that could make vaginal birth less likely.
- Give antacids regularly if prescribed. These encourage reduced acidity and improved emptying of stomach contents, which may reduce risks to the mother if a caesarean is required.
- Discuss any augmentation with the obstetrician. Oxytocin and artificial rupture of the membranes (ARM) may be indicated when the progress of labour appears slow. Monitor carefully the strength, frequency, and length of the uterine contractions so that hyperstimulation may be avoided.
- Support the woman during the second and third stages of labour according to her birth plan. The third stage may be conducted physiologically.
- Be aware that a rare complication of pregnancy following caesarean is placenta accreta (see Placenta accreta, p. 389).
- Keep the obstetrician informed of progress throughout, document key decisions, and care given.

1 National Institute for Health and Clinical Excellence (2004). Caesarean section. Clinical guideline 13. London: NICE. Available at: www.nice.org.uk/cg13.

2 Enkin M (2000). Labour and birth after previous caesarean. In: Enkin M, Keirse M, Neilson J, et al. (eds). *A Guide to Effective Care in Pregnancy and Childbirth*, 3rd edn. Oxford: Oxford University Press, p. 267.

3 Johnson C, Keirse M, Enkin M, et al. (2000). Hospital practices—nutrition and hydration in labor. In: Enkin M, Keirse M, Neilson J, et al. (eds). *A Guide to Effective Care in Pregnancy and Childbirth*, 3rd edn. Oxford: Oxford University Press, pp. 255–66.

Obstructed labour

If progress in labour is limited in the first stage (i.e. no increase in cervical dilatation in 3–4h) consider the following:
- The woman is not in established labour: proceed as for normal labour
- Labour may be prolonged by psychological stress, support is paramount
- The uterine contractions are not effective: the woman may benefit from oxytocin augmentation (☐ see Intravenous oxytocin, p. 368). Never arrange to use oxytocin to augment labour without gaining the consent of the woman and the obstetric registrar
- The labour is obstructed: there is no advance of the presenting part in the presence of strong contractions.

Causes
- Obstruction at the pelvic brim may be apparent if the fetus is large in relation to maternal size. Contracted pelvis or previous pelvic injury could be a factor.
- Obstruction at the outlet may occur, for example, when deep transverse arrest complicates the second stage. A fetus in the occipito-posterior position may occasionally be unable to rotate and becomes wedged at the level of the ischial spines.
- Obstruction may occasionally occur as a result of:
  - Fetal abnormalities, e.g. the hydrocephalic fetus
  - Fetal malposition
  - Fetal malpresentation—shoulder or brow presentation
  - Persistent mentoposterior position
  - Rarely, locked twins
  - Rarely, fibroids or tumour.

Prevention
- Refer to the consultant obstetrician:
  - All women with suspected malpresentation
  - Some units require referral of primigravidae with non-engagement of the fetal head at term.
- Be alert to a history of previous prolonged labour or difficult delivery.
- Monitor labour carefully to detect a slow/no descent of the presenting head.

Signs of obstructed labour
In the first stage:
- On abdominal palpation, assess for failure of the presenting part to engage
- The cervix dilates slowly
- The presenting part remains loosely applied to the cervix
- The forewaters may rupture early or form a loose bag before the presenting part.
  In later first or second stage (late signs of obstruction):
- Maternal pyrexia and rapid pulse
- Maternal pain and anxiety

- Dehydration and poor urine output, ketotic, sometimes bloodstained urine
- Non-reassuring fetal heart recording
- Tonic contractions
- Rarely the retraction ring may be seen abdominally and marks the junction between the upper and stretched lower segment (Bandl's ring)
- On vaginal examination the vagina feels hot and dry, the presenting part is high and caput succedaneum and/or moulding are present on fetal skull.

Management

- Help to relieve anxiety by giving information and explanation.
- The obstetric registrar must be contacted if:
  - There is no progress in the first stage of labour despite the administration of intravenous oxytocin
  - There is no progress in descent in the second stage of labour.
- Take FBC and G&S in case of need at delivery.
- An IV infusion will correct dehydration and prepare for operative delivery.
- When the woman is pyrexial (temperature 38°C) the obstetrician will request antibiotic therapy.
- Under instruction from the registrar, prepare the woman for emergency caesarean section (☐ see Emergency LSCS, p. 379).
- The woman may be transferred to obstetric theatre for trial of instrumental delivery. If this is unsuccessful, a caesarean section can be performed immediately.
- Ensure that neonatal resuscitation facilities and personnel are available at delivery.

Complications

Maternal
- Infection
- Trauma to the bladder due to pressure from the fetal head, or bruising during forceps delivery
- Severe neglect may cause rupture of the uterus, haemorrhage, morbidity, and mortality.

Fetal
- Asphyxia
- Trauma at delivery
- Infection
- Meconium aspiration.
All of the above may lead to morbidity, stillbirth, neonatal death.

Delivery care for twins and other multiple births

Twin and multiple pregnancies carry a higher risk of antenatal complications. This is especially true of monochorionic twins, due to:
- Unequal growth
- Polyhydramnios
- Fetal abnormalities
- Intrauterine death of one or both twins
- Spontaneous abortion
- Pre-eclampsia
- Preterm labour.

- There is a higher risk of complications during labour, due to:
  - Malpresentation of either twin
  - Asphyxia
  - PPH.
- As a result, the following intervention may be necessary:
  - Intrauterine manipulation
  - Episiotomy and instrumental delivery
  - Caesarean section for one or both twins.

These factors will affect the mode of delivery. Caesarean section is usual:
- If there is only one amniotic sac
- For multiple births (triplets and more).

A plan for delivery will be made antenatally in discussion with the parents and obstetric consultant.

Management of labour

- When the first twin is cephalic and no other complications are present, expect to deliver the babies vaginally.
- If a vaginal delivery is anticipated, encourage the woman to telephone and attend the delivery suite as soon as possible after the onset of labour, especially if she is multiparous, since labour may progress rapidly.
- On admission, inform the senior obstetrician.
- Consider the progress of the pregnancy, review the hospital records and assess maternal blood pressure, urinalysis, pulse, and temperature, ensuring general maternal well-being. Obtain IV access and send blood samples to the laboratory for FBC and G&S.
- Confirm the growth and presentation of the fetuses by abdominal palpation and ultrasound scan.
- If the woman is in early labour and the membranes are intact, continuous monitoring of the fetal hearts, movements, and uterine contractions for a short period may provide some assurance of fetal well-being.
- During early labour the woman may find comfort from being able to change her position and walk around, and from the use of TENS or water.

- Encourage her to follow consultant guidelines on diet during labour. In early labour light snacks and fluids are usually recommended. If prescribed by the anaesthetist give ranitidine 150mg orally, three times a day.

Established first stage

- As labour establishes, monitor the fetal hearts continuously, alongside uterine contractions.
- Epidural anaesthesia is often recommended for pain relief. It provides adequate analgesia if intrauterine manipulation of the second twin, forceps delivery, or caesarean is necessary in the second stage. However, be sensitive to individual choice.
- Whatever the woman's choice, an infusion of normal saline may help to keep her hydrated and maintain IV access.
- Make regular assessment of the woman's blood pressure, pulse, temperature, and fluid balance.
- If an epidural is in place and if the presenting head of the first twin is well engaged in the pelvis, after obtaining the consent of the woman artificially rupture the membranes, and place a fetal scalp electrode on the first twin, to facilitate monitoring.
- Care should be taken to ensure the woman's comfort, regularly easing her position and paying attention to hygiene. Encourage her to choose lateral positions to avoid supine hypotension.
- Assess progress and keep the obstetric registrar, anaesthetist, and paediatric team informed. If possible, introduce all personnel to the parents.

Second stage of labour

- When delivery is imminent, call the obstetric registrar in case manipulation of the second twin is necessary.
- The anaesthetist on call should be immediately available outside the delivery room.
- The paediatric team should be present and additional resuscitation equipment prepared to receive both babies.
- Maintain a calm environment and minimize stress for the parents.
- A portable ultrasound scanner should be ready.
- An oxytocin infusion (e.g. oxytocin 5IU added to 250mL of normal saline set to run at 6mL/h) should be prepared to run via a pump. It should be connected to the IV cannula already *in situ* by a dual tap. Initially it remains turned off.
- The woman may prefer not to deliver in the lithotomy position, but the potential for this should be available. An upright position will facilitate pushing and descent of second twin.
- Proceed with the delivery of the first twin:
  - NEVER give Syntometrine® because the second stage is not yet concluded.
  - Episiotomy may not be necessary.
  - Clamp and cut the cord.
  - If the baby is in good condition, encourage the father and mother to hold the baby.

- Occasionally, but not usually, the first placenta may deliver next.
- The registrar should remain present while the midwife performs the second delivery. The midwife should:
  - Palpate the abdomen or scan to determine the lie of the second twin, which must be longitudinal
  - Monitor the heart rate continuously
  - With the woman's consent, gently perform a vaginal examination The midwife will be able to feel the bulging membranes (unless the twins are monozygotic) and a cephalic presentation. Confirm descent
  - Leave the membranes intact
  - Encourage the woman to continue pushing and, if necessary, administer the oxytocin infusion to help contractions
  - When the presenting head is well engaged and progressive descent is obvious, the membranes may rupture spontaneously or the midwife may perform ARM
  - The second twin should be delivered within approximately 30min of the first
  - Mark the cord of the second twin with an extra clamp or ligature, to distinguish it from the first.
- If the babies are well on delivery, encourage skin-to-skin contact between babies and parents. If there is concern on delivery, the paediatric team will assess the babies.
- Samples of cord blood may be taken for assessment of pH.

Complications with the second twin

If the second twin does not take up longitudinal lie following the delivery of the first twin, the obstetric registrar will take over care. With the woman's consent, the following may be performed.
- A catheter will be placed *in situ*.
- External cephalic version may be attempted.
- If not successful, but the fetal heart is reassuring, analgesia is adequate and the second twin is no larger than the first, internal podalic version and breech extraction may be attempted.
- Internal podalic version is performed by the obstetric registrar. The ultrasound scanner is used to assess the position and locate the feet of the second twin. If the feet are easily accessible vaginally, between contractions the obstetrician should reach into the uterine cavity and grasp the foot through the membranes. At the onset of a contraction the fetal foot is pulled downwards with one hand whilst ARM is performed with the other hand. The fetus should then be longitudinal lie and it should be possible to grasp the other foot and encourage maternal effort to push. A vaginal breech birth should ensue.
- However, because of the perceived risks of breech birth, protocols recommend emergency caesarean section.

Third stage of labour
- Allowing the third stage to progress unaided is not usually recommended because of the risk of excessive blood loss from two placental sites.

- Obtain the mother's consent to proceed to active management of the third stage, and give 1mL of Syntometrine® intramuscularly.
- Once delivered, the placenta should be sent for histological examination.
- An oxytocin infusion continued for 4h following delivery will help to minimize PPH.

Rare scenarios with twin pregnancies

Monoamniotic twins

- Vascular anastomoses can occur between the placental vessels of the twins.
- One twin may be small, pale and anaemic and the other large, plethoric and polycythaemic.
- As a result of twin–twin transfusion, fetal asphyxia can occur in either twin.
- These twins are usually diagnosed prior to labour and caesarean section performed to avoid the complications of fetal asphyxia.

Locked twins

- This situation may arise when the first twin is in the breech position and the second twin is a cephalic presentation.
- The head of the first twin can become locked above the head of the second.
- Caesarean section is now recommended for twins with this presentation.

Hypertensive disorders

Definitions of hypertension during pregnancy

- *Essential hypertension* is raised arterial blood pressure, 140/90mmHg or more, before 20 weeks' gestation. No proteinuria is present.
- *Gestational hypertension* (pregnancy-induced hypertension, PIH) is blood pressure raised above 140/90mmHg after 20+ weeks' gestation. No proteinuria is present. It can be classified as a blood pressure of 20–25mmHg above the baseline diastolic reading, sustained over 24h.
- *Pre-eclampsia* is a multisystem disorder. The classification of severity depends on levels of maternal blood pressure and proteinuria: blood pressure, 140/90mmHg; proteinuria, a dipstick reading of 1+, or 0.3g in a 24h urine collection.
- *Eclampsia* is defined as the occurrence of convulsions alongside signs and symptoms of pre-eclampsia.

  Hypertensive disorders can worsen or flare up suddenly during labour or up to 10 days post natally.
- All affected women should be considered to be at high risk:
  - Access consultant-led care
  - Deliver at a unit with neonatal facilities.
- Untreated hypertensive disorders in pregnancy can progress to pre-eclampsia, eclampsia, HELLP syndrome (📖 see p. 408), DIC syndrome (📖 see Disseminated intravascular coagulation, p. 410), and fetal/maternal death.
- Eclampsia is the leading cause of maternal death.
  - Death may occur from acute respiratory distress syndrome (RDS), intracerebral haemorrhage, hepatic, renal, or cardiovascular failure.
  - Fetal death may occur from asphyxia, compromise in labour or placental abruption.
- The only known cure for worsening pre-eclampsia is delivery of the baby. The decision to deliver depends on the condition of the mother and fetus and the length of gestation.

Principles of midwifery care

An experienced midwife should:

- Provide continuous care to the woman and liaise with all the team.
- Monitor the maternal and fetal condition closely.
- Be aware of abnormal clinical findings/complications.
- Refer changes in maternal and fetal condition immediately to the consultant/senior obstetrician for early treatment.
- Carry out the obstetrician's plan of care or assist the obstetrician and multidisciplinary team to perform actions necessary to achieve optimum outcome, considering appropriate time and route for delivery of the fetus. Attentive intrapartum care according to a management plan by a consultant obstetrician is paramount.
- Facilitate communication between all members of the multidisciplinary team, including the senior midwife, obstetrician, anaesthetist, paediatrician, neonatal intensive care and laboratory staff.

- Ensure documentation of care and management decisions.
- Be sensitive to/supportive of the woman's psychological needs and attempt to minimize stress.

Mild hypertensive disorder

A pregnant woman with mild hypertensive disorder may be admitted labouring to the delivery suite. On admission:
- Ensure the woman is/has been transferred from midwifery-led to consultant care, and liaise with the obstetric registrar.
- Review the general well-being of the woman and exclude symptoms of pre-eclampsia (📖 see p. 332).
- Ensure accurate blood pressure measurement. Hypertension >150mmHg systolic or >100mmHg diastolic requires treatment. Discuss this with the obstetrician.
- Assess maternal renal function: take a clean mid-stream sample (MSU) for proteinuria and to exclude infection.
- Assess temperature, pulse, respirations, and oxygen saturation. This assessment on admission may be performed using a maternity early warning scoring system.
- Obtain IV access with a large-bore cannula and take a venous blood sample for urea and electrolytes (U/E), liver function tests (LFTs), FBC, and G&S. The results should be reviewed by a senior obstetrician as soon as they are available and will give indication of the severity of the condition.
- Review fetal well-being: abdominal (or ultrasound) assessment of fetal growth. Commence continuous monitoring of fetal heart alongside uterine contractions, also assess for fetal movements.
- Report and record any deviations from the normal (📖 see Cardiotocograph monitoring, p. 236).

During established labour

- Keep the woman and her partner informed at all times of options available for care, and consider the woman's choices for coping in labour. Try to provide a relaxed environment.
- Encourage as much position change as practical.
- When a woman diagnosed with hypertensive disorder is immobile as in labour she should be encouraged to wear anti-embolic stockings.
- Pain may increase the blood pressure further. Epidural analgesia could help, it causes vasodilation which may reduce the blood pressure.
- Observe the balance between fluid intake and output.
- Assess urine with reagent strip every 2h. Note that a show/blood may contaminate the sample. If proteinuria is +2, obtain a catheter specimen to confirm the reading.
- Measure the blood pressure every 30min in the established first stage, and every 15min during the second stage of labour. Report rising diastolic pressure; if the readings are over 100mmHg in the second stage, the obstetrician may perform an assisted delivery.

Avoid active second-stage pushing, which may affect blood pressure. Allow descent of the fetal head to the perineum then encourage spontaneous efforts at pushing.

Avoid ergometrine/Syntometrine® for the third stage of labour. It may aggravate hypertension. Syntocinon® 10IU IM is preferred.

Pre-eclampsia

- A woman with pre-eclampsia may be admitted to the delivery suite for assessment and possible induction of labour or caesarean section.
- Alert the consultant obstetrician, who will perform a full examination of woman and fetus. This includes neurological assessment.
- Prepare a quiet private examination room for the woman and her partner. Ensure it is equipped with:
  - A suitable sphygmomanometer (the manual sphygmomanometer gives a more accurate reading than an automated machine, which sometimes under-records hypertension)
  - Stethoscope
  - Thermometer
  - Patella hammer
  - Ophthalmoscope
  - CTG monitor
  - Ultrasound scanner
  - Equipment to site IV infusion and to take blood samples, MSU, and to perform vaginal examination.
- Try to alleviate any stress the woman may experience. Listen to preferences, explain procedures, and answer questions.

Maternal assessment

Observe the signs of pre-eclampsia:

- Measure the woman's blood pressure accurately.
  - Use the appropriate cuff size. The standard cuff may be too small and may give an overestimation. If the arm is >33cm in circumference, use a large cuff.
  - Ensure a correct sitting position, with the machine at the level of the woman's heart.
  - Use Korotkoff phase 5 (disappearance of the sound) and note the final digit. It should be recorded accurately and not rounded up or down.
  - Note that the mean arterial pressure (MAP) is used by some obstetricians: a value >125mmHg must be reported.
  - Study the present findings alongside the woman's previous antenatal record. 20–25mmHg above the baseline diastolic reading may be significant.
- Assess urine accurately for proteinuria.
  - Ask the woman to produce a clean MSU. If positive to 2+(>1g/L) on the reagent strip, exclude infection:
    — Assess maternal temperature
    — Send the urine sample to the laboratory for culture and assessment of antibiotic sensitivity
  - Review previous records: 24h urine collection, a value of >300mg/24h suggests that the woman is at risk.
- Take a careful history and enquire about the following symptoms:
  - Headaches: usually frontal and occipital; worse on standing
  - Visual disturbances: flashing lights, loss of patches of visual field (scotomata), photophobia
  - Epigastric pain: probably due to liver oedema, stretching of the capsule
  - Facial oedema (general oedema is no longer rated as a symptom)

- Sometimes no symptoms are discernable
- In severe cases:
  - — Nausea, vomiting, and generally feeling unwell
  - — Irritability, on edge, occasionally drowsy (because of cerebral oedema).
- Discuss the haematological investigations required with the obstetrician. Site large-bore IV access, take and dispatch the required samples for:
  - FBC:
    - — Haemoglobin: enables red blood cells to transport oxygen. A low count indicates anaemia
    - — White cell count: a high count is indicative of stimulation of the immune system and may suggest infection.
  - Clotting screen:
    - — Platelets, thrombin, prothrombin time; these indicate the clotting time of plasma
    - — D-dimer/fibrinogen degradation products; detect the breakdown of fibrin and may suggest thrombosis.
  - U/E: indicate renal function since waste products of metabolism are excreted via the kidneys
  - Creatinine; may be raised when filtration of blood by the glomeruli in the kidneys is impaired
  - LFTs: will assess the extent of liver damage
  - G&S: to assess Rh grouping and save serum in case of bleeding.
- Perform an abdominal assessment to exclude:
  - Abdominal tenderness: fundal tenderness might suggest abruption, hepatic tenderness might indicate a worsening condition
  - Blood loss via the vagina (per vaginam, PV)
  - Uterine contractions indicative of labour.

Fetal assessment
- Perform an abdominal assessment of fetal well-being, especially:
  - Symphysis—fundal height, for growth
  - Fetal movements
  - Begin continuous fetal monitoring (CTG).
- Review antenatal notes to determine the clinical picture and assess any IUGR and placental insufficiency: previous CTG, ultrasound scans for growth, size assessment, fetal breathing movements, amniotic fluid index, and umbilical artery Doppler analysis.

Maternal and fetal assessment by the obstetrician
The obstetrician will:
- Monitor this assessment and review findings
- Carry out a neurological assessment of the woman: in severe pre-eclampsia the reflexes are brisk (clonus), there may be difficulty in focusing and papilloedema may be present
- Determine the presentation of the fetus, by ultrasound scan
- Make a decision on the mode of delivery
- Perform a vaginal examination to assess for possible induction (□ see Induction of labour, p. 364).

Maternal monitoring, management, and treatment
Monitor blood pressure every 15min. Aim to achieve a slow reduction in both systolic and diastolic blood pressure and stabilize. The blood pressure must be stable before a decision about delivery is made.

- Admission to a high dependency unit (if available) may be necessary if the woman's blood pressure is ≥160/110mmHg.
- Oral labetalol, a β-blocker, may be prescribed in milder cases.
- Labetalol should be avoided when a woman is known to be asthmatic.
- The obstetrician may recommend 200mg oral labetalol, if there is time and no immediate risk to woman or fetus. The woman's BP should fall by 10mmHg within 1h. If the response is positive and adequate, maintain the dose orally: 200mg three times a day. 1200mg daily is maximum dose.
- Oral nifedipine 10mg can be given as an alternative. If the BP remains >160/110mmHg after 30min the consultant may prescribe a further 10mg orally.
- If the BP does not fall in 1h, an IV infusion of labetalol may be prescribed: 300mg (5mg/mL) via a 60mL syringe and pump, beginning at 10mL/50mg per hour. The maternal diastolic blood pressure should be maintained at 95–105mmHg. The rate can be changed (increased or reduced) by 2mL/10mg hourly. The maximum rate is 32mL/160mg hourly.
- Hydralazine may also be used. It acts directly on smooth muscle in arteriolar walls, causing vasodilatation. The dose is 5mg as a slow bolus. It may be repeated at an interval of 20min, depending on the woman's BP, or after giving a loading dose an infusion via a syringe driver pump may be prescribed according to local protocol. However, side-effects can be troublesome, e.g. nausea/vomiting, tachycardia, headache. Maternal and fetal condition should be carefully monitored.

In all circumstances, follow the instructions of the medical staff carefully, and abide by local protocols.

IV antihypertensive drugs may cause fetal compromise if the blood pressure is reduced too rapidly. Monitor the fetal heart rate continuously.

Monitor the woman's progress and report any side-effects or changes in condition to the obstetrician. Note that lowering the BP may mask symptoms and does not remove the risk of eclampsia.

- Monitor and restrict IV/oral fluids to approximately 85mL/h, measured via an electronic monitor.
- Measure the oxygen saturation and respiratory rate, using a pulse oximeter. Report levels <95% to medical staff. Low oxygen saturation may indicate pulmonary oedema due to fluid retention.
- Observe the woman's colour and level of consciousness.
- Measure her temperature every 2h.
- Monitor and record her urine output and fluid balance:
  - A bladder catheter is usually recommended. Output is measured hourly using a urometer; 30mL/h is acceptable.
- A doctor should assess tendon reflexes hourly.
- A central venous pressure (CVP)/arterial line may be indicated for accurate measurement of maternal BP.

- Obtain the results of laboratory tests. The following may be indicative of severe hypertensive disorder:
  - Platelet count <100×10^9/L
  - Rising aspartate transaminase (AST) >50IU/L
  - Increasing uric acid levels.
- While the woman is resting in bed, take measures to avoid deep vein thrombosis:
  - Encourage deep breathing and leg movements
  - Provide anti-embolic stockings
  - Enoxaparin sodium, for the prophylaxis of thrombo-embolism is usually prescribed
  - Attend to the woman's hygiene needs, ensure sheets are kept fresh and crease-free. Monitor pressure points and skin integrity.
- Attention to details of comfort may reduce anxiety and pain. Be sensitive to the abdominal discomfort resulting from continuous monitoring of the fetal heart. When movement is restricted, encourage changes of position (especially right or left lateral positions or sitting upright), massage back, hands, or feet. Pay attention to patient preferences for light and sound, peace and space for rest.
- Observe for uterine contractions and ensure adequate pain relief.
- It may be necessary to deliver the baby prematurely.
  - If the fetus is 23–35 weeks, the mother is given corticosteroids (e.g. betamethasone 12mg, repeated in 12/24h if possible according to hospital protocol) to help mature the baby's lungs and reduce respiratory distress.
  - Alert the paediatrician and special care baby unit (SCBU) team to ensure availability of cot and personnel. It may be possible for the parents to visit SCBU or for the staff to describe and explain neonatal special care to the parents prior to delivery.
- Give ranitidine 150mg orally every 6h (according to protocol). This may be requested by anaesthetist. It reduces the production of hydrochloric acid in the stomach and may help to avoid the patient inhaling regurgitated stomach contents (Mendelson's syndrome) which are lethal to the lung tissue and can cause chemical pneumonitis.

Delivery

- All pregnant women requiring IV hypotensives should be delivered as soon as blood pressure is sufficiently controlled. The antihypertensive therapy should be continued during labour. If possible, she should be delivered at a unit with neonatal intensive care facilities.
- An urgent caesarean may be necessary (see Emergency LSCS, p. 379).
- Blood pressure can return to more normal levels soon after delivery but may rise again within 24h. It should be monitored and therapy continued as necessary.

Care of the diabetic mother and fetus

When diabetes is present during pregnancy, risks of the following complications during intrapartum care are increased:

- Preterm labour
- Unstable lie
- Cord prolapse
- PPH—may occur as a result of polyhydramnios
- PIH occurs earlier in the pregnancy than in non-diabetic women and in a more severe form; it may complicate labour
- Large baby (macrosomic)—may result in shoulder dystocia (📖 see Shoulder dystocia, p. 446) in the second stage of labour
- Fetal abnormality (usually excluded by antenatal ultrasound scan)
- IUD when diabetes is inadequately controlled.

It is recommended that woman with diabetes and a fetus which is normal size for dates should be offered elective birth at 38 weeks gestation to prevent complications of fetal macrosomia.[1] This would mean induction of labour or elective caesarean. However, each woman should be treated individually and given information and choice.

Management during the first stage of spontaneous labour[1]

When a woman who has insulin-dependent diabetes is admitted to the delivery suite and found to be establishing in labour:

- Inform the obstetric registrar or consultant on call
- Treat the woman as high risk and follow the plan of care documented in the notes; offer vigilant and continuous care
- Recognize that when the diabetes is well controlled, progress may be normal
- Consider the progress of the pregnancy, review the hospital records, and assess the woman's blood pressure, urinalysis, pulse, and temperature, ensuring general maternal well-being. Any moderate ketonuria should be reported to the obstetrician[2]
- Obtain IV access and send blood samples to the laboratory for FBC—haematocrit and white cell count/U/E, urates, and bicarbonate/G&S
- Review the woman's record of blood glucose readings. Ask the woman to take a capillary sample for immediate assessment. The reading should be in the range 3–7mmol/L
- Gain the woman's consent to assess the fetus and her contractions by abdominal palpation and to monitor the fetus continuously by CTG. Any non-reassuring patterns should be reported to the obstetrician
- Begin an IV regimen (when insulin dependence prior to pregnancy (classified as type 1) is present IV sliding scale is always indicated) that aims to keep the blood sugar level stable, for example:
  - An IV infusion with 500mL 10% dextrose saline + 10mmol KCl is set to run at 100mL/h
  - An insulin pump with soluble insulin 50IU in 49.5mL saline is set to run according to a standard regimen (Table 18.1)
  - Assess blood sugar every 30min. The woman or her partner may be happy to do this. Control the sugar level at 4–7.9mmol/L. If this is not achieved, consult with the obstetric registrar to consider use of the augmented regimen (Table 18.1)

Table 18.1 Insulin sliding scale

Blood glucose (mmol/L)	Insulin dose (IU/h); standard regimen	Insulin dose (IU/h); augmented regimen
<4	0	0
4–5	1	2
6–7	2	4
8–12	3	6
13–17	4	8
>17	6	12

- If the blood sugars are >17mmol/L, obtain a maternal IV sample for measurement of U/E and bicarbonate, the results of which should be reviewed by the obstetrician
- Once stable at 7mmol/L, assess blood glucose hourly.
- During labour, test all urine for ketones and protein, measuring the amount as part of careful fluid balance monitoring. Dehydration and ketosis (which is dangerous to the fetus) can thus be avoided.
- Recommend the drinking of only clear fluids during labour, and give ranitidine 150mg three times a day.
- Blood glucose levels may be more erratic in labour. The body has greater needs for energy. In addition, pain causes catecholamine release, which may make glucose control more difficult.
- Use of patient-controlled epidural anaesthesia in established labour may be recommended to the woman. Mobility is quite limited by this technique and the woman will have difficulty in finding comfortable positions as labour progresses. However, the midwife and obstetric team should be sensitive to the woman's choice if the diabetes is not beset by any of the complications listed above.
- If labour is proceeding normally, support the parents and observe progress to ensure a safe labour and delivery. No intervention is needed.
- If it is essential to aid progress, ARM may be necessary. This should be performed with caution, ensuring that the fetal head is well engaged. The colour and quantity of liquor should be noted. An oxytocin regimen may be requested by the registrar.

Management in the second stage of labour

- Towards the end of the first stage, inform the obstetric registrar of progress.
- If the woman has an effective epidural, the fetal head may be allowed to descend and rotate in the second stage. Oxytocin is recommended for a primigravida with epidural anaesthesia, as it helps to achieve a normal rather than assisted delivery.
- The registrar and paediatrician should be immediately available in case of fetal compromise or shoulder dystocia.

- The baby should be classed as high risk for hypoglycaemia (📖 see Hypoglycaemia, p. 592).

Post-delivery

- Continue the insulin pump with 2h measurements of blood sugar levels until a normal diet can be resumed.
- When the mother is ready to eat, give subcutaneous insulin as for her pre-pregnancy regime, then discontinue the insulin pump after 1h.

Gestational diabetes

Use of the insulin pump and the IV insulin infusion may be discontinued after delivery since the condition usually resolves. Assessment of blood sugar approximately 2h later and during the subsequent morning will exclude an establishing diabetes.

1 National Institute for Clinical Excellence (NICE) (2008). *Diabetes in Pregnancy, Management of Diabetes and it's Complications From Preconception to the Post Natal Period.* Guideline 63. London: NICE. Available at: 🔎 www.nice.org.uk.

2 The Practice Development Team (2010). *Jessop Wing Labour Ward Guidelines 2009–2010.* Sheffield: Sheffield Teaching Hospitals NHS Trust.

Drug and alcohol misuse

Intrapartum care

- Most women who are known to be drug or alcohol dependent will have normal labour and deliveries. They should receive the same information and choices in labour as other women.
- Ideally the woman should be cared for by a midwife known to her.

On admission

- Ensure that you are familiar with any plan for social care and child protection, and inform the appropriate agencies/workers involved of the client's admission to the delivery suite. Ensure that the plan is documented in the hospital notes.
- Inform the obstetrician (although if there are no complications, the obstetrician need not be the lead professional), paediatrician, and SCBU of admission.
- A woman with a history of drug addiction may have veins that prove difficult to cannulate. If she is considered to be at risk of bleeding, the anaesthetist may site a cannula early in labour as a precaution.

The methadone programme

- Women who have opted for a methadone programme to facilitate withdrawal from their habit should continue this drug according to the dose currently prescribed.
- If caring for a woman who is an addict who has withdrawn from treatment, it should be assumed that she is taking drugs. Encourage her to disclose her most recent use. Aim to achieve cooperation and involvement of the woman and partner.
- Respect confidentiality.
- Do not tolerate illicit drug use on the hospital premises.
- Symptoms of withdrawal may occur during labour.
- Women with a history of previous addiction may wish to avoid narcotics. However, they are not contraindicated for pain relief. Unless stated otherwise in the management plan, higher doses of opiates may be necessary because of tolerance.
- Epidural analgesia can be offered.
- Avoid cyclizine, it may increase the effect of methadone and is a central nervous system (CNS) irritant. It is also a misused drug with significant street value.

Infection risk[1]

If the woman is, or has been, an IV drug abuser, then she is at risk of carrying HIV and hepatitis B or C (📖 see Infections, p. 164). If this is a concern, to avoid vertical transmission:
- Membranes should not be ruptured
- A fetal scalp electrode should be avoided
- Fetal blood sampling is contraindicated.

Care[1] of the fetus and neonate[2]

- Placental insufficiency may have occurred in pregnancy. IUGR is common. There is a risk of fetal compromise and intrapartum asphyxia.
- Meconium staining of the liquor, and meconium aspiration are sometimes present as a result of fetal compromise due to periods of intrauterine drug withdrawal.
- During established labour, if the above are noted, monitor the fetal heart continuously via abdominal ultrasound transducer. However if there are no other concerns (apart from known drug/alcohol dependency) midwifery-led care protocols (intermittent monitoring of the fetal heart) may be followed.
- If there are concerns, alert the paediatrician and prepare for resuscitation of the neonate: sometimes breathing may be depressed at delivery.
- Avoid giving naloxone to reverse the effect of opiates during neonatal resuscitation, since this can result in rapid withdrawal which is associated with increased perinatal morbidity and death.
- The baby should be carefully assessed following delivery. Alcohol-related birth defects (📖 see Alcohol, p. 82) should be excluded as far as possible.
- The baby's condition should normally be stable at delivery, if the mother chooses, encourage her to place the baby in skin-to-skin contact and initiate early breastfeeding.
- Transfer the baby to the postnatal ward with the mother.
- Postnatal ward staff should monitor the baby for signs of drug withdrawal. Ensure that the mother recognizes and knows to report the symptoms (📖 see Neonatal abstinence syndrome, p. 648).
- A Common Assessment Framework (CAF) plan may document an agreed care pathway. The following professionals may be involved in care and need to be kept informed:
  - Paediatrician
  - Specialist midwife for drug/alcohol use
  - Community midwife
  - Liaison health visitor
  - Social worker
  - Specialist midwife for child protection
  - Supervisor of midwives.

1 Sheffield Teaching Hospitals NHS Trust (2009). *Jessop Wing, Labour Ward Guidelines 2009–2010*. Sheffield: Sheffield Teaching Hospitals NHS Trust.

2 Martin M (2005). *Guidelines for Practice, Babies Born to Substance Misusing Mothers*. Sheffield: Sheffield Teaching Hospitals NHS Trust.

Epilepsy

Epilepsy affects about 0.5% of pregnant women. Some experience an increase in fits during pregnancy. This may be because women discontinue their medication or they experience nausea/vomiting. Also, a haemodilution and increased metabolism of anticonvulsant drugs may lead to a fall in the concentration of the drug in the plasma. Only 1–2% of women with active epilepsy will have a seizure in labour.[1]

A brief isolated fit is unlikely to be dangerous to the fetus, only occasionally will a seizure cause morbidity, but status epilepticus is a cause of maternal and fetal death.

Women with epilepsy are frequently anxious and require much reassurance. Ideally they should be cared for in labour by a midwife who is known to them and they should have met the consultant overseeing care.

Prevention of seizures

- The midwife should listen to the woman's assessment of her own needs. She will be familiar with the factors which stimulate her seizures and she may experience warning of an attack.
- Anticonvulsant medication should be given as normal during labour. Anticonvulsants include:
  - Phenytoin
  - Primidone
  - Sodium valproate
  - Carbamazepine
  - Phenobarbital.

  Missed doses will cause a drop in plasma levels which should be avoided. Malabsorption during labour may also increase risk of a seizure. If excessive nausea and vomiting occurs an IV regimen of phenytoin may be necessary.
- The midwife should help the woman to achieve a good night's sleep during early labour and prolonged labour should be avoided— exhaustion may cause a seizure.
- Anxiety and stress should be minimized. The midwife can help by encouraging support from the partner and discussing the plan of care fully with the woman.
- Pain or hyperventilation related to pain or stress may cause seizure so adequate analgesia is paramount. The midwife should offer the same range of pain relief (including epidural) as available to other women.
- The midwife should ensure adequate hydration and nutrition since dehydration or hypoglycaemia can trigger seizures.
- The midwife and/or partner should be in attendance throughout the labour.

Signs of epileptic seizure

Epileptic seizures occur in a variety of forms. The most dangerous are tonic clonic seizures.

- Tonic clonic seizure: the woman may experience aura: a strange feeling, taste, or smell. She will suddenly stiffen and if standing fall backwards. She may cry out or bite her tongue. Her muscles will relax and tighten causing the body to convulse. She may be incontinent of urine.

Her breathing may be laboured. The colour of her skin may change to blue-grey. She cannot hear. The episode may last just a few minutes.
  • Following the seizure: the colour of the woman's skin returns to normal. The woman may feel tired and confused. She may have a headache and want to sleep.
• Tonic seizure: the woman's muscles suddenly become stiff. She may fall backwards. Recovery after a tonic seizure is quick.

In the event of an epileptic seizure

• Call for emergency help from obstetric registrar and anaesthetist.
• Note time of onset.
• Turn the woman to left lateral position if possible.
• Ensure clear airway/breathing.
• Give oxygen.
• Remove items which might cause harm.
• Wait at least 3min as most epileptic seizures are self limiting.
• Talk reassuringly to the woman as she regains consciousness.
• Assess maternal and fetal well-being.

Status epilepticus can occur in any type of seizure. If it happens with tonic clonic seizure it is a serious emergency. If the fit continues the anaesthetist will administer 10mg IV diazepam (Diazemuls®) slowly. A further 10mg diazepam may be given. If seizure control is not then achieved the anaesthetist will induce general anaesthesia.

The baby will be delivered by caesarean.

Immediate postnatal care for epileptic mother and her baby

• The midwife should recommend to the parents intramuscular vitamin K (1mg) for the baby at birth since anticonvulsant drugs (carbamazepine, phenytoin, primidone, phenobarbital) are known to increase the risk of haemorrhagic disease of the newborn caused by deficiency in the mother and fetus of vitamin K dependent clotting factors.
• The midwife may safely encourage initiation of breastfeeding since the resulting dose of medication received by the baby is small and is unlikely to cause sedation. The baby's progress should be kept under review.

1 The Royal College of Obstetricians and Gynaecologists: Scottish Executive Committee (1999). *The Management of Pregnancy in Women with Epilepsy. A clinical Practice Guideline for those involved in Maternity Care.* Aberdeen: Scottish Programme for Reproductive Health.

Cardiac conditions

Women with cardiac conditions should have individualized plans made for their care by a team including cardiologist, anaesthetist, obstetrician and midwife. All women should be assessed for exercise tolerance and cardiac function prior to labour and birth.

The aim of care is to reduce the risk of cardiac failure. There are a number of haemodynamic changes taking place in the cardiovascular system during labour and birth which will affect a pregnant woman with significant cardiac disease.

- Increase in cardiac output by 34%.
- Rise in blood pressure from early first stage to the end of second stage. There is a marked increase during second stage contractions when this is accompanied by the mother's pushing efforts.

First stage of labour

- Spontaneous labour and vaginal birth are preferable and there is no significant benefit from elective caesarean section.
- Epidural analgesia is a good option because it decreases cardiac output by increasing peripheral dilatation and reducing the need for fluid pre-load. Care must be exercised in those with a fixed cardiac output.
- Fluid balance requires particular attention and care must be taken not to overload as this may precipitate pulmonary oedema.
- Maternal and fetal well-being must be continuously and carefully assessed.

Second stage of labour

- The second stage of labour can be shortened by elective instrumental delivery to minimize the dramatic rise in blood pressure observed when the mother is pushing.
- In mild heart disease where there have been no antenatal problems it would not be necessary to intervene if progress is rapid and a short second stage anticipated.

Third stage of labour

- Ergometrine and Syntometrine® should be avoided as they can cause generalized vasospasm and hypertension resulting in a 500–800mL bolus of blood returning to the venous circulation.
- Use of oxytocin infusion avoids the problems of bolus and PPH. However, oxytocin should be used with caution in women with severe disease because it can cause profound hypotension.
- Physiological management results in a return of 200–300mL of blood to the circulation. As no oxytocic is given this occurs over a period of minutes rather than during one contraction.
- Women with cardiac disease should be closely monitored for at least 24h following birth.

Cardiac conditions classified into groups according to risk[1]

Low-risk conditions
- Uncomplicated septal defects
- Mild or moderate pulmonary stenosis

- Corrected tetralogy of Fallot
- Corrected transposition without any other significant defects
- Acyanotic Ebstein's anomaly
- Mild mitral or aortic regurgitation
- Hypertrophic cardiomyopathy.

Conditions with some risk
- Coarctation of the aorta
- Cyanosed mother with pulmonary stenosis
- Univentricular circulation after Fontan operation or Rastelli conduits
- Marfan or Ehlers–Danlos syndrome (serious threat if aortic root dilated <4cm)
- Prosthetic cardiac valves.

High-risk conditions
- Pulmonary hypertension (primary), in Eisenmenger's syndrome, (residual) after closure of non-restrictive ventricular septal defect
- Tight mitral stenosis
- Severe aortic stenosis
- Myocardial infarction
- Cardiomyopathies with a low ejection fraction (<35%).

Any case where there is heart failure which is difficult to control. The fetus may be at particularly high risk when maternal cyanosis or heart failure is present.

Some cardiac conditions may require antibiotic cover prophylactically for the prevention of endocarditis, at the onset of spontaneous labour or for obstetric procedures such as induction of labour.

1 Siu SC, Colman JM (2001). Heart disease and pregnancy. *Heart* **85**, 710–15.

Pyrexia

- Pyrexia is defined as a persistent temperature above 38°C.
- It is often associated with coincidental maternal infection, such as upper respiratory tract infection, or may be due to chorioamnionitis.
- Epidural analgesia is often accompanied by a rise in maternal temperature but it cannot always be assumed that this is the cause and an infective agent must be ruled out.
- Fever exceeding 38°C is associated with an increased risk of cerebral palsy in the baby.
- Be aware of maternal sepsis developing, especially if there are predisposing factors such as prolonged rupture of membranes, surgical delivery, pyelonephritis (inflammation of the kidney and renal pelvis). Both maternal and fetal infection must be considered.
  Women who develop pyrexia should receive the following care.
- Sepsis screen: blood culture, catheter specimen of urine and high vaginal, introital, and rectal swabs should be sent for laboratory analysis.
- Cooling strategies: use of a fan, paracetamol, and tepid sponging of the skin.
- The registrar on call should be informed of the woman's pyrexia.
- Broad-spectrum IV antibiotics will be prescribed as per unit protocol. (e.g. cefuroxime 750mg–1500mg IV 8h and metronidazole 500mg IV 8h)
- Be alert for septic shock. It usually presents with pyrexia and hypotension. Inform the obstetrician of any deterioration in the woman's condition.

A wide variety of organisms have been implicated in septic shock during pregnancy, including *Escherichia coli*, *Staphylococcus aureus*, and β-haemolytic streptococcus.

Suspected septicaemia is an indication for transfer of the woman to a high-dependency care facility, and the intensive care medical team, consultant obstetrician, and anaesthetist need to be involved prior to transfer.

Infections

Care of the mother with an infection during pregnancy, labour, and the postnatal period should be individualized according to the needs of the woman and her family. Information shared among carers should be on a need-to-know basis in order to protect the woman's confidentiality.

Hepatitis B

A woman newly diagnosed during pregnancy should have had the opportunity to discuss her management and been given written information about the condition. The Public Health Laboratory should have been informed of the diagnosis and a full hepatitis B serology obtained.

If the woman is antigen positive, neonatal hepatitis B immunoglobulin is indicated as there is a high risk of neonatal transmission. This can be obtained in advance on a named patient basis.

During labour, if possible:
• Do not apply a scalp electrode
• Do not perform fetal blood sampling.

Options for analgesia are the same as for the woman who is hepatitis B negative.

Hepatitis C

As for hepatitis B, do not perform fetal blood sampling or attach a fetal scalp electrode.

There is a small risk of transmission to the neonate and the baby will need paediatric follow-up, as detection of transmission may require more than one blood test over a 6–12-month period.

HIV

Make arrangements for the birth in advance and liaise with the infectious disease specialist and pharmacy, who need to know the expected date of delivery in advance in order to ensure enough stock of antiviral therapy.

Most transmission is known to occur around the time of delivery, and elective caesarean delivery before the membranes rupture is known to lower vertical transmission rates compared with emergency section or vaginal delivery.[1]
• Some women choose to have a vaginal delivery, and for these women do not apply a fetal scalp electrode or perform scalp sampling.
• Offer the same analgesia as would be offered to other women in labour.
• Zidovudine infusion can be commenced prophylactically during labour, to help prevent maternal–fetal transmission of the virus.[2]
  • A continuous infusion of 2mg/kg over 1h followed by 1mg/kg/h until the umbilical cord is clamped.
  • For an elective caesarean section, the infusion can be started 4h prior to the operation at 2mg/kg for 1hr, followed by 1mg/kg/h until the umbilical cord is clamped.
• Procedures at birth include obtaining blood samples from the baby, after washing, to test for antibodies and the potential effects of zidovudine treatment during pregnancy.

Herpes

Neonatal herpes is a severe systemic viral infection with high morbidity and mortality. The risks are greatest when a woman acquires a primary infection during late pregnancy, so the baby is born before the development of protective maternal antibodies.[3]

- Consider any woman developing lesions within 6 weeks of birth for caesarean section, as the shedding of virus during labour is high.
- There is a 40% risk of vertical transmission, which increases with the length of time that the membranes have been ruptured. If vaginal birth is unavoidable, or it is more than 4hr since the rupture of membranes, give the mother and baby aciclovir.[4]
- In these cases, do not use scalp electrodes and avoid fetal blood sampling and instrumental birth.
- An alternative approach for women who develop primary lesions within 6 weeks of birth is to offer them suppression therapy with aciclovir and vaginal birth. Discuss this with a genitourinary medicine physician.
- In recurrent herpes, management is controversial and most would advise vaginal birth.

1 Read JS (2000). Preventing mother to child transmission of HIV: the role of caesarean section. *Sexually Transmitted Infections* **76**, 231–2.

2 Sheffield Teaching Hospitals NHS Trust (2009). *Jessop Wing Labour Ward Guidelines 2009–2010.* Sheffield: Sheffield Teaching Hospitals NHS Trust.

3 Low-Beer NM, Smith JR (2002). *Management of genital herpes in pregnancy.* Green Top Guideline 30. London: RCOG Press.

4 MacLean A, Regan L, Carrington D (2001). *RCOG 40th Study Group 'Infection and Pregnancy'.* London: RCOG Press.

Group B haemolytic streptococcus

Women who are at risk of giving birth to a baby with GBS infection should be offered antibiotics in labour. If the woman accepts, the treatment must be administered at least 4h before the birth in order to have maximum effect. Timely intrapartum treatment with antibiotics reduces the incidence of GBS infection in the neonate occurring in the first 7 days after birth. There are a number of other circumstances to consider:[1]

- If a woman is admitted with prelabour rupture of the membranes after 36 weeks' gestation and is known to carry GBS, she should not be treated conservatively but advised induction of labour and intrapartum antibiotic prophylaxis.
- If a woman is known to have GBS vaginal colonization and gives birth by elective caesarean section with intact membranes, there is no evidence that antibiotic prophylaxis is beneficial.
- A woman admitted in preterm labour should have introital, rectal, and high vaginal swabs on admission. If any show positive for GBS and the result is available before labour is advanced then intrapartum antibiotics should be offered.
- Prolonged rupture of membranes after 37 weeks. Antibiotics are not indicated unless GBS has been detected antenatally, or the woman has had a baby with neonatal GBS, or she becomes pyrexial in labour. She should have a rectal and introital swab to screen for GBS.
- GBS vaginal colonization and home delivery. The same GBS prevention strategy should be offered to all women regardless of place of birth. Risks and benefits of home birth in these circumstances should be discussed and an agreed plan of action documented.
- A woman known to have GBS colonization should be offered rectal and introital swabs at 37 weeks' gestation. If the swabs are negative the risk of being colonized before the birth is low. If the swabs are positive she could be offered a course of oral antibiotics and a follow-up swab taken after treatment. If this is negative the risk is low.
- The woman should be aware that if she goes into labour before the follow-up swab result is available, the oral antibiotics may not have cleared the infection. In either case the woman may be willing to accept these risks and give birth at home.
- Attending labour ward for a dose of antibiotics and then returning home for the birth. This option would only be practical in isolated cases where the woman lives close by and has safe, reliable transport. The drawbacks of this are that she may give birth while travelling to and from hospital and if the labour is long she will require a second dose of antibiotics. A recommended regimen is benzylpenicillin 3g (5 mega units) IV stat followed by 1.5g (2.5 mega units) at 4h intervals until delivery. When a woman has a penicillin allergy, give clindamycin 900mg IV every 8h until delivery. Follow local preferences for treatment.

1 Royal College of Obstetricians and Gynaecologists (2003). *Guideline No. 36 Prevention of Early Onset Neonatal Group B Streptococcal Disease*. London: RCOG Press.

Preterm labour

Definitions
- *Threatened preterm labour*: pregnancy complicated by clinically significant uterine activity but without cervical change.
- *Preterm labour*: the occurrence of regular uterine contractions which cause cervical effacement or dilatation prior to 37 completed weeks of pregnancy.

Preterm, prelabour rupture of the membranes
This occurs in more than one-third of preterm labours. Most women so affected will deliver within 1 week. Prelabour rupture of the membranes (PPROM) is often associated with maternal infection.

Incidence of preterm delivery
- Just under 7% of UK births are preterm.
- Less than one-quarter of UK preterm births are <32 weeks' gestation.

Some predisposing factors
- Pre-eclampsia, eclampsia
- APH, placental abruption, placenta praevia
- Intrauterine growth retardation
- Disease or infection in the woman or fetus
- PPROM
- Intrauterine death
- Multiple pregnancy
- Polyhydramnios
- Congenital abnormalities
- Previous preterm labour (in selected cases cervical suture may have been placed to reduce the risk of a second preterm delivery)
- Cervical incompetence (may be a result of cervical surgery or surgical termination of pregnancy).

Risks of preterm delivery
- Major problems occur for babies born after 24 weeks' (when the baby is viable) and before 33 weeks' gestation.
- Fetal death may occur as a result of intraventricular haemorrhage, RDS, infection, jaundice, hypoglycaemia, or necrotizing endocolitis.
- In cases of PPROM, survival rates are linked to the gestation at membrane rupture rather than duration of rupture. There is a high risk of chorioamnionitis.
- The prognosis depends on the antenatal administration of steroids to the mother, the gestation, and birthweight, condition at birth, and the immediate care after birth, including the availability of a neonatal intensive care unit (NICU).

Diagnosis and management of preterm labour

A woman may present to the delivery suite with regular painful contractions before 37 weeks' gestation.

The midwife should:

- Inform an obstetrician. If necessary transfer from midwifery to consultant care
- Acknowledge the woman's anxiety and explain the rationale for care
- Review and summarize her obstetric history and the history of her current pregnancy. Note her Rh status and blood grouping
- Record a history of the recent episode
- Ask the woman whether she has had any recent injury
- Assess her respirations, temperature, pulse, oxygen saturation and blood pressure (cf maternity early warning scoring). Request an MSU sample and dispatch it to the laboratory for urgent culture and antibiotic sensitivity to exclude urinary tract infection
- Perform a gentle abdominal palpation and assessment. Assess especially fetal size, lie, and presentation. There is a risk of cord presentation if the fetus is breech or the lie oblique. Listen for the fetal heart with Doppler and ask about the frequency of fetal movements.
- Assess abdominal tenderness, tension, and irritability. Sit beside the woman for a while, allowing time to assess the length, strength, and frequency of uterine contractions. Regular contractions lasting 30s, at least once every 10min, may be significant
- Ask about any discharge PV (blood or fluid)
- Ask about pain other than the pain from contractions (e.g. renal pain)
- Monitor the contractions and fetal heart and movements via a CTG monitor:
  - Monitoring is not indicated if the gestational age is assessed to be <25 weeks
  - If the gestational age is estimated to be 27 weeks, discuss with the consultant obstetrician the action to take if the pattern is abnormal (🕮 see Cardiotocograph monitoring, p. 236).
  - At <34 weeks the fetal heart is less likely to demonstrate sleep/wake patterns; accelerations to 10 beats are considered normal in this context
- Document the findings and discuss them with the obstetrician

Careful monitoring and assessment by the midwife will assist an accurate diagnosis.

Further assessment will be made by the obstetrician.

- Perform speculum examination (rather than digital assessment which may introduce infection and may augment labour) to assess cervical effacement/dilatation, exclude infection and perform fetal fibronectin test if indicated.
  - Ensure privacy for the woman, obtain consent, and explain the procedure.
  - Ask the woman to rest on the bed for 30min and to wear a sanitary pad. This is to allow the collection of any fluid, 'pooling of liquor' in the vagina prior to the assessment.
- Diagnosis of preterm labour is made if cervical dilatation is as much as 2cm in a nullipara or 3cm in a multipara, or a change in the cervix (length and dilatation) is noted over two speculum examinations, preferably performed by the same practitioner, 2–3h apart.

- Exclude vaginal bleeding/PPROM/discharge.
- Exclude infection and take swabs for culture and antibiotic sensitivity: a high vaginal swab and endocervical swab for *Chlamydia*, a rectal and introital swab for GBS. If infection is suspected, send blood cultures urgently to bacteriology.
- An ultrasound scan may be necessary, e.g. to assess fetal size, presentation, breathing movements, or liquor volume. (The early pregnancy ultrasound scan will be most accurate when establishing gestation.)
- An IV line should be sited. Take blood samples for FBC and U/E; G&S if labour seems to be establishing or there is any bleeding. If the cervix is <2cm in a primigravida or <3cm in a multigravida, commence 500mL normal saline over 4h and give oral analgesia.
- If the woman's blood group is Rh-negative, take blood for Kleihauer's test. This test detects whether any (potentially Rh-positive) fetal cells have crossed over into the maternal circulation. This may happen, for example, as a result of injury or placental bleeding. In cases of threatened preterm labour this cannot be excluded. Anti-D 500IU (which coats and eliminates any Rh-positive fetal cells in the mother's blood and so prevents maternal sensitivity) may be prescribed.

Threatened preterm labour <34 weeks (without PPROM)

- The plan of management aims to delay the delivery of a preterm baby for 24–48h, to allow for the administration of intramuscular steroid therapy to the mother or to facilitate intrauterine transfer (see below). Tocolytics, drugs which may delay established labour and delivery, are not usually given if the woman has already received the required steroid therapy.
- The plan to treat a woman who appears to be experiencing threatened preterm labour may be based on the use of the fetal fibronectin test (fFt). The fFt may facilitate diagnosis of women at minimal risk of progressing in preterm labour. This is a negative fFt and can prevent unnecessary treatment.
  - The test involves taking a swab of cervicovaginal secretions from the posterior fornix and ectocervix during a speculum examination.
  - Fetal fibronectin is a glycoprotein found in the secretions. When present at levels which are detectable on the test between 24–34 weeks of pregnancy it is associated with preterm delivery.
  - fFt negative: 0.8% risk of delivery in 7–10days. If symptoms persist repeat test in 24h. Seek senior obstetric advice before transferring the woman or discharge home.
  - fFt positive: 14% risk of delivery in 7–10 days. Administer tocolytics and steroids and ensure neonatal provision.[1]
- Indications: 24–34 weeks' gestation with intact membranes and symptoms of preterm labour with the intention to treat with tocolytics and steroids.
- Contraindications: multiple pregnancy, coitus in previous 24h, moderate bleeding PV or ruptured membranes,

- The test needs to be performed at the beginning of a speculum examination using water only as lubricant and following the testing kit procedure.
- Steroid therapy: *Corticosteroids* may reduce the risk of RDS by 40–60%. Other complications of the neonatal period may also be reduced, e.g. necrotizing enterocolitis and intraventricular haemorrhage.
  - Give two doses of betamethasone 12mg IM 12 or 24h apart.
  - After the initial course the baby will benefit after approximately 24h and for up to 7 days.
  - However, repeated doses to a woman who remains undelivered but still at risk may be less beneficial, because corticosteroid administration may be associated with endocrine defects in infants.
  - Systemic infection in the mother is a contraindication to administration.
- Tocolytics: a variety of *tocolytics* have been used to delay delivery:
  - Betamimetics: ritodrine, salbutamol, terbutaline
  - Prostaglandin synthetase inhibitors: indometacin
  - However, since these may have serious side-effects and much careful monitoring of the mother and fetus is required. The oxytocin antagonist atosiban is preferable.
- Contraindications include:
  - Fetal heart pattern irregularities
  - Placental abruption or active bleeding
  - Infection/chorioamnionitis
  - PPROM
  - Severe pre-eclampsia, since delivery is necessary.
- *Atosiban* works by blocking the oxytocin receptors sites in the myometrium and preventing the influx of calcium necessary for a contraction.
  - Atosiban may be used when a diagnosis of uncomplicated preterm labour has been made between 24 and 33 (+6 days) weeks' gestation.
  - It may also be used if a woman with a history of spontaneous preterm delivery at less than 34 weeks' gestation presents with uterine contractions without cervical changes.
  - Measure the woman's blood pressure and pulse to provide a baseline. Hourly observations are then adequate.
  - Continuous monitoring is indicated throughout the treatment period, especially if there is any bleeding or concern for fetal well-being. If contractions stop and there are no other concerns, intermittent auscultation for 2min every hour may be performed until treatment is complete.
  - Atosiban is not associated with serious side-effects and is well tolerated. It is quickly cleared from the body after the infusion is discontinued. Nausea, vomiting, headache, fever, tachycardia, hyperglycaemia, hypotension, and injection site reaction have been reported.
  - Treatment can be repeated if regular uterine contractions recur.

PPROM <34 weeks' gestation

Following diagnosis, provided it is safe to do so, the woman should be transferred to a hospital with neonatal intensive care facilities. She should be treated conservatively, with admission to an antenatal ward for observation.

The midwife should:
- Observe the woman's temperature and pulse 4h
- Give medications as prescribed: steroid therapy and broad-spectrum antibiotics (erythromycin 500mg four times daily for 10 days) if required
- Assess the woman's discomfort and be vigilant for any onset of uterine contractions
- Assess the amount, colour, and smell of PV loss
- Perform CTG as requested by the obstetrician
- Take blood for a FBC (for white cell count) and C-reactive protein estimation (CRP levels increase to >10mg/L during acute inflammation). These blood samples, taken on alternate days, will help to assess for infection
- Arrange ultrasound scanning as requested by the obstetrician, to measure remaining amniotic fluid and assess the growth of the fetus
- Report promptly any changes in maternal/fetal condition to the obstetrician.

Delivery is indicated if
- There is evidence of infection:
  - *Chorioamnionitis*, indicated by:
    — A rising maternal temperature and pulse
    — A tachycardic fetal heart
    — Maternal abdominal pain, especially on palpation of the uterus
    — An offensive discharge PV
    — The maternal white cell count and CRP may be raised.
  - *β-Haemolytic streptococci*
    — If there is definite infection recorded from microscopy on the vaginal swab, the woman should be delivered with IV antibiotic cover.
- Labour occurs spontaneously. It should be allowed to progress without the use of tocolytic drugs.
- The fetus is mature enough at approximately 34 weeks' gestation.
- The decision to deliver has been made by a consultant/senior obstetrician.
- The paediatrician and NICU have been informed of the full case history.

PPROM >34 weeks' gestation
- PPROM is frequently associated with infection, and the risks associated with infection are higher than the risks of prematurity. Therefore, following a definite diagnosis and if the woman is not in labour, induction may be indicated.

- After a period of waiting to see if the woman establishes (72h) this may be performed using an oxytocin infusion.
- This decision should be made by the consultant obstetrician.

Management of preterm delivery

- One-to-one midwifery care is especially recommended.
- Liaise with other members of the team. The plan of care should be discussed between obstetric, anaesthetic and theatre, neonatal, senior midwifery staff, and parents.
- Monitor documentation of the plan in the woman's notes.
- Ensure that corticosteroids and antibiotics are given if necessary.
- Arrange an ultrasound scan, to:
  - Confirm the fetal lie and presentation
  - Give an estimated fetal weight
  - Exclude serious abnormality.

If the fetus is between 22 and 26 weeks' gestation

- When a cot is not available locally, *in utero* transfer will be considered by the obstetrician for all threatened preterm deliveries above 22 weeks' gestation. Sometimes it may be that delivery, assessment, and postnatal transfer is more appropriate.
- Before delivery, communication with parents is especially important. They need to understand, discuss, and agree what care is appropriate. They should be made aware of the morbidity and mortality risks to their baby. Survival rates are poor below 24 weeks' gestation.
  - Follow the agreed management plan when discussing the family's needs. Be a sympathetic listener and encourage the parents to seek psychological support from family, friends, and other networks.
  - Help the parents to understand how their baby may look at delivery. Discuss the approximate size, features of prematurity, and possible bruising which may be present after delivery.
  - The parents should understand the procedure that will be followed. Be prepared to repeat explanations. Distressed and anxious parents may not remember information.
  - Check that the content of the paediatrician's discussions with the parents are documented in the woman's notes.
  - If the plan is to resuscitate the baby, the parents should understand that the baby's condition will be continually assessed and care will be provided in the NICU as long as this is appropriate.
- Initial assessment of gestational age by ultrasound is important, alongside the mother's menstrual history. It may help determine the action necessary.
- Caesarean section is rarely appropriate below 25 weeks' gestation. There are significant risks of complications for the mother when the lower uterine segment is not formed. Each case should be considered individually. The consultant may seek a second obstetric opinion.
- Monitor the fetal heart unobtrusively and intermittently, unless requested to monitor continuously by the obstetrician. At early gestation an abnormal fetal heart trace would not necessarily be acted

upon. It is also sometimes difficult and time consuming to attempt to obtain a continuous trace when the fetus is very preterm.
• Once established, labour may progress quickly. The cervix may not need to dilate to the traditional 10cm before delivery! Early preparation for delivery and confirmation of availability of personnel will minimize anxiety and help the delivery run smoothly.
• Call the paediatrician to attend all births thought to be >22 weeks' gestation, to assess the condition of the baby at birth and to make a decision about resuscitation.
• At >23 weeks' gestation the paediatrician and neonatal nurse team should attend the birth, to assess the baby's condition and resuscitate actively if appropriate.
• The response of the baby to resuscitation determines whether the baby is transferred to the neonatal unit for further intensive care and assessment.
• If there has been no time to discuss a plan of action with the parents, it is acceptable to offer intensive care 'provisionally' pending further assessment and discussion.
• The placenta may be sent to histology for examination.

If the fetus is >27 weeks' gestation
• When a diagnosis of preterm labour is made, arrange for the parents to visit a NICU and to discuss the plan of action with the paediatrician and neonatal team.
• Ensure that the parents understand what will happen at delivery.
• The environment of care is particularly important when labour is preterm. If psychological stress is reduced, the woman may labour more effectively, with better tolerance of pain. The midwife can help provide a peaceful environment by minimizing the numbers of staff, interruptions, intrusive noise, or light.

During the first stage of preterm labour
• Monitor the woman as for a normal first stage.
• Encourage the intake of light snacks and fluids. (The anaesthetist may suggest oral ranitidine 150mg 6 or 8h as an antacid in the case of emergency anaesthesia.)
• Enable the woman to mobilize. This will enhance the normal descent and well-being of the fetus. The woman's comfort may be improved with mobility. Supine positions may increase the FHR.
• If possible, provide one-to-one support with a variety of coping strategies. This may enhance the woman's experience of labour and reduce her needs for analgesia.
  • Choices for analgesia include TENS, Entonox®, and patient-controlled analgesia.
  • If opiates must be used for maternal analgesia, explain possible side-effects to the woman: opiates can make the baby slow to breathe at delivery, or sleepy, with limited interest in suckling.
• Monitor the fetal heart according to the obstetrician's recommendations and parents' preference. When considering continuous monitoring (CTG) remember that the preterm fetus may demonstrate a different heart pattern:

- The baseline may be higher than 160bpm
- The variability may be reduced
- Bradycardia and variable decelerations may occur more frequently.
- Although the CTG may appear non-reassuring, fetal blood sampling (FBS) frequently does not demonstrate any acidosis in the fetus.
- However, if the fetus is >34 weeks' gestation and if there is no obvious maternal infection, FBS will be considered.[1] If performed, provide support for the mother during the procedure.
- Take particular care to minimize the number of vaginal examinations, which may increase the risk of infection.
- ARM should also be avoided:
  - There is a risk of infection to the fetus
  - Cord compression or prolapse may occur
  - It may precipitate variable decelerations in the fetal heart.
- The midwife's role in the first stage of preterm labour is to observe maternal and fetal progress, support the parents, coordinate care, and report deviations from normal.

The second stage of labour

- Prepare a warm environment, with warm towels ready. Switch off fans and close windows.
- Check that resuscitation equipment is complete and functioning, and that the heater is on. Inform neonatal staff of the impending delivery, allowing time for them to be prepared.
- The unit supervisor and the obstetrician may wish to be informed.
- If the fetal condition appears satisfactory and descent is evident, there is no necessity to limit time in the second stage.
- Pushing should be spontaneous. Encourage the woman to push as she wishes. If the woman has chosen epidural anaesthesia do not allow it to wear off in the second stage, but let the head descend to the perineum then encourage pushing. Directed active pushing may cause fetal compromise.
- Episiotomy is only necessary as an emergency when fetal compromise is evident.
- Forceps and ventouse will be avoided by the obstetrician (especially at <34 weeks' gestation) because they may cause trauma to the fetal head.
- At delivery the low-risk preterm baby may benefit from being wrapped in a warmed towel and held below the level of the uterus for 30s. This may allow the normal physiological changes to take place and the optimum transfusion of blood via the cord.
- Then, while gently drying the baby, place the baby on the mother's abdomen and encourage the mother to keep the baby in skin-to-skin contact. The baby's head and body should be well covered with warmed towels to prevent heat loss.

The third stage of labour

- The third stage may be managed physiologically or actively.
- Clamp and cut the cord only if the baby is in need of urgent resuscitation and this is required by the neonatal team.

- Delayed clamping and cutting may be applied even when the third stage is managed actively. It may reduce anaemia in the preterm neonate and the red cell transfusion requirements. It may also reduce the duration of the baby's need for oxygen therapy.
- The obstetrician may ask the midwife to double clamp the cord so that cord venous and arterial blood samples can be taken for pH analysis. This provides a baseline and may aid neonatal management.
- When clamping and cutting the cord, leave approximately 6cm at the baby's end in case of a later need for umbilical catheterization.
- Although a baby may be compromised at delivery, it is important to encourage the parents to look at and touch their baby before transfer to the NICU.
- Where possible, encourage the maintenance of skin-to-skin contact, since this maintains the baby's temperature and may reduce the baby's stress response. It promotes bonding between the mother and baby. These may be important memories for the parents after the baby's transfer to NICU. It may improve the duration of breastfeeding.
- It is the midwife's responsibility to ensure that baby identity labels are *in situ*—one on each ankle—before transfer to NICU.
- Take surface swabs from ear, axilla, and umbilicus of the baby if the membranes have been ruptured for longer than 72h. These will be sent for culture and determination of antibiotic sensitivity.
- Ensure that the neonatal team has access to the mother's notes.
- A photograph may be taken in NICU and given to the parents.
- Encourage the parents to visit as soon a mutually acceptable time can be arranged.
- The obstetrician may request histological examination of the placenta.

Recommended reading

Written with reference to: The Practice Development Team (2009). *Jessop Wing Labour Ward Guidelines 2009–2010*. Sheffield: Sheffield Teaching Hospitals NHS Trust.

1 National Institute for Health and Clinical Excellence (2001). *Electronic Fetal Monitoring*. London: NICE.

Induction of labour

Definition: labour is initiated using mechanical and/or pharmacological methods. The intervention is necessary when the well-being of the mother or baby may be at risk if the pregnancy is continued. The parents should be in agreement and fully informed of procedures.[1]

Some indications

- Post maturity
- PROM (>37 weeks)
- PIH, pre-eclampsia
- APH
- Placental insufficiency and IUGR
- Large fetus, twins
- Diabetes, renal disease, or other underlying condition
- IUD.

Method of induction

Prostaglandin gel is used to soften/ripen the cervix. When this is achieved, the membranes are ruptured (amniotomy) and an oxytocin infusion commenced to stimulate regular uterine contractions and dilatation of the cervix.

Management

- If a consultant-booked woman requires induction of labour, always act under the instructions of the obstetric consultant or registrar.[2]
- The obstetric consultant or registrar should authorize the induction and write the indication and method in the woman's notes.
- The woman will be admitted to the delivery suite.
- If she is a primigravida and is likely to need induction using vaginal prostaglandin, she may be admitted at 5pm, given treatment, and allowed to progress over night.
- A multigravida who may already have a cervix favourable for induction, and may not need prostaglandin before amniotomy is possible, may be admitted at 7am.
- Carefully explain the length of time that induction may take and the procedures involved and possible outcomes. This will help to alleviate the prospective parents' anxiety and enable them to make appropriate arrangements for hospital admission.
- Before commencing the induction, ensure that:
  - The woman and her partner understand and consent. If induction fails, a caesarean section is indicated. NICE has produced a booklet about induction of labour[3]
  - The rationale for induction is documented and current
  - The estimated date of delivery is correct and, if possible, confirmed on early pregnancy scan
  - The presenting part is engaged (3/5 palpable abdominally)
  - The fetal heart (CTG) has been monitored for 30min and is reassuring
  - The obstetric registrar has prescribed the treatment
  - The woman is comfortable and has passed urine.
- Ensure that the woman's dignity and privacy are preserved at all times.

Bishop score

You should be experienced in assessing the state of the cervix.

* The Bishop score (see Table 18.2) is a frequently used system of assessing the cervix which can give a clear indication of progress. The score should be recorded in the woman's notes each time an assessment is made, i.e. at the time of administration of prostaglandin gel and amniotomy.
* The higher the initial score, the more successful induction.
 If the Bishop score is:
* <5: the cervix is unfavourable for induction and prostaglandin gel will be necessary to soften the cervix
* 5–8: the cervix is moderately favourable (1mg prostaglandin may suffice)
* >8: the cervix is very favourable and prostaglandin is not required.
 Variations on this scoring include one recommended in the NICE guidlines.[4]

Sweeping the membranes

When a woman's care during pregnancy has been midwifery-led, induction of labour should be discussed by the midwife towards term. The community midwife may arrange with the delivery ward for the induction to be planned for a mutually convenient time.

Prior to induction of labour in hospital, offer the woman a vaginal examination to assess the state of the cervix and to perform a sweeping of the membranes. This has been shown to increase the possibility of labour occurring naturally with in the following 48h.[4]

The NICE antenatal guidelines[5] recommend that this should form part of the antenatal consultation at 41 weeks' gestation. If the membrane sweep is discussed at a previous appointment, the woman has the opportunity to arrange support for the visit if she wishes.

This procedure may be performed in the woman's home or at an antenatal clinic visit. It may be a preferable first step to stimulate labour and sometimes may pre-empt formal induction.

Table 18.2 Modified Bishop (Calder) score

Score	0	1	2	3
Dilatation (cm)	<1	1–2	2–4	5 or more
Cervical length (cm)	5 or more	2–4	1–2	<1
Station above spines (cm)	–3	–2	–1/0	+1/+2
Consistency	Firm	Average	Soft	
Position	Posterior	Central/anterior		

- The pregnancy should be uncomplicated.
- The gestational age should be term, 41 weeks.
- The membranes must be intact.
- Warn the woman that she may experience some discomfort as a result of the procedure and that she may have a mucoid/bloodstained 'show' and should wear a light sanitary pad.
- Reassure her that membrane sweeping is not associated with increased maternal or neonatal infection.
- Perform a vaginal examination and locate the cervix. A finger is inserted through the internal os, stretching the cervix slightly, and the membranes are palpated. Use a sweeping circular movement of the finger to separate the fetal membranes from the decidua/lower uterine segment.
- There is potential for a natural rapid increase in prostaglandin production in late pregnancy. Sweeping of the membranes is a mechanical stimulant to tissue prostaglandin release in the cervix and lower segment. This, in turn, can initiate the onset of labour.

Prostaglandins for induction of labour

- Obtains consent from the woman, perform a vaginal examination and assess the cervix using the Bishop score.
- If the cervix is not favourable (Bishop score <5), use vaginal prostaglandin dinoprostone (PGE2) gel to soften/ripen the cervix, as follows:
  - Nulliparous women: 2mg prostaglandin gel.
  - Multiparous women: 1mg prostaglandin gel.
- The gel should be placed in the posterior fornix of the vagina.
- Record the Bishop score, amount of prostaglandin gel, and time of procedure in the notes.
- Encourage the woman to rest on the bed for an hour following the procedure, during which time the fetal heart is monitored continuously. If the recording is reassuring, the woman should mobilize and eat/drink as normal.
- Warn the woman that she may experience mild discomfort/ soreness in the vagina as a result of prostaglandin, or painful uterine contractions caused by the prostaglandin prior to the onset of the regular contractions of labour. Oral or intramuscular analgesics may be prescribed.
- Repeat the vaginal examination to assess progress in 6–12h. Nulliparous women admitted for post-dates induction may rest overnight and be reviewed the following morning.
- If the cervix is still firm in consistency and in a posterior position (Bishop score <5), a second dose of prostaglandin gel should be given and the fetal heart monitored as previously.
- The total dose of prostaglandin gel given should not exceed 4mg for nulliparous and 3mg for multiparous women.
- Vaginal (PGE2) tablet preparations are also available and the recommended dose is 3mg PGE2 6h. The maximum dose is 6mg for all women.
- Propess® vaginal insert 10mg (PGE2) may be preferred by women to help soften the cervix as it is a slow release preparation and delivers

about 0.4mg/h of active agent in 24h. Propess® should be inserted into the posterior fornix of the vagina using a water-soluble lubricant. It has a tape to aid removal after 24h. Follow local protocols for use.

Risks of induction with prostaglandin

- The consultant or registrar must always authorize prostaglandin and time of insertion for:
- Grandmultiparous women
  - Women with severe asthma
  - Non-reassuring fetal heart pattern
  - IUGR
  - Previous precipitate labour
  - Previous caesarean section, myomectomy, hysterotomy.[2]
- Never use prostaglandins if the woman is already experiencing painful contractions. Either perform an amniotomy or allow the woman to progress and review later.
- Never perform amniotomy within 6h of giving prostaglandin gel, because uterine activity may become excessive. If the membranes rupture after administering prostaglandin gel, an interval of 6h should be allowed before commencing IV oxytocin.
- PGE2 may cause mild pyrexia, due to its effect on cerebral thermoregulatory centres.

Artificial rupture of the membranes

- If the cervix is favourable (i.e. Bishop score >6), then it may be possible to perform amniotomy for induction of labour.
- Amniotomy may be performed if:
  - The senior registrar authorizes/performs the procedure in the high-risk client
  - The woman understands the procedure and consents
  - The fetal head is engaged or 3/5 palpable abdominally
  - 6h have elapsed since the last insertion of prostaglandin gel
  - The CTG is reassuring.

Management

- The woman may value the support of a partner/friend. She should understand that she can withdraw consent to the procedure at any point if she so wishes.
- The procedure is performed using sterile pack, gloves, lubricant, amnihook, protection for couch, and clothing.
- Monitor the fetal heart continuously.
- Entonox® should be available in case the woman experiences discomfort.
- The woman should pass urine prior to the procedure.
- Perform a vaginal examination, assess the Bishop score, insert a finger through the internal os and palpate the membranes and forewaters. Introduce the amnihook along the examining fingers and perform the amniotomy.
- Address the woman's hygiene needs.
- Document the Bishop score, time of amniotomy, colour and volume of liquor.

- Monitor the fetal heart
  - Continuously following the procedure
  - For 60min when the induction is in a low-risk woman; thereafter the fetal heart should be monitored intermittently (each 15min) until contractions occur regularly or IV oxytocin is commenced.
- If the woman is not experiencing regular contractions, administer an oxytocin regimen:
  - Immediately after ARM for all primigravidae and multigravidae with urgent indication for induction, such as pre-eclampsia
  - 2h after ARM if regular contractions have not commenced and if multiparous and non-urgent indication for delivery.

Complications of ARM

- Prolapsed cord may occur if the fetal head is not engaged when the membranes are ruptured, or if it has not been recognized that the cord is presenting prior to the procedure.
- Non-reassuring fetal heart pattern may occur following ARM. This may be due to compression of the fetal head or placenta. It should settle to normal soon after.
- Increased infection risk once the membranes have been ruptured. It is important that effective progress in labour is achieved.

Intravenous oxytocin

- Syntocinon® is a synthetic oxytocin. It is effective in stimulating uterine activity and promoting dilatation of the cervix.
- Before commencing Syntocinon®, ensure that:
  - The drug is prescribed by the registrar
  - The woman understands the procedure for administration, the restriction it will place on her mobility, and the analgesia available
  - 6h have elapsed since the last administration of vaginal prostaglandins
  - Spontaneous rupture of membranes is certain or that ARM has been performed
  - You are fully conversant with client's obstetric history, since extreme caution is indicated in clients with a uterine scar or grand multiparity
  - You are aware of the current state of maternal observations, contractions, and cervical dilatation as a baseline
  - The fetal heart is monitored continuously and is reassuring.
- Check the medication with a colleague: it can be given via IV infusion using an Alaris® pump and a dilution of 5IU of Syntocinon® in 250mL of normal saline.
- Siting of an IV cannula is a good time to take FBC/platelets and G&S in case of later need. A double Luer catheter will allow an infusion of 1000mL normal saline to be sited to run slowly alongside 250mL of normal saline/5IU of Syntocinon® via an Alaris pump. The initial dose is 6mL/h. Titrate the dose against uterine activity.
- The aim is to achieve three or four regular contractions in 10min. There should be 1min relaxation between each contraction. To achieve this, the dose may be increased every 30min as shown in Table 18.3.

Table 18.3 Syntocinon® regime

2mU/min	6mL/h
4mU/min	12mL/h
8mU/min	24mL/h
16mU/min	48mL/h

- Further increases should be discussed with the obstetric registrar.
- NICE guidelines suggest other similar regimens.[3]

Risks/complications of Syntocinon® administration

You should remain in attendance, ensuring the safety of mother and fetus, and observe for the following:

- The uterus may be hyperstimulated. This may cause FHR irregularities. Stop the infusion temporarily and observe the FHR. If the abnormality persists, inform the registrar, who may perform fetal blood sampling. If the FHR becomes reassuring, the Syntocinon® may be restarted at half the preceding rate.
- Hyperstimulation of the uterus could cause rupture. This rarely happens in primigravidae but care is needed in multiparous women.
- Postpartum haemorrhage is more common following induction.
- Syntocinon® may be ineffective on the cervical dilatation so that labour does not progress. Caesarean section may be necessary.
- Syntocinon® tends to encourage water retention. This is minimized by diluting it in normal saline. Care should be taken to monitor IV fluids infused and assess maternal observations.
- Amniotic fluid embolism is not now thought to be precipitated by Syntocinon® induction.

1 Arulkumaran S, Symonds IM, Fowlie A (2004). *Oxford Handbook of Obstetrics and Gynaecology.* Oxford: Oxford University Press.

2 The Practice Development Team (2009). *Jessop Wing, Labour Ward Guidelines 2009–2010.* Sheffield: Sheffield Teaching Hospitals NHS Trust.

3 National Institute for Health and Clinical Excellence (2001). Induction of labour. Inherited Clinical Guideline D. London: NICE. Available at ✍ www.nice.org.uk.

4 Boulvain M, Fraser WD, Marcoux S, *et al.* (2001). Stripping/sweeping the membranes for inducing labour or preventing post-term pregnancy (Cochrane review). In: *Cochrane Library*, Issue 3. Oxford: Update Software.

5 National Institute for Health and Clinical Excellence (2003). Antenatal care guideline 6. London: NICE. Available at: ✍ www.nice.org.uk.

Augmentation of labour: active management

A variety of protocols exist which are aimed at avoiding a long labour and maternal exhaustion and achieving delivery of the baby within 12–18h.

Augmentation of labour may be initiated if the normal progress of labour appears slow. You may consider active management in a normal labour without previous obstetric or antenatal complications if:

- The woman is definitely in established labour (changes in the cervix demonstrating progressive effacement and dilatation) but is making slow progress because the uterine activity appears limited
- The woman states that she understands the concept, interventions, and mobility restraints and prefers active management
- You have discussed the plan and obtained the agreement of the delivery suite coordinator and the obstetric registrar.

Management

- Careful observation of maternal and fetal condition is necessary.
- Accurate documentation of the interventions on the partogram is essential.
- Monitor the FH continuously.
- Monitor the length, strength, and number of uterine contractions.
- Site an IV infusion.
- If the membranes are intact, following abdominal assessment, perform a vaginal examination and ARM. This may shorten the ARM delivery time if used in conjunction with an oxytocin infusion. Remember, however, that hydrostatic pressure no longer cushions the placenta. There is a higher risk of fetal cardiac irregularities. There is also a risk of infection to the fetus.
- Note the current cervical dilatation, state of descent of the presenting part, and colour of the liquor.
- Some authorities suggest a cervicograph guide may be used to measure progress. Action is recommended if cervical dilatation is 2h behind the cervicoragh curve. The oxytocin regimen may be commenced as for induction of labour (🕮 see Induction of labour, p. 364).
- Vaginal examination (using a sterile procedure) may be performed at regular intervals, for example 2–3h, to ascertain progress.
- Assess maternal blood pressure and pulse half hourly.
- Monitor maternal temperature and urine output 2h.
- Encourage the woman to take fluids and light snacks. However, narcotics used for analgesia in labour seem to delay stomach emptying.
- Be guided by the woman's choice for analgesia. Assist the woman to use upright positions and some non-pharmacological methods of pain relief. However, contractions augmented by oxytocin may be experienced as more painful than those of spontaneous labour.
- If a normal delivery is not achieved within the set time frame, inform the obstetric registrar.

Measures to assist birth

The midwife may be required to assist the obstetric team when an instrumental (ventouse or forceps) or caesarean delivery is necessary.

When caring for a woman in labour, the midwife should report the following to the obstetric registrar:

- FHR irregularities or abnormalities of the CTG occurring in the first or second stage of labour. The registrar may request FBS
- Delay in the first or second stage when the labour does not respond to oxytocin
- Deterioration in the woman's condition.

It may be necessary to deliver the baby quickly. Caesarean section will be necessary to expedite birth in the first stage, after full dilatation ventouse or forceps delivery may be possible. If there is doubt about achieving delivery by forceps, trial in theatre may be arranged, with the anaesthetist and theatre team present. Caesarean section can follow immediately if forceps delivery fails.

Instrumental delivery: forceps

The decision to deliver by forceps is made by the registrar or consultant. Indication for forceps delivery, explanation of the procedure, and possible problems should be discussed with the parents, and their consent obtained. Provide support for the woman during the delivery by further explanation, prompting her as appropriate, and monitoring her needs.

Indications for forceps delivery include:

- Delay in, or no progress during the second stage, related to limited maternal expulsive effort and exhaustion
- Absence of the urge to 'push' because of epidural administration
- When excessive pushing may worsen pre-eclampsia or cardiac conditions
- When CTG is non-reassuring, the fetal head is below mid-cavity and delivery can be more quickly achieved with forceps
- If there is suspected mild malposition or asynclitism which might be corrected and delivery facilitated.

The obstetric registrar will want to know the following:

- Does the fetus feel, on abdominal palpation, to be a normal size? Could there be disproportion present? Is the fetal head 'well down'? Is there <1/5 fetal head palpable above the pelvic brim?
- On vaginal examination, is the cervix fully dilated? Is the station of the head below the spines (+1cm)? Is the moulding or caput minimal? Is the position occipito-anterior (OA)? Is the liquor clear and the FHR reassuring?
- Does the woman experience strong and sustained regular uterine contractions which achieve some descent of the head with maternal 'pushing' effort?
- Does the woman have adequate pain relief? Is the epidural effective? Is a pudendal block needed?

Preparation for the delivery:

- The birthing bed needs preparation, with facility for lithotomy position
- Delivery pack

- Eye protection
- Gown and gloves
- Instruments
- Local anaesthetic
- Syringes and sutures
- Catheterization pack
- Good light
- Stool
- Syntometrine® for the third stage, if appropriate
- Protection for the birthing bed
- Sanitary pads for the mother.
  There are three different types of forceps (Table 18.4).

Table 18.4 Types of delivery forceps

Wrigley's	Small size, for 'lift out' from lower cavity
Neville Barnes	Straight, mid-cavity, at least pudendal block required
Kielland's	Mid-cavity rotational forceps, epidural essential

Procedure
- If the woman has had an epidural, and there is no emergency, a top-up in the sitting position will give good perineal analgesia.
- Help the woman into the lithotomy position. Supine hypertension can be avoided if a cushion is placed to lift the woman slightly off her back. The partner may choose to sit beside her and give support.
- The registrar performs the procedure as a clean/sterile technique:
  - The bladder is emptied
  - Effectiveness of analgesia is assessed
  - The appropriate forceps are applied between contractions
  - Rotation of the fetal head is attempted if needed
  - When the forceps are safely in place, traction is applied with contractions and the woman encouraged to push
  - The obstetrician may perform an episiotomy as the fetal head distends the perineum
  - The baby should be delivered within two or three contractions
  - The forceps are removed when the head is delivered and the baby can be delivered on to the mother's abdomen.

Risks and complications
The baby
- Examine the baby for bruising and/or abrasions to the skin of the scalp and face caused by the curved blades of the forceps. If bruising is severe, jaundice may develop.
- Occasionally, VIIth nerve paralysis will occur and facial palsy will be apparent. This is due to pressure on the nerve as it is compressed against the ramus of the mandible.
- Reassure the parents that these complications will usually resolve within a few days.

- In a traumatic forceps delivery, cerebral irritability may occur due to cerebral oedema or haemorrhage. Cephalhaematoma may occasionally form as a result of trauma from forceps delivery (📖 see Examination of the newborn, p. 304).

The mother

- The mother may experience vaginal tears caused by the forceps.
- Perineal bruising, oedema, and occasionally haematoma may occur.
- Perineal trauma may be caused by extended episiotomy.
- Bruising and trauma to the urethra may cause retention or dysuria, haematuria, or incontinence.

Ventouse delivery

The application of a suction cup to the fetal scalp to facilitate delivery by traction is associated with less maternal trauma than forceps delivery.

The indications for ventouse delivery are the same as for forceps. The obstetrician will need the same information before proceeding and the midwife will make similar preparations for delivery. Training is now available for specialist midwives to become ventouse practitioners.

Selection of the ventouse extractor

- Electric pumps are efficient at maintaining the optimum vacuum pressure and are easy to operate, with a variety of cups available.
  - The usual size is 5cm silicon/rubber cup for a normal occipito-anterior presentation.
  - A posterior cup (which is metal and flatter in shape) is available for occipito-transverse or posterior positions.
- Hand-operated vacuum pumps may appear less anxiety provoking for the woman.
  - Examples are the Mityvac®, a cup for single use which can be attached to a handheld pump, and the Kiwi Omnicup, a small, totally disposable device.

Procedure

- Explain the procedure carefully to the woman and partner, and obtain consent. Keep them informed of progress.
- The maternal position used for delivery is lithotomy, as for forceps.
- Perform a vaginal examination and determine the position of the fetal head.
- Select an appropriate cup and apply to the fetal head at the midline, just in front of the occiput. The obstetrician will ensure that no cervix or vaginal tissue is trapped under the cup before applying suction.
- The vacuum is built up gradually from 0.2kg/cm to 0.8kg/cm (0.2kg/cm at 2min intervals).
- Once the optimum pressure is achieved, with a strong uterine contraction and maternal expulsive pushing, steady traction is exerted gently on the fetal head following the line of the pelvic axis (curve of Carus). Descent should occur and, if necessary, rotation to an anterior position may be achieved.
- An episiotomy is not usually needed. The head is controlled carefully during crowning. As soon as the head is delivered the vacuum is released. The body is delivered as normal.

Complications
- The cup may slip off and the procedure may fail.
- The baby will have trauma to the scalp as a result of the suction. A chignon develops, which is an area of bruising and oedema the approximate shape of the suction cup. This usually resolves without problem in a few days.
- Cephalhaematoma may occur and neonatal jaundice may develop.
- Retinal haemorrhage is a rare complication in the neonate.

Caesarean section

Types of caesarean section

Classical caesarean section
- This is used only in an emergency or when there is obstruction (placenta/fibroids) in the lower segment.
- It may be necessary to perform a caesarean section prematurely when the lower segment is not fully formed (before 32 weeks' gestation).
- The incision is made longitudinally in the upper segment of the uterus. Since the upper segment has a thick muscular structure, there is a higher incidence of excessive blood loss and rupture of the scar subsequently.

Lower-segment caesarean section
- This is the most common type of caesarean section.
- The lower segment is thinner and not so vascular, therefore blood loss can be less, with better healing, and lower infection rate. Cosmetically the 'bikini line' scar is more discrete and acceptable to women.

Caesarean section and hysterectomy
Very occasionally, in a severe emergency such as massive haemorrhage, uterine rupture, or an adherent placenta (placenta accreta) this might be necessary.

Some indications for planned/elective caesarean section
- Singleton breech presentation when ECV was ineffective or contraindicated.
- Transverse lie or malpresentation (such as brow presentation).
- Placenta praevia.
- A twin pregnancy when the first twin is breech.
- Triplets.
- HIV and hepatitis C.
- Genital herpes is present during the third trimester of pregnancy.
- Maternal request, for example, where there has been a previous delivery that caused physical or psychological trauma.

Plan of care
- Organize a consultant appointment to discuss the mode of delivery when the woman's pregnancy has reached about 36 weeks' gestation.
- The final decision should be made by a consultant obstetrician in conjunction with the parents.
- Give information clearly, in a way that can be understood by the parents.

Difference of opinion
- If a consultant declines a request for a caesarean section, the woman can request a second opinion.
- A competent pregnant woman can refuse a caesarean section even if she puts herself and her baby at risk.[1]

Arrangements for planned LSCS

- The timing of the caesarean section should ideally be after 39 weeks' gestation, to decrease risks of respiratory morbidity to the baby.
- The day before the planned caesarean section, the woman and her companion/partner may attend a clinic appointment or they may be seen on the antenatal ward.
  - At this visit the obstetrician verifies the rationale for the operation, clearly documents this in the woman's hospital notes, and obtains written informed consent from the woman. Document the information given to the woman.
  - Assess baseline observations of blood pressure, pulse, temperature and urinalysis. Review fetal well-being, this may include an ultrasound scan.
  - The anaesthetist reviews the general health of the woman. The type of anaesthetic is discussed and confirmed with the woman—usually spinal/regional anaesthesia. If a spinal anaesthetic is accepted, the partner may accompany the woman in theatre to provide support. General anaesthetic may occasionally be requested by the woman or be necessary if the regional anaesthesia proves inadequate.
  - Obtain FBC and G&S and send for testing. However, NICE guidelines suggest that G&S is not necessary for a healthy woman with an uncomplicated pregnancy.[1]
  - During the caesarean section antibiotics should be given to the woman, therefore carefully document any allergy.
  - Low-molecular-weight heparin (enoxaparin) will be prescribed prophylactically to help prevent deep vein thrombosis.
  - Ranitidine 150mg is prescribed 8h. Usually two doses prior to caesarean section. This minimizes the amount of gastric acid produced. Ensure that the woman understands the need to take no food/drinks for at least 6h before the caesarean section.
  - Explain the procedure, the immediate postoperative care, and the probable length of hospital stay. It should be recognized that while some women will feel content to experience caesarean section, others may miss the sense of achievement a normal delivery can afford. Be sensitive to this, listen, and answer questions.
  - Give the woman and her partner an appropriate time at which to attend the ward prior to the caesarean section.
  - If the woman has a BMI >35 theatre staff should be made aware.

On the day of the caesarean section

  - Ideally, the woman and her partner should be welcomed by a midwife who is known to them. Throughout the procedure, the midwife should keep the couple informed of events affecting care.
  - The midwife should prepare the woman for theatre. The woman may wish to have a bath. A shave of the skin area affected by the caesarean section scar might be considered necessary. Provide a clean theatre robe, cap, and anti-embolic stockings. Place an identity label on the woman's wrist and remove all jewellery or cover it with adhesive strapping. Reassess maternal observations and listen to the fetal heart.

- Give sodium citrate, 30mL orally, prior to transfer. This neutralizes the gastric acid.
- Prepare documentation according to local protocol.
- Escort the woman and her partner to theatre where the theatre staff, obstetrician, and anaesthetist should welcome them.
- The anaesthetist sites an IV infusion and spinal anaesthetic. When the woman is positioned for the operation, the theatre table is tilted, or a wedge placed to facilitate a slight left lateral position, to prevent supine hypotension.
- When the woman is comfortable and the spinal anaesthetic is effective, insert an indwelling urinary catheter, since the bladder must be empty prior to the caesarean section. This will remain in place for 24h.
- Seat the partner so that support may be given to the woman during surgery. Sensitively describe and explain the proceedings while preparing baby resuscitation equipment and warm towels.
- Note the time of the start of the operation. The surgeon divides the skin, fat, rectus sheath, abdominal muscle, abdominal and pelvic peritoneum, and uterine muscle. Once the uterus is opened, the amniotic fluid is aspirated and the baby is quickly delivered. Occasionally it is necessary to use forceps to deliver the head. The operator places the baby on a sterile towel. Dry him or her well, note the time of delivery, assess the Apgar scores, wrap the baby and, if in good condition, give to the parents to cuddle. If there is concern about the baby, call the paediatrician.
- IV oxytocin is given to the woman to facilitate the delivery of placenta and membranes. Prophylactic antibiotics (e.g. 1.2g co-amoxiclav) are given IV.
- The surgeon then repairs the wound using dissolvable sutures or clips to the skin.
- Diclofenac 100mg per rectum may be given for effective analgesia when the spinal anaesthetic wears off.
- If the woman's blood group is Rh-negative, take samples from the cord and from the woman 1h following delivery, as usual.

Immediately post delivery
- The midwife accompanies the family to a recovery area. One-to-one care is maintained.
- Assess maternal blood pressure, pressure, respirations, colour, and oxygen saturation (using pulse oximetry) every 15min until stable. Take her temperature 2h. MEWS may be used.
- Every 30min, assess:
  - Is there any oozing from the wound?
  - Is the uterus well contracted?
  - Is the vaginal loss of blood excessive?
- Monitor fluid balance. Continue the IV infusion (e.g. 1000mL Hartmann's solution) as prescribed by the anaesthetist. Urine output from the catheter drainage should be at least 30mL hourly.
- Ensure that the woman is comfortable and give analgesia as prescribed by the anaesthetist. Diamorphine 5mg hourly may be given via a

subcutaneous cannula (NICE guidelines suggest epidural/intrathecal diamorphine).[1]

- Attend to the woman's hygiene needs. The woman should continue to wear anti-embolic stockings.
- The woman may take sips of water orally, if the observations are within the normal limits and the woman is well. Further fluids can be given at 1h and thereafter food as the woman feels hungry.[1]
- As soon as it is practical, the baby is placed in skin–skin contact with the mother and she should be given opportunity to initiate breastfeeding.

Emergency LSCS

Complications can occur in pregnancy and labour which may necessitate an emergency caesarean section.

Some indications

In pregnancy:
- Severe pre-eclampsia
- Severe IUGR
- Haemorrhage related to placental abruption when the fetus is still alive.

In labour:
- There is no/limited progress
- Induction of labour fails
- There is apparent scar dissonance during a trial of labour after previous caesarean section
- There is apparent fetal compromise
- There is a prolapse of the cord.

The urgency of the caesarean section

- Immediate threat to the woman or fetus.
- Maternal or fetal compromise which is not immediately life-threatening.
- Needs early delivery but no maternal or fetal compromise.
- Delivery to suit the woman and partner or staff/unit.[1]

In cases of suspected acute fetal compromise, delivery should be achieved in 30min.[1] A general anaesthetic may be necessary in acute emergency, or when the woman requests it.

During emergency LSCS, prioritise:

- Explanation to the parents of the need for caesarean section and informed consent.
- Communication with, and support for, client, obstetrician, anaesthetist, theatre staff, porters, support staff, and paediatrician.
- IV access using large-bore cannula and blood for FBC/G&S or cross-match.
- Medication: sodium citrate 30mL, to neutralize stomach acid.
- Matters of hygiene, privacy, and safety.
- Catheter to bladder.
- Positions of comfort for the woman and measures to reduce risk of deep vein thrombosis.
- A call to the paediatrician if opiates have been given to the woman (within 4h), the woman has a general anaesthetic, there is meconium liquor, or suspected fetal compromise.

- A cord blood sample for assessment of fetal pH post delivery (📖 see Cord blood samples: fetal pH at delivery, p. 437).
- Clear documentation of urgency, time of decision, and delivery.
- High-dependency support for a woman immediately following general anaesthesia.

Complications of caesarean section

- Haemorrhage that could lead to shock. This may be manifest during the surgery, immediately post delivery, or may result from a slow, initially undetected blood loss due to internal bleeding or PV trickle. Occasionally retained products may cause bleeding.
- There is a risk of deep vein thrombosis which can result in pulmonary embolism.
- Damage/bruising during the operation is possible and may include bladder and ureters. Urinary tract infection may occur or urinary tract trauma may cause a fistula and leaking urine.
- Trauma to the colon is possible.
- There is a risk of infection, endometritis, or breakdown of the wound.
- Complications of general anaesthesia may occur. The effects of progesterone on the gastrointestinal tract lead to delayed emptying of the stomach. During induction of general anaesthesia, silent regurgitation may occur and cause aspiration into the lungs and chemical pneumonitis. This impairs breathing and can be serious—a cause of maternal death.

1 National Institute for Health and Clinical Excellence (NICE) (2004). Caesarean section. Clinical guideline 13. London: NICE. Available at: 🔗 www.nice.org.uk/cg13.

Breech delivery

A breech delivery will usually take place in a hospital maternity unit with experienced obstetricians and facilities for operative measures should this become necessary. It is customary for most known cases of breech to be delivered by elective LSCS.[1] ECV may be offered at 36–38 weeks, depending on parity and the position of the placenta. An undiagnosed breech in labour is usually delivered by emergency LSCS. However, it may sometimes be necessary to perform a vaginal breech birth, or the woman may choose to give birth vaginally. 📖 See Breech presentation, p. 160.

Management of labour: first stage

- The first stage often proceeds normally as with a cephalic presentation, particularly if the breech is engaged in the pelvis.
- Sometimes the breech may not be well applied to the cervix resulting in a long latent phase.
- Augmentation of labour is not recommended. If progress during established first stage is limited, caesarean section might be considered.
- Where the breech is not engaged, it is probably in a flexed position. This poses a risk of early rupture of the membranes and cord prolapse. IV access should be established and FBC and G/S taken.
- In either situation, perform a vaginal examination to exclude cord prolapse and assess progress.
- Monitor the fetal heart continuously and observe carefully maternal condition and progress in labour. Encourage maternal mobility as much as possible.
- Epidural anaesthesia may be recommended for pain relief but those caring for the woman should give consideration to maternal choice. The breech may tend to slip through the cervix before full dilatation. This may result in a premature urge to push, so that the larger diameter of the fetal head gets delayed because of the partially dilated cervix. This could lead to serious delay in the second stage. If epidural anaesthesia is in place, descent may occur more steadily and slowly and the woman will not use her pushing instincts prematurely. However, epidural may restrict mobility and inhibit positions for comfort and facilitation of a breech delivery.
- Where an epidural is not *in situ*, the woman may be helped with inhalational analgesia to avoid premature pushing. She may wish to adopt alternative positions.
- Ranitidine may be prescribed throughout labour in view of the possibility of a general anaesthetic.
- On vaginal examination, the breech feels soft and irregular with no palpable sutures. This may be mistaken for a face presentation. The anus or external genitalia may be felt. In a flexed breech, a foot may be felt. The fetus may well pass meconium.

Mechanism of labour

- The lie is longitudinal.
- The attitude is one of complete flexion.
- The presentation is breech.

- The position is the right/left sacro-anterior/posterior.
- The denominator is the sacrum.
- The presenting part is the anterior buttock.
- The bitrochanteric diameter of 10cm enters the pelvis in the right or left oblique diameter of the brim.

Movements
- Descent occurs with compaction due to increased flexion of the limbs.
- The anterior buttock meets the resistance of the pelvic floor and undergoes internal rotation through 45° to the anterior. The bitrochanteric diameter is then in the antero-posterior of the outlet.
- With lateral flexion of the trunk, the anterior buttock escapes under the pubic arch, the posterior buttock sweeps the pelvic floor and the body is born. The shoulders are entering the brim at this stage in the same oblique diameter as the bitrochanteric diameter. The diameter of the shoulders measures approximately 11cm.
- The buttocks undergo restitution and external rotation. This is accompanied by internal rotation of the shoulders, bringing the bisacromial diameter into the antero-posterior diameter of the outlet. The anterior shoulder escapes under the pubic arch, the posterior shoulder sweeps the pelvic floor, and the shoulders are delivered.
- The head enters the pelvis in the transverse diameter and internal rotation of the occiput through 90° to the anterior is accompanied by forward rotation of the back. The occiput escapes under the pubic arch and the mentum, face, sinciput, and vertex sweep the perineum and the head is born.

Obstetric management of the second stage

- It is crucial that full dilatation is confirmed by vaginal examination prior to allowing the woman to push. Await the descent of the presenting part. It should be visible at the perineum before active pushing begins.
- Inform the obstetrician, anaesthetist and paediatrician of the impending birth.
- In a multigravida or a small preterm fetus, the delivery may be spontaneous with minimal intervention.
- The lithotomy position may be adopted and sterile field prepared with drapes.
- Catheterization may be carried out to prevent delay and maximize the pelvic space.
- Preparation and equipment for a forceps delivery should be to hand but intervention should only be when strictly necessary. Allow spontaneous descent and birth.
- Infiltrate with local anaesthetic if needed when the buttocks distend the perineum.
- An episiotomy should only be performed if necessary to facilitate the birth.
- The buttocks should be born spontaneously.
- The baby then descends up to the umbilicus without intervention, if the legs are flexed they will deliver quite easily.
- If the cord is under tension, ease a loop down to avoid unnecessary traction.

- With the next contraction, the shoulder blades appear, if the arms are flexed they will deliver easily.
- The shoulders rotate into the antero-posterior diameter of the outlet the body can be tilted towards the mother's sacrum to facilitate delivery of the anterior shoulder. The posterior shoulder sweeps the perineum and is aided by lifting the buttocks towards the mother's abdomen.
- It is important that the baby is held only around the pelvic girdle and handled as little as possible, to avoid trauma to internal structures.
- The head enters the pelvis in the transverse diameter, therefore the back is in a lateral position until restitution and internal rotation takes place.
- When the back has turned uppermost, allow the body to hang by its own weight, this encourages flexion of the head and rotation into the antero-posterior diameter of the outlet, when it meets the resistance of the pelvic floor.
- When the nape of the neck becomes visible, deliver the head. It is essential that the head is delivered in a controlled manner. Many obstetricians apply forceps, otherwise it the following techniques may be used.

Mauriceau–Smellie–Veit manoeuvre (Fig. 18.1a)

This technique is used when the head is extended and therefore flexion needs to be maintained.

- The baby's body is straddled over the operator's arm, the operator's hand is passed into the vagina and a finger is placed on each malar bone.
- The middle finger of the opposite hand is placed on the baby's sub-occipital region and the other fingers over the shoulders.
- Steady traction is then applied in the axis of the pelvis—first downwards and backwards, then downwards and forwards.

The Burns–Marshall technique (Fig. 18.1b)

- The baby's ankles are grasped and a steady traction is exerted as the baby's body is lifted upwards in the arc of a circle.
- When the nose and mouth are free, clear the airway.
- The perineum is supported so that the head can be delivered slowly.
- This method if used incorrectly may lead to over extension of the baby's neck. Its use is therefore not recommended.

Extended legs

- If the buttocks are not expelled, the operator's finger is inserted into the fold of the baby's anterior groin or both groins and slight traction applied during uterine contractions.
- When the popliteal fossae appear at the vulva, two fingers are placed along the length of one thigh, with the fingertips in the fossa.
- The leg is swept to the side of the abdomen and the knee is flexed by the pressure on its under surface.
- This is then repeated to deliver the second leg.

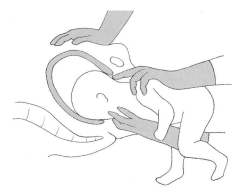

Fig. 18.1a Mauriceau–Smellie–Veit manoeuvre.

Extended arms, the Lövsett manoeuvre

If the arms are not across the chest as the trunk is delivered, they must be extended, this complication needs to be dealt with immediately as this will prevent delivery. This manoeuvre is the technique now used for dealing with extended arms. It is based on the premise that as a result of the curvature of the birth canal, the posterior shoulder must be at a lower level than the anterior shoulder, and that the subpubic arch is the shallowest part of the pelvis.

- The fetus is grasped by two hands around the pelvic girdle, the thumbs on the back and the fingers in the groins.
- By downward traction, the anterior shoulder is brought to lie behind the symphysis pubis and the posterior shoulder will then lie below the promontory of the sacrum, and therefore below the pelvic brim.
- The fetus is rotated through 180° so that the back always remains upwards.
- Moderate traction is used during rotation and by this manoeuvre the posterior shoulder is brought to the anterior and appears beneath the pubis.
- The arm may deliver spontaneously; if not, it may be hooked out by digital pressure.
- The shoulder that was previously anterior now lies posteriorly in the hollow of the sacrum.
- The fetus is then rotated 180° in the opposite direction, the back being kept uppermost.
- The other arm is then delivered.
- Syntometrine® must not be given until the head has been delivered.

Midwives and breech birth

- Occasionally the midwife may experience a planned or unexpected breech birth at home.

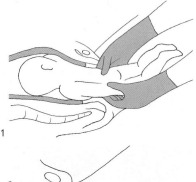

1

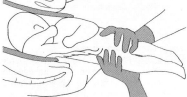

2

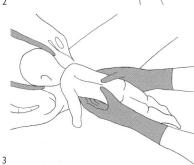

3

Fig. 18.1b Burns–Marshall technique.

- Expect meconium to be present. When fetal heart rate irregularities are present contact help from emergency obstetric services.
- Hands and knees ('all fours') position facilitates delivery. Also squatting and standing have been used according to maternal preference and comfort. Allow spontaneous pushing.
- The progress of the delivery should be observed and no touching of the breech is recommended unless there is a complication.
- Episiotomy may be performed if the midwife perceives this is needed.
- Extended legs should be allowed to birth spontaneously and the body to the umbilicus. Only handle the cord (very gently) if it is compressed or under tension.
- Let the baby's body take some of the weight and the chin will come to the perineum. After this the head will be born.
  - Gentle support might be given to the baby allowing the buttocks to rest on the midwife's cupped hands. This may slow the birth of the head a little and prevent sudden decompression.
  - The midwife should be familiar with the above manoeuvres.
  - A breech baby may be slower to breathe at delivery and resuscitation equipment should be ready.
  - Conduct third stage according to maternal preference.

Complications of breech delivery
- Increased risk of early membrane rupture.
- Increased risk of cord prolapse.
- Sometimes women experience premature urge to push.
- Hypoxia, anoxia, cord compression.
- Premature separation of the placenta.
- Intracranial haemorrhage: rapid decompression of the after-coming head.
- Fractures, nerve/muscle damage, rupture of internal organs.
- Oedema/bruising of feet and genitalia.
- Increased risk of operative delivery.
- Increased risk of perinatal morbidity and mortality.

1 Hannah ME, Hannah WJ, Hewson SA, et al. (2000). Planned caesarean section versus planned vaginal birth for breech presentation at term: a randomised multicentre trial. Lancet 356, 1375–83.

Retained placenta

The third stage is concluded when the placenta is delivered complete. If bleeding is not excessive, it is reasonable to wait for delivery of the placenta. If the placenta is undelivered after 30min (active management) or 1h (physiological) a diagnosis of retained placenta is made.

Causes

- The physiological third stage may be longer.
- During the active third stage, unless the placenta is delivered quickly by controlled cord traction, Syntometrine®/ergometrine may cause a constriction of the muscles of the lower segment and os, which prevents delivery until the action has worn off.
- The placenta may still be partially attached.
- Placenta accreta is when the placenta is morbidly adherent to the uterine wall.

Immediate management

- Inform the obstetrician if there is heavy blood loss. A partially adherent placenta where there is bleeding is an obstetric emergency.
- Assess by abdominal palpation whether the uterus feels contracted. If it feels 'boggy', lacking tone on palpation, and a contraction is not easily stimulated and intramuscular Syntometrine® has been given, inform the obstetrician. Otherwise:
  - Take any cord bloods required
  - Explain the problem to the mother. She may be pleased to breast feed the baby, which will encourage oxytocin release and stimulate uterine contractions. This may expel the placenta naturally
  - Ask the woman, if she is able, to sit upright on a bed pan and blow sharply into her fist (causing sudden downward movement of the diaphragm) or encourage maternal effort
  - Obtain permission from the woman to ensure an empty bladder by passing a urinary catheter.
  - If Syntometrine® has been used for active third stage, wait 30min and attempt controlled cord traction again.
  - If this fails or the cord snaps, manual removal in theatre is usually indicated.

Manual removal of the placenta

- Contact the registrar, theatre, and anaesthetist.
- Good analgesia is required. This means topping up an existing epidural, siting a spinal anaesthetic, or possibly a general anaesthetic.
- The procedure is explained to the woman and consent obtained.
- Accompany the woman during transfer to theatre.
- An IV infusion is sited using a large cannula and bloods taken for FBC and to cross-match two units of blood.
- The woman is placed in lithotomy position, aseptic precautions taken, and the bladder is catheterized. The obstetrician controls the fundus with the left palm on the abdomen and the right hand is passed into the uterus. The placenta is sheared off the uterine wall and removed on the palm of the hand.

- It is carefully examined to ensure it is complete.
- Prophylactic antibiotics should be given (e.g. cephalosporin and metronidazole).
- An IV infusion of oxytocin 20 units in 500mL normal saline over 4h is given.
- The woman is observed on the labour ward.
- An indwelling catheter should be inserted and left until the woman regains feeling in the lower limbs following anaesthetic and until she is fit for transfer to the postnatal ward.

Placenta accreta

Very rarely, if the placenta cannot be separated, it may be morbidly adherent.

- If it is totally adherent and bleeding has not occurred, it can be left *in situ* to absorb during the postnatal period.
- If partially adherent, there is a high risk of prolific haemorrhage.
- Operative treatment, and possibly hysterectomy, may be unavoidable.

Chapter 19

Emergencies during pregnancy, labour, and postnatally

Major obstetric haemorrhage

The definition of a major haemorrhage is an estimated blood loss of >1000mL or a blood loss which causes clinical shock in the woman.

Conditions that increase the risk of haemorrhage

- Placenta praevia
- Placental abruption
- Large or multiple uterine fibroids
- Previous PPH with complications
- Grand multiparity
- Multiple pregnancy
- Prolonged labour
- Polyhydramnios
- Precipitate labour.

Causes

- Uterine atony
- Trauma—lacerations and uterine rupture
- Retained placenta/morbidly adherent placenta[1]
- Rarely:
  - Uterine inversion
  - Coagulation problem.

Prevention and preparation

- Haemorrhage is a major cause of maternal morbidity and mortality in the UK and is increasing.[2]
- Women known to be at high risk should attend antenatal clinic to discuss prevention.
- Antenatal anaemia should be treated.
- Prepare a major haemorrhage pack and a well-rehearsed haemorrhage drill should be in place on the labour ward.
- Under certain circumstances (e.g. severe placenta praevia) cross-match several units of blood and have them immediately available before the woman's estimated delivery date (EDD).
- Ensure that blood is available when the woman at high risk of bleeding has been admitted to labour ward.
- Inform the obstetric and anaesthetic team and haematologist immediately on the arrival or delivery of a patient known to be at high risk.

Signs and symptoms

- Signs may be obvious:
  - Deterioration in the woman's condition
  - Visible copious bleeding vaginally
  - Bulky or soft, uncontracted uterus (postpartum).
- Sometimes signs are less apparent:
  - The woman looks pale
  - She feels cold and clammy
  - Her pulse is rising
  - Her blood pressure is falling.

- She may have nausea/fainting and be restless/drowsy
- Blood loss vaginally could be concealed.

Immediate care

- Call for the help of colleagues and the emergency obstetric/anaesthetic team and access the prepared pack.
- If undelivered, the woman should be laid flat, in the left lateral position, or lateral tilt, to minimize the effects of aorto-caval compression.
- Assess the airway and respiratory effort.
- Give oxygen via a facemask and monitor maternal oxygenation using a pulse oximeter.
- Site IV infusions (one in each arm) using large-bore (16 gauge) cannulae. Use normal saline followed by up to 1.5L of colloid (e.g. Gelofusine® or Haemaccel®) until blood is available. Increase the speed of IV infusion using a pressure bag. The aim is, over the first hour of care, to replace fluid lost and thereafter to replace continuing loss and maintain normal vital signs.
- Take blood samples and urgently request FBC, clotting screen, D Dimer, Kleihauer (if Rh-negative) and cross-match 4–6 units. If the oxygen saturation is low (<95%) in spite of oxygen given, an arterial sample may also be taken by the anaesthetist for blood gases.
- It might be necessary to give ABO- and Rh-compatible blood until fully cross-matched blood is available for the woman. It should be given via warming equipment, and a pressure bag can aid speedy administration.
- The haematologist will be involved. DIC may complicate obstetric haemorrhage and must be corrected (📖 see Disseminated intravascular coagulation, p. 410). If blood clotting irregularities are present, fresh frozen plasma (FFP, containing fibrinogen and all clotting factors), cryoprecipitate (containing fibrinogen and factor VIII), or platelets may be indicated.

Stabilization

- Record maternal pulse, blood pressure, oxygen saturation, and respiratory rate every 5min.
- Pass a urinary catheter. Monitor all fluid input, revealed blood loss, and urinary output.
- Document all drugs given and timing of events using a high-dependency recording chart.
- Support the anaesthetist to establish a central venous pressure (CVP) line and document readings. The CVP line avoids under-transfusion or fluid overload. The pressure is measured in the superior or inferior vena cava. An indication of the venous return is obtained.
- During stabilization, the obstetric team will investigate the cause and intervene to arrest the haemorrhage.
- A consultant obstetrician should be present for any elective or emergency surgery.
- Any anaesthetic should be administered or supervised by a consultant anaesthetist.
- Transfer to obstetric high-dependency unit (HDU) is always required when the patient is stable.

Major antepartum haemorrhage

- This is bleeding from the genital tract (after 20 weeks and before delivery) of greater than 500mL (or causing deterioration in the maternal or fetal condition).
- The haemorrhage is usually from the placenta. A placental abruption or bleeding placenta praevia is present. It may sometimes be concealed within the abdominal cavity.
- The aim is to resuscitate and stabilize the woman (as above), and assess fetal well-being as soon as possible.

If, on examination of the abdomen, you find that:

- The uterus is woody hard
- The woman is in continuous pain/experiencing strong contractions
- The fetal heart is heard;

the woman should be transferred immediately to theatre and the consultant obstetrician and team, anaesthetist, and paediatrician called.

- Prompt action is needed to save the fetus.
- Management depends on the maternal and fetal conditions and gestation.

Major postpartum haemorrhage

- This is bleeding from the genital tract of more than 500mL (or bleeding causing maternal compromise).
- In cases where there is a loss of 1000mL, admission to HDU is indicated.
- The primary PPH occurs immediately following delivery. Uterine atony is the most common cause. The uterus is soft, the fundus difficult to palpate, or high and full of blood clots.

Immediate care

- Call for help from the obstetric team.
- Explain briefly to woman and partner. Direct relatives to a suitable waiting point.
- Rub up a contraction:
  - Feel for the fundus of the uterus
  - If it is soft/relaxed, massage the fundus using a circular movement
  - A contraction should occur.
- Prepare for and start an IV infusion of normal saline 500mL with 40 units oxytocin at 125mL/h via a pump. The prescription may vary with local policy. FBC and cross-match 2–4 units blood urgently.
- Consider giving 250micrograms ergometrine IV.
  Avoid in hypertension, asthma, cardiac disease, impaired pulmonary, renal, or hepatic function.
- Or (in the above cases) use IV oxytocin 5 units slowly. IV oxytocin should be used with care when the woman is hypovolaemic. Given as a bolus it may cause dangerous profound hypotension.
- Catheterize the bladder and measure all fluid intake/output.

Investigate cause

- Deliver the placenta and expel blood clots with gentle pressure at the fundus.
- Consider whether any retained products remain, causing uterine atony.

- If measures fail to arrest bleeding, consider bimanual compression of the uterus, which will apply pressure to the placental site:
  - With the fingers of the right hand bent over, they are inserted into the vagina and the hand is made into a fist at the anterior vaginal fornix
  - The palm of the left hand is placed abdominally, using the tips of the fingers to lift the uterus slightly forward, to position the hand behind the uterus
  - The uterus is compressed between the left and the right hands.
- If the bleeding continues, accompany the woman with the obstetric team to theatre for exploration of the vagina, cervix, and uterus to exclude genital tract trauma, uterine inversion, or retained placental tissue.
- Inform the consultant obstetrician.
- If the haemorrhage continues, the consultant may prescribe/give Hemabate® (prostaglandin $F_2\alpha$) 250micrograms intramuscularly or directly into the myometrium.
  - Additional doses may be given up to a maximum of 2mg but always more than 15min apart.
  - Intramyometrial Hemabate® is given via a spinal needle trans-vaginally or trans-abdominally.
  - Side-effects include pyrexia, vomiting, hypertension.

❶ Caution in hypertension, asthma, cardiac disease, impaired pulmonary, renal, or hepatic function. Prostaglandins may be fatal if administered IV.

- Surgical procedures that may be attempted by the consultant obstetrician include the insertion of a Rusch balloon catheter into the uterine cavity:
  - The balloon is filled with warm saline
  - This packs the cavity and may arrest bleeding, and is left in place for 24h
  - Oxytocin 40 units in 1L of normal saline is given over 24h to maintain the uterine tone
  - Antibiotic cover is indicated.
- The obstetrician may call on vascular radiologist to perform pelvic arterial embolization.[2]
- A brace (B-Lynch) suture may be considered.[2]

In the most severe cases of bleeding, when other surgical techniques have been unsuccessful[3] and the patient is severely shocked, hysterectomy may be the only option.

Further reading

Arulkumaran S, Symonds IM, Fowlie A (2004). *Oxford Handbook of Obstetrics and Gynaecology*. Oxford: Oxford University Press.

1 Confidential Enquiry into Maternal and Child Health (2007). *Saving Mother's Lives: 2003–2005. The Seventh Report of the Confidential Enquiry into Maternal Deaths in the UK*. London: RCOG.

2 Confidential Enquiry into Maternal and Child Health (2004). *Why Mother's Die 2000–2002. The Sixth Report of the Confidential Enquiry into Maternal Deaths in the UK*. London: RCOG.

3 The Practice Development Team (2009). *Jessop Wing, Labour Ward Guidelines 2009–2010*. Sheffield: Sheffield Teaching Hospitals NHS Trust.

Table 19.1 Postpartum haemorrhage patient label

Action or observation	Time and recording
Time of delivery	
Time of bleed	
Time help arrived	
Airway—give O_2	
Breathing	
Circulation—blood pressure and pulse	
Site 2 large bore IV infusions	
Gelaflex®	
FBC, clotting, cross-match 2 units	
Check placenta is complete	
1. Rub up a contraction	
2. Catheterize bladder	
3. 20IU oxytocin in 500mL normal saline at 250mL/h	
4. IV ergometrine	
5. Hemabate® 250micrograms intramuscularly (senior opinion)	
Bimanual compression	
Check for trauma	
Check clotting screen	
Preparation for theatre	
Transfer to theatre	
Blood pressure and pulse	
Blood pressure and pulse	
Blood pressure and pulse (5 min intervals)	

Source: The Practice Development Team (2005). Sheffield Teaching Hospitals NHS Trust.

Uterine rupture

Definition
This is a dangerous complication of pregnancy and labour when there is a laceration of the uterine wall. Tears may extend to uterine vessels and haemorrhage ensue. Uterine rupture is a cause of maternal and fetal death.

Types
Incomplete
- The depth of the myometrium may be torn. The perimetrium remains intact.
- The external myometrium may be torn but the laceration does not extend into the body of the uterus. This may lead to intraperitoneal haemorrhage.

Complete
All layers of the uterus involved. There is direct communication between the uterine and abdominal cavity and the fetus may be expelled from the uterus into the abdominal cavity.

Factors associated with risk of rupture during labour
- Scar rupture following caesarean section (both lower and upper segment incision), hysterotomy, myomectomy, previous rupture repair. Scar dehiscence is the most common cause of rupture.
- Spontaneous rupture resulting from strong uterine contractions. It is sometimes associated with use of oxytocin, especially in multiparous women or with obstructed labour.
- Traumatic rupture from instruments, e.g. a high rotational forceps delivery or from manipulation (e.g. internal podalic version and breech extraction of second twin) when there is previous scarring.
- Trauma may occur as a result of accident.

Prevention
For women with a uterine scar
- On admission to labour ward the midwife should ensure that a birth plan discussion is documented in the notes by a senior obstetrician and that the woman is satisfied with the plan.
- If VBAC is anticipated good progress in labour should be observed and any fetal heart abnormalities reported to the obstetrician by the midwife.
- If augmentation of labour is indicated IV oxytocin must be prescribed by the registrar and administered with care.
- Induction should be overseen by a consultant obstetrician and proceedings documented carefully in the case notes. Amniotomy is the preferred method. However, one or two doses of dinoprostone gel 1mg PV (prostaglandin) may be given but repeat doses should preferably be avoided and further management discussed. Propess pessary may be used with caution—remove after 12h.[1]

Spontaneous rupture
- If oxytocin is used to induce or augment labour the midwife should be vigilant that contractions occur no more than four in 10min and last approximately 60s. The amount of oxytocin given should be carefully monitored in multiparous women.
- The midwife should consider disproportion or abnormal presentation when labour is delayed.

Signs and symptoms
Silent rupture
- Associated with previous caesarean section and partial scar separation: perhaps some blood loss PV but no haemorrhage at site of scar dehiscence.
- Mildly raised maternal pulse (>100bpm), pale.
- Some abdominal pain, scar tenderness. Epidural may sometimes mask the pain.
- Contractions may continue but no progress in labour.
- Irregularities of fetal heart, but, if diagnosed, fetus born alive.

Typical signs
- Develops over an hour or two
- Low abdominal pain, unlike contraction pain, continuous
- Tenderness on abdominal palpation
- Vomiting
- Faintness, pale
- Blood loss PV, variable amount
- Rising pulse
- Signs of fetal compromise, variable decelerations, bradycardia.
- If undiagnosed—hypotension and shock, absent FHR.

Violent rupture
- Strong uterine contraction. The woman reports 'something giving way' and sharp pain in lower abdomen.
- Contractions cease and the abdominal pain is continuous.
- The woman has a sense of foreboding that something serious has happened. She becomes anxious.
- Blood loss PV/haematuria.
- On abdominal palpation the fetus is felt close to the fingers and the presenting part can be moved easily and may not be in the pelvis.
- Maternal tachycardia, shock, and collapse soon occur.
- The FHR is profoundly bradycardic or absent.

Management
- Briefly explain to the woman and partner.
- Alert senior obstetric and anaesthetic team.
- The consultant should be called.
- Ensure IV access with large bore (16 gauge) cannula and commence IV infusion; infuse quickly.
- Give the woman oxygen via a face mask.
- Alert theatre staff to prepare urgently for laparotomy.

- Follow protocol for major obstetric haemorrhage. Cross-match six units (📖 see Major obstetric haemorrhage, p. 392).
- Transfer the woman to theatre immediately in the hope of delivering a live baby if the FHR is still recordable.
- 📖 See Emergency LSCS, p. 379.

Postnatally
- Admit the woman to HDU.
- Close monitoring of maternal condition especially fluid balance and oxygen saturation.
- Prescribe broad spectrum antibiotics for 5 days.

1 The Practice Development Team (2009). *Jessop Wing, Labour Ward Guidelines 2009–2010.* Sheffield: Sheffield Teaching Hospitals NHS Trust.

Eclampsia

- Eclampsia is rare: <1% of pre-eclamptic women have fits.
- Eclampsia can occur at any time in the second half of pregnancy. It may occur in labour or post partum.
- Cerebral oedema and spasm, clots, or haemorrhages in small arteries may be causative.
- Most women make a good recovery. However, some die or are left with permanent disability. The fetus is at risk of acute asphyxia and may die. Repeated or continuous fits carry high morbidity/mortality for mother and fetus, therefore prompt treatment and control is vital.

Signs and symptoms

- Headache and blurred vision, epigastric pain, nausea, and vomiting, drowsiness, or confusion may precede the onset of a fit. However, sometimes these types of symptoms occur after the fit, with no forewarning.
- Eclamptic convulsions appear similar to epileptic fits: repetitive, jerky, violent muscle spasms. Loss of consciousness occurs, the woman may hold her breath, bite her tongue, or be incontinent of urine.
- Convulsions last about a minute. If the fit continues status eclampticus ensues.

The midwife's response

- Call for senior obstetrician, anaesthetist, midwifery, and support staff.
- Ask for emergency eclampsia drugs and resuscitation equipment. You should know the location of these in your unit.
- Note the time of onset.
- Try to maintain a private, safe physical environment.
- Turn the woman to her left side and ensure a clear airway.
- Give oxygen at 4L/min via face mask.
- When possible, observe respiration, oxygen saturation, pulse and blood pressure and level of consciousness (see also Table 19.2).
- Talk to the woman, reassuring her of the presence of help and support.

Immediate management by the obstetric team

If a fit occurs, the mother must be stabilized before urgent delivery of the baby.

- Site an IV large-bore cannula and take blood for FBC, clotting, G&S, U/E and urates, LFTs.
- Seizures are controlled with a loading dose of magnesium sulphate 4 gm IV over 20min. Women treated with magnesium sulphate have fewer recurrent seizures than those treated with diazepam or phenytoin. However the latter may be used if the former is unavailable. The obstetrician may give 5–10 mg IV Diazemuls® over 2–5min.
- After the initial episode, transfer the woman, accompanied by the emergency team, to the HDU, to stabilize her condition further.
- The fetal heart should be monitored continuously—eclampsia and antihypertensive agents may cause abnormal fetal heart patterns.

- Give IV magnesium sulphate slowly to prevent further fitting:
  - After the initial loading dose of 4g IV; e.g. a bag of 50mL IV 5% glucose is used and 8mL of IV 50% magnesium sulphate added. It is infused over 20min.
  - Follow with a continuous IV regimen: magnesium sulphate 1g/h for 24h (e.g. use 150mL of 5% glucose and add 48mL of 50% magnesium sulphate; infuse at 8.3mL/h via an Alaris® pump).
- Monitor the woman for signs of toxicity:
  - Warm/flushing, slurring of speech, visual disturbance, nausea
  - Weakness, drowsiness, hypotension
  - Loss of deep tendon reflexes
  - Respiratory depression (14–16 respirations per min is minimum)
  - O_2 saturation reducing below 95%
  - If Diazemuls® and magnesium sulphate are administered in succession there is a risk of maternal respiratory depression.
- Refer side-effects to the consultant, discontinue infusion, and give oxygen. The obstetrician may wish to monitor $MgSO_4$ blood levels: therapeutic range is 1.5–2.5mmol/L.
- If the woman's diastolic blood pressure is >100mmHg, labetalol 20mg may be given by slow IV injection. Then maintenance therapy may be given:
  - The maternal diastolic blood pressure should be maintained at 95–105mmHg.
  - If the woman is asthmatic hydralazine may be used (🕮 see Maternal monitoring, management, and treatment, p. 336). Follow local protocols.

Occurrence of an eclamptic fit is the end-stage of the condition and the risks to the woman and fetus are too great to justify prolonging pregnancy.

- Urgent delivery, usually by caesarean section, will be arranged by the consultant obstetrician as soon as the woman's condition allows. However, induction may be attempted if the woman's condition remains stable with no further fits, the cervix is favourable for induction (Bishop score >6, 🕮 see Bishop score, p. 365), and delivery is likely to occur quickly—the presentation is cephalic and the CTG is reassuring.
- Make every effort to support the obstetric team in keeping the woman and family informed about care decisions.
- If the woman's condition deteriorates and fitting recurs or continues, the anaesthetist may sedate and ventilate the patient.

**Eclamptic seizure: example of chart
for emergency recordings**

Table 19.2 Eclampsia recordings

Action or treatment	Time and recording
Time of seizure	
Time help called	
Time help arrived	
Airway-left lateral, O_2	
Breathing	
Circulation—blood pressure, pulse, large bore IV infusion	
FBC, Clotting, G&S, U&E, LFTs	
Eclampsia tray	
Drugs (state)	
Blood pressure and pulse:1	
2	
3	
Time of transfer to HDU	
Monitoring fetal heart	

Source: The Practice Development Midwives (2009). Sheffield Teaching Hospitals NHS Trust.

Amniotic fluid embolism

- This is a rare condition affecting pregnant women, typically occurring during labour but can occur antenatally and up to 48h post partum. It may happen at amniocentesis, termination of pregnancy, or caesarean section.[1] It carries a high maternal mortality rate.
- Amniotic fluid enters the maternal circulation. Fetal skin cells or meconium in the amniotic fluid cause platelet thrombi to form blocking the pulmonary vessels. Pulmonary hypertension ensues ultimately leading to right-sided heart failure. Amniotic fluid may also cause DIC.

Possible predisposing factors or cause

- It cannot be predicted or prevented.
- There are similarities in blood pattern and clinical findings in anaphylactic and septic shock and amniotic fluid embolism.
- Intrapartum placental abruption.

Signs and symptoms

- A sudden change in the woman's behaviour or mood may be an early feature of the onset of hypoxia
- Maternal anxiety and feelings of doom
- Dyspnoea, tachypnoea, cyanosis
- Pink frothy sputum
- Hypotension
- Convulsions may occur (can precede respiratory symptoms)
- Bleeding PV/haemorrhage
- Shock/collapse.

Subsequent picture and complications

- Hypoxia may cause permanent neurological damage.
- Massive haemorrhage may occur as a result of DIC
  (📖 see Disseminated intravascular coagulation, p. 410).
- Acute renal failure as a result of hypotension.
- Anoxia and neurological damage to fetus.
- Death of both mother and fetus.

Management[2]

- The woman's life may depend on early detection and immediate action by the midwife.
- Call for emergency resuscitation team including obstetrician, anaesthetist. Inform haematologist and chest physician on call.
- Assess airway and breathing: give 100% oxygen via face mask initially. Use pulse oximeter.
- Assess blood pressure and pulse. For the maintenance of circulation and to combat hypotension site/help site an IV infusion. Diuretics and drugs which support the cardiac muscles to contract effectively (dopamine and digoxin) may be given to the woman.
- Take bloods and dispatch for FBC, cross-match 4 units, coagulation screen, U/E, blood glucose, blood culture, blood gases.
- Organize electrocardiogram (ECG) and portable chest X-ray.

- The anaesthetist may insert a pulmonary artery catheter to aid fluid replacement and monitor for fluid overload.
- After initial IV infusion has been given to improve the blood pressure the midwife may be asked to restrict fluids to prevent pulmonary oedema and respiratory distress.
- A urinary catheter is sited and strict fluid balance maintained. Output should be 25–30mL/h.
- Treat DIC: FFP and platelets should be administered immediately, or whole blood if available.
- It may be necessary for the anaesthetic team to intubate the woman to maintain adequate oxygenation.
- The team may need to deliver the baby by emergency caesarean section within 15min to minimize anoxia and prevent neurological damage to the baby and to facilitate maternal resuscitation.
- Cardiopulmonary arrest may occur which has a low rate of survival but if the woman survives, her condition will be monitored in intensive care.

Any suspected or proven case of amniotic fluid embolism should be reported to the UK register.

1 Arulkumaran S, Symonds IM, Fowlie A (2004). *Oxford Handbook of Obstetrics and Gynaecology*. Oxford: Oxford University Press.

2 The Practice Development Team (2010). *Jessop Wing, Labour Ward Guidelines 2010*. Sheffield: Sheffield Teaching Hospitals NHS Trust.

HELLP syndrome

(**H**, haemolysis; **EL**, elevated liver enzymes; **LP**, low platelets)
- This is an uncommon but severe complication of pre-eclampsia, although it is sometimes seen when hypertension is not present. It is a manifestation of impaired liver function.
- It may occur during the later stages of pregnancy, during or up to 48h after delivery. Diagnosis is confirmed by laboratory assessment of the blood coagulation pattern. There is a risk of maternal/fetal morbidity/mortality due to:
  - Impaired clotting, or bleeding
  - Severe liver damage, leading to failure or rupture
  - Severe kidney damage, leading to failure
  - Respiratory difficulties
  - Cerebral haemorrhage/convulsions
  - IUGR: premature delivery may be needed and intrauterine death may occur.
- Be aware of, and assess for:
  - Epigastric pain (severe, not relieved by antacid; liver tenderness)
  - Nausea and vomiting, headaches
  - Haematuria, jaundice
  - Blood slow to clot.
- Discuss management plans with a consultant obstetrician.

Diagnosis

- Blood samples to send for laboratory assessment include:
  - FBC/platelets
  - U/E
  - Clotting and DIC screen
  - LFTs
  - G&S and cross-match.
- Laboratory reports demonstrate the altered blood pattern:
  - *Haemolysis* (the breakdown of red blood cells). This process begins to occur faster than it would naturally. Severe pre-eclampsia causes damage to the vascular system. Changes occur in the liver. Platelets collect as the initial step of repair and fibrin networks form. Haemolysis results from damage that occurs as the circulating red cells are pushed through the fibrin networks. A reduction in red cell numbers occurs. Haematocrit (a measure of red cell concentration) may therefore decrease; bilirubin (a by-product of red cell breakdown) may increase.
  - *Elevated liver enzymes*. Intravascular fibrin deposits obstruct the flow of blood in the liver. The liver is under stress, therefore the liver enzyme levels become raised. Liver damage is indicated by raised alkaline phosphatase (APT), alanine transaminase (ALT), and AST.
  - *Low platelets* (<100×10^9/L). Platelets initiate and are essential to blood coagulation. In HELLP syndrome, clotting factors are mopped up and platelet levels in the blood decrease (thrombocytopenia). This is only treated if bleeding occurs.

Treatment

- Urgent delivery may be indicated.
  - Transfusion of platelets or blood may be necessary if the woman is bleeding.
  - Caesarean may be performed under general anaesthesia since regional anaesthesia may be contraindicated because of low platelets; however, intubation may increase blood pressure further.
- The aim of management is to support hepatic and renal function until the condition resolves.
  - IV glucose may be needed (10% glucose/500mL in 6h) to maintain blood glucose at 5+ mmol/L.
  - Accurate assessment of intake and output of fluids is paramount.
  - A CVP or arterial line will facilitate accuracy.

Be aware that the woman may have haemorrhage during and/or post caesarean. Ensure an adequate local supply of suitable cross-matched blood.

Disseminated intravascular coagulation

- DIC may occur as a secondary to severe pre-eclampsia and HELLP syndrome.
- Because of injury to vessel walls, blood clotting activity is abnormally increased. Fibrin is formed, resulting in a large number of small thrombi in the capillary circulation.
- As a normal reaction to clot formation, to maintain equilibrium, the body initiates a process of clot breakdown (fibrinolysis).
- In DIC, because clot formation is widespread a large number of fibrin degradation products (FDPs) are produced. These are also anticoagulants. Clotting factors and platelets are mopped up as the large number of microthrombi form.
- As a result, uncontrolled bleeding may occur, without clot formation.

Diagnosis

- Report:
  - Any unexpected bleeding from the nose or mucous membrane and oozing from a venepuncture site
  - Cyanosis of the extremities (fingers/toes).
- Laboratory tests of venous blood samples should demonstrate when a case of severe pre-eclampsia is beginning to be affected by DIC. Discuss the required frequency of testing with the obstetrician. It is usually daily.
  - The *D-dimer test* detects fibrin derivatives and therefore breakdown. FDPs should normally be 200ng/mL but in DIC can be >2000ng/mL. This is the most specific test for DIC.
  - *FBC and platelets.* Platelets are essential factors for coagulation of the blood and will be decreased in DIC (<100×10^9/L).
  - *Prothrombin time* (PT) measures the coagulation time of plasma (extrinsic clotting pathway). The normal range is 11–15s. In DIC this time may be increased.
  - *Activated partial thromboplastin time* (APTT) measures plasma coagulation (intrinsic clotting pathway). The normal range is 29–37s. This time may also be increased in DIC.
  - *Fibrinogen levels* detect the coagulation capacity of the blood. Fibrinogen is a protein formed in the liver. Thrombin activates fibrinogen to form fibrin. The normal range is 0–40g/L. It may be decreased in DIC.

Treatment

This is aimed at prevention and correcting the underlying problem, and therefore removing the trigger mechanism for DIC. If the blood pattern demonstrates rising FDPs, this would form part of the rationale for a speedy delivery.

- Unless FDP levels are very high, the presence of some clotting factors should stop bleeding.
- If treatment is considered necessary, for instance to prepare a woman for caesarean, a senior haematologist should be consulted.
- Treatment involves replacement of clotting factors in order to restore equilibrium.

Acute uterine inversion

Definition
This is a rare complication of labour. The uterus turns inside out and pro-lapses into the vagina. It happens suddenly during the third stage of labour. It can be a cause of maternal death because of shock and haemorrhage.

Factors associated with acute uterine inversion
- Adherent placenta
- Fundal placenta
- Short umbilical cord
- More common in primiparae
- Macrosomic fetus
- Atonic uterus (sometimes with sudden cough or sneeze)
- Distended uterus suddenly emptied.

Types of acute inversion
- Incomplete inversion when the body of the uterus does not extend beyond the cervical rim.
- Complete inversion when the body of the uterus extends as far as the introitus.
- Prolapse of the uterus through the introitus.

Prevention
- The reason why inversion happens is not fully understood. However, acute inversion may sometimes be aggravated by mismanagement of the third stage of labour.[1]
- The midwife should *never*:
  - Use fundal pressure to expel the placenta (Crede's manoeuvre)
  - Use excessive controlled cord traction (CCT)
  - Attempt to deliver the placenta without signs of separation
  - Use CCT when the uterus is relaxed
  - Use CCT omitting to guard the uterus with the left hand above the symphysis pubis.

Signs and symptoms
- The placenta may/may not be separated.
- Haemorrhage is usually present whether or not the placenta is separated.
- Shock due to:
  - Blood loss
  - Pain.
- On abdominal palpation the fundus of the uterus cannot be located or if inversion is incomplete a concave shape may be felt.
- A bluish, bleeding mass may be present in the vagina or at the introitus. It is the interior of the fundus of the uterus.
- Incomplete inversion is more difficult to identify. Extreme shock and pain (possibly caused by tension on the peritoneum, ovaries, and nerves of the broad ligament) may be out of proportion to the amount of haemorrhage and may be a clue to diagnosis.

Management
- Call for the obstetric and anaesthetic team.
- The best opportunity for replacing the uterus is as soon as the inversion occurs. This is especially important in the community situation. This will avoid blood loss and shock.
- The woman should be laid flat. The foot of the bed should be raised.
- The woman should be given an explanation to gain her consent and cooperation and have adequate analgesia.

Johnson's manoeuvre
- It may be possible to speedily reduce an inversion if the midwife recognizes the condition immediately and applies gentle pressure to the uterus starting at the point nearest to the cervix and working towards the fundus. Thus the inverted uterus is pushed back, following the angle of the vagina, through the cervix then directing the push upwards towards the umbilicus to restore the normal position.
- If the placenta is not delivered, and not bleeding it should be left *in situ* to avoid haemorrhage. The inverted uterus cannot contract.
- If the woman's condition is stable, there is some bleeding because of apparent separation and she has adequate analgesia the placenta can be removed if this facilitates repositioning.
- IV ergometrine 0.25mg or 5 units of oxytocin slowly administered will secure a good contraction once the uterus is established in place.

Shock
- If there is severe bleeding and hypotension the woman must be treated immediately and urgently for shock.
- Two IV infusions are sited using a large bore cannula, and IV fluid commenced to help fast replacement of fluid and allow administration of drugs.
- Respirations, pulse and blood pressure, and oxygen saturation are monitored.
- Bloods are obtained for FBC and platelets, G&S and cross-match, coagulation.
- Analgesia should be given urgently.
- Catheterize the bladder and monitor output.
- Transfer to theatre at the earliest opportunity.

Other methods to help replacement
- Manual replacement of the uterus may be complicated by the development of a retraction ring between upper and lower segments or a tight cervix. The anaesthetist may give IV drugs to relax the uterus such as terbutaline 0.25mg or ritodrine 6mg before the obstetrician attempts replacement. However, this relaxation of the uterus may also be achieved by giving the woman a general anaesthetic.
- Under general anaesthetic hydrostatic repositioning may be effective. The obstetrician replaces the inverted uterus in the vagina and 'seals off' the external labia with one hand. Several litres of warm saline are infused into the posterior vaginal fornix via an IV giving set. The fluid exerts pressure evenly over the uterus and pushes it back into position. The manual and hydrostatic methods may be used together.

- Operative procedures are successful as a last resort. Laparotomy may be necessary under general anaesthetic. Forceps are placed on the round ligaments. The obstetrician pulls gently on the ligaments while a second operator pushes the uterus upwards from the vagina.
- The hand is kept inside the uterus until oxytocin (for example: Syntocinon® 5U IV) has produced a firm effective contraction.
- Oxytocin (e.g. IV Syntocinon® 20U in 500mL normal saline via a pump over 4h), should then be administered to keep the uterus contracted and to prevent recurrence.
  ❶ IV oxytocin should be used with caution in hypovolaemia.

Post partum

- The woman should be observed in a high dependency area until stable.
- Broad-spectrum antibiotics should be given for 5 days minimum.

1 Arulkumaran S, Symonds IM, Fowlie A (2004). *Oxford Handbook of Obstetrics and Gynaecology.* Oxford: Oxford University Press.

Shock

Collapse, due to failure of the woman's circulatory system; the body is unable to receive oxygen and nutrition and to excrete waste. Acute shock must be reversed quickly to avoid chronic conditions and death.

Causes specific to childbearing
- PPH
- Uterine rupture or inversion
- Undiagnosed intra-abdominal or genital tract haematoma
- Amniotic fluid embolism
- Eclampsia.

Causes that may complicate childbearing
- Thromboembolism
- Pulmonary embolism, pulmonary oedema, Mendelson's syndrome
- Sepsis (endotoxic/bacteraemic shock)
- Allergy (anaphylactic shock)
- Metabolic or endocrine (e.g. diabetic collapse)
- Haemorrhage from organ rupture or aneurysm
- Epilepsy, cerebrovascular accident, subarachnoid haemorrhage
- Heart failure, arrhythmias, myocardial infarction (📖 see also Cardiac conditions, p. 182)
- Substance misuse or overdose.

Signs and symptoms
- Pale, cold, clammy, fingernails blue grey
- Dry mouth, thirsty
- Initially blood pressure is maintained then it falls
- Increasing pulse rate: thready and weak
- Increased respiratory rate: fast and shallow
- Oliguria, anuria if low blood pressure (systolic <80mmHg) continues
- Dizzy, restless, lethargic, sometimes in acute pain
- Mood change, altering consciousness.

Management
The first priority is resuscitation, but, at the same time, it is necessary to think about cause, so that treatment can be given.
- Call for emergency equipment and help from the obstetric and anaesthetic team.
- Explain briefly to the woman's partner, and acknowledge anxiety. Give information as available.
- Position the woman flat or in recovery position if semi-conscious.
- Assess breathing and give oxygen via face mask.
- Assess vital signs, blood pressure, pulse, oxygen saturation.
- Site, or help site, large-bore (14 gauge) IV cannulae, enough to replace fluids.
- Take blood as indicated and requested by the obstetrician for FBC, G&S or cross-match, U/E, LFTs, coagulation screen, blood cultures, or blood glucose.

- Support the anaesthetist to take and dispatch any arterial bloods for blood gases, to site a CVP line, and monitor readings.
- Catheterize the woman and measure urine output hourly. Anuria, oliguria, and blood staining of the urine indicate low renal blood flow.
- Help the team to facilitate speedy delivery of the baby if necessary.
- Assist the obstetrician to perform a full clinical, including neurological, examination.

Addressing the cause of shock

Be ready with the following information at the onset of collapse, to help with diagnosis of the cause:

Has the woman:
- Delivered baby and placenta?
- Had excessive blood loss?
- Been in pain, if so what area of the body?
- Had a fit?
- Any medical history of, for example, PIH, diabetes, epilepsy, heart condition?
- Been given any medication?
- Had pyrexia?

Haemorrhage

Diagnosis of haemorrhage (see p. 392).

Septic shock

Diagnosis of septic shock during labour may depend on careful observation and documentation of signs by the midwife. Document and report any persistent temperature >38°C. Such pyrexia is associated with cerebral palsy in the infant.
- It usually begins with pyrexia, a restless mental state with warm, flushed complexion. Then hypotension, tachycardia, cold extremities, cyanosis, tachypnoea, jaundice, and coma may occur as late signs.
- Predisposing factors include prolonged rupture of membranes, operative delivery, manual removal of placenta, and pyelonephritis.
- Organisms associated with septic shock include:
  - *Escherichia coli*
  - *Klebsiella* sp.
  - *Proteus mirabilis*
  - *Pseudomonas aeruginosa*
  - *Staphylococcus aureus*
  - *Bacteroides* sp.
  - Streptococcus
  - Group A β-haemolytic streptococcus.
- When sepsis is a possible cause of shock in labour, obtain MSU, high vaginal swab, and introital and rectal swabs and send for urgent culture.
- Obtain blood cultures. Take venous blood samples for FBC and platelets, clotting, U/E, and LFTs and send for screening.
- Arrange chest X-ray.
- Commence IV antibiotics (e.g. piperacillin, tazobactam, netilmicin) after taking cultures. Consult the microbiologist.

- Severe septic shock may precipitate DIC (📖 see Disseminated intravascular coagulation, p. 410).
- Admit to high dependency area for observation and care by a midwife. Very rarely, you may see the following.

Anaphylactic shock

- This occurs because the woman has been exposed to an antigen against which she has been previously sensitized. The body releases histamine when challenged with the antigen, which dilates arteries and makes capillaries more permeable.
- The blood pressure falls and signs of shock are present.
- Typically this may occur following the administration of medicines such as anaesthetic agents or antibiotics.
- Adrenaline or ephedrine may be given by the anaesthetist.

Cardiorespiratory collapse

- A fall in cardiac output occurs as a result of heart failure. Venous return is reduced. The lungs become congested with blood.
- Arrange chest X-ray, arterial gases, ECG, FBC, U/E.

Neurological conditions

- Indicated by an alteration in consciousness when cardiorespiratory signs are not present.
- A magnetic resonance imaging (MRI) scan of the brain may be needed.

Diabetic collapse

- The woman will typically be an insulin-dependent diabetic.
- The woman may become uncooperative, distant, and confused.
- She will feel faint, sweating but clammy.
- Give a drink with sugar if possible—unconsciousness will not then occur. If it does, it is quickly reversed by a glucagon injection or IV glucose fluids.

Maternal resuscitation

Cardiopulmonary arrest is estimated to occur once in every 30 000 late pregnancies;[1] the outcome can be poor for both mother and unborn child. Basic resuscitation skills are an essential requirement of all midwives, who should be familiar with resuscitation guidelines and the location and use of resuscitation equipment provided.

Although the incidence of arrest is low, there are emergency situations that may result in cardiopulmonary arrest necessitating resuscitation:

- Anaphylaxis
- Amniotic fluid embolism
- Cerebral aneurysm
- Eclampsia
- Embolism
- Epilepsy
- Haemorrhage
- Cardiac disease
- Placental abruption
- Pulmonary embolism
- Ruptured liver/spleen
- Septic shock
- Thromboembolism
- Total spinal
- Uterine rupture
- Uterine inversion.

Responsibility of the midwife

- Provide effective basic life support to ensure adequate circulation and perfusion of vital organs.
- Participate in, and often initiate, advanced life support.

In pregnancy

- Oxygen consumption is increased, therefore oxygen supply to the brain will diminish more rapidly than in a non-pregnant person.
- To optimize fetal outcome, support should be given to the mother.
- Basic life support should be initiated immediately.

Resuscitation in a hospital setting

If a woman collapses or is found collapsed:

- Pull the emergency buzzer/shout for help.
- Assess responsiveness. Gently shake her shoulders and shout.
- If she **responds**:
  - Send for medical assistance
  - Position in left lateral
  - Maintain airway
  - Give oxygen
  - Monitor vital signs
  - Consider venous cannulation
  - Stay with her until medical review and investigations.

- If there is **no response**, check breathing and circulation. This can be done simultaneously. Take no more than 10s.

Airway

With your hand on the woman's forehead, gently tilt her head back, remove any visible obstruction from the mouth, place your fingertips on the point of her chin and lift the chin to open the airway. If trauma to the head or neck is suspected, avoid this head tilt manoeuvre. Instead jaw thrust should be performed.

Breathing

- **Look** for chest movements.
- **Listen** for breath sounds.
- **Feel** for air on your cheek.

Circulation

- Feel for a carotid pulse.
- If she is not breathing, ensure that the cardiac arrest team has been called, and the defibrillator and emergency equipment have been sent for.
- If pregnant, position on to back and support the woman using pillow or wedge in a left-sided 30° tilt.
- Commence cardiopulmonary resuscitation (CPR).
- CPR should be commenced with 30 chest compressions, observe chest movements.
- If no definite pulse was felt, commence chest compressions at a rate of 100/min.

  To perform chest compressions: place the heel of one hand over the lower half of the sternum, place the heel of the other hand on top of the first hand, and extend or interlock the fingers. Do not apply pressure over the ribs, upper abdomen, or tip of the sternum. From above the woman, with arms straight, press down to depress the sternum 4–5cm. Release the pressure and repeat at a rate of about 100/min. Take equal time with compression and release to allow the chest to recoil.

- After 30 compressions check the airway position and give two more breaths. Continue this ratio of two breaths to 30 compressions until advanced life support is in place. In the ideal situation it would be advisable to deliver cardiac compressions continuously without pauses as this increases the chances of survival. This is only possible once an endotracheal tube or advanced airway has been placed.
- If other staff are present while waiting for the arrest team to arrive they should:
  - Apply ECG monitor/defibrillator pads
  - Monitor pulse oximetry
  - Monitor blood pressure
  - Cannulate using ×2 large bore Venflon®
  - Obtain bloods for urgent cross-match, FBC, coagulation screen, U/E, blood glucose, LFTs, and arterial blood gas
  - Make notes of times, actions, and any fluid/drug treatment.

Considerations in pregnancy

Airway

It may be difficult to maintain an airway, and intubation may be difficult due to:

- Neck obesity
- Enlarged breasts
- Glottic oedema.

A bag-valve-mask is preferred, with two staff working together; one holding the mask and maintaining the airway and the other giving inflation breaths and chest compressions. If a pocket mask is nearby, use this until more help and equipment arrives, connect to oxygen as soon as possible. If the woman is unconscious a Guedal airway can be used to help maintain the airway.

Breathing

Due to delayed gastric emptying, reduced tone of stomach muscle sphincter, and increased pressure on the stomach from gravid uterus, there is an **increased risk of regurgitation and pulmonary aspiration**. Early intubation using cricoid pressure is preferable.[2] Until the airway is protected by the insertion of a cuffed tracheal tube, aspiration can occur. Give each ventilation slowly over 2s, with volumes just sufficient enough to produce a visible chest rise (400–600mL). Allow the chest to deflate following each breath.

Circulation

There is an increased circulatory demand in pregnancy.

- Prevent aorto-caval compression: pressure on the major vessels should be relieved by left lateral displacement of the uterus. This will improve venous return and cardiac output. Placing a Cardiff wedge or pillow under the right side will achieve this by tilting the woman by approximately 30°. Alternatively, raising her right hip, or manual displacement of the uterus to the left and upwards, will suffice until suitable equipment arrives.
- Chest compression may be more difficult in this position.

Advanced life support

Treat arrhythmias according to standard protocols.

- Avoid lidocaine when epidural anaesthesia has been used, as high levels of local anaesthetic may be present in the blood. Amiodarone is an alternative antiarrhythmic drug.
- If 5min of in-hospital resuscitation is unsuccessful, emergency caesarean section is indicated to save the fetus (in the third trimester) and improve the prognosis for the mother. Advanced life support should continue during and after the procedure.[2]

Resuscitation out of the hospital setting

Follow basic life support guidelines, assess responsiveness and breathing. If no response and no breathing, send for medical assistance. An emergency ambulance should be sent for, clear instructions are important stating 'I have an unconscious, pregnant woman who is not breathing, we are at [address]', as this should influence the type of assistance that is sent.

In the home setting a partner, friend, or neighbour could be given clear instructions and asked to call an ambulance. If alone and without the use of a phone, you will have to decide whether to start resuscitation or go for help. This might be influenced by the condition/cause of collapse and available equipment; however, if there is no breathing and/or pulse it is advisable to call medical assistance before attempting resuscitation, to ensure that advanced life support and defibrillation are available as soon as possible. If the likely cause of unconsciousness is a breathing problem, i.e. drugs/alcohol, 1min of CPR should be performed before going for help. If you are alone, you may need to use your knee to tilt the woman onto her left side; a cushion or clothing might have to be used while you call for assistance. On arrival of the ambulance basic life support should continue. Advanced life support may be initiated, depending on the skills of the team that arrives, and the woman should be transferred to hospital as soon as possible. The hospital should be notified of her pending arrival so that preparations can be made.

Cross-infection

All community midwives should carry equipment that will protect them when performing basic life support. Key fobs are available containing a single-use mask which, when placed over the victims mouth to perform mouth-to-mouth resuscitation will give some protection against cross-infection. Pocket masks are also available with one-way valves, which will prevent transmission of bacteria. In the hospital the midwife should wait for equipment to arrive before attempting ventilations. Chest compressions can be performed while waiting. Gloves and eye protection must be worn, and considerable care taken with needles and sharp instruments.

Jaw-thrust manoeuvre

Used to open the upper airway with minimal movement of the cervical spine. Using both hands, place the forefingers behind the angle of the jaw. Keeping the head and neck still, push the jaw forward and upwards, this will push the tongue forwards and away from the pharynx.

Further reading

Resuscitation Council (UK). (2010). *Resuscitation Guidelines 2010*. Available at: http://www.resus.org.uk/pages/guide.htm (accessed 28.2.11).

1 Jevon P, Raby M (2001). *Resuscitation in Pregnancy. A Practical Approach*. Oxford: Reed Educational and Professional Publishing.

2 The Practice Development Team (2010). *Jessop Wing HDU Skills Development* (2010). Sheffield: Sheffield Teaching Hospitals NHS Trust.

Guidelines for admission to HDU

Policy for admission may vary between units depending on facilities and available personnel. Admission to the HDU should be considered in the following situations:

- Ante- or postnatal hypertensive women whose condition is deteriorating. For example, when the blood pressure is difficult to control, LFTs are abnormal, and signs of fulminating pre-eclampsia or cerebral agitation are present
- Women who experience major haemorrhage which is causing maternal compromise
- Women who experience blood loss of 1000mL or more
- Women suspected of having pulmonary embolism or having signs of respiratory distress, hypoxia, tachycardia
- Following LSCS, when the woman has insulin-dependent diabetes mellitus and a sliding scale with insulin and glucose is in progress
- Any woman having had general anaesthesia
- Women who receive diamorphine via epidural catheter
- Women showing signs of shock, septicaemia, anaphylaxis
- Status epilepticus
- Women diagnosed with pulmonary oedema or suspected amniotic fluid embolism
- Any woman requiring continuous oxygen therapy
- Women suffering from HELLP syndrome or DIC (☐ see Disseminated intravascular coagulation, p. 410)
- Any woman with an underlying medical or surgical condition which is compromising maternal condition, e.g. known symptomatic heart condition
- Cardiac arrhythmia requiring continuous ECG monitoring
- Women requiring CVP or arterial line
- Woman transferred back from a general ITU.

Guidelines for transfer out of HDU to ITU

The woman requiring intensive care is unstable and requires multiple organ monitoring/support. The level of dependency is an important factor in determining appropriateness of intensive care. A woman needs urgent attention in the following situations (if there is no improvement in 2h, seek consultant review for transfer to ITU):

- Women with chronic impairment of one or more organ systems, sufficient to restrict daily activities, and who require support for an acute reversible failure of another organ system
- A woman not responding to commands
- The woman with deteriorating respiratory rate not responding to treatment:
  - Inability to maintain own airway
  - Requiring advanced respiratory support
  - Oxygen saturation of <90% despite 60% inspired oxygen.
- Pulse of <40bpm or >130bpm
- Oliguria: urine output of less than 30mL/h for 3 consecutive hours.

Maternal mortality

The *Confidential Enquiry Into Maternal and Child Health*[1] (CEMACH) reported 391 maternal deaths between 2000 and 2002. The purpose of the enquiry is to assist in identifying factors that may be detrimental to maternal health and to assist in improving the care that mothers receive in pregnancy and when they are newly delivered. The most common cause of direct death was thromboembolism, with an increased rate as a result of haemorrhage and those associated with anaesthesia. The most common cause of indirect death, and the largest cause of maternal deaths overall, was psychiatric illness.

The CEMACH report[1] aimed to evaluate all the factors playing a part in women's deaths, and further analysis reinforces the need to ensure that maternity services are designed to meet the needs of all women and, in particular, those who are vulnerable or disadvantaged in any way. Risk factors for maternal deaths are identified as follows.

- Social disadvantage: women were up to 20 times more likely to die if they lived in families where both partners were unemployed, compared to those from more advantaged groups. Single mothers were three times more likely to die than those in stable relationships.
- Poor communities: in the most deprived areas of England, women had a 45% higher death rate compared with women from more affluent areas.
- Minority ethnic groups: women from groups other than white were three times more likely to die. Black African women, including asylum seekers and newly arrived refugees, had a seven times higher mortality rate than white women and had problems accessing the service.
- Late booking or poor attendance: 20% of the women who died booked for care after 22 weeks, or had missed over four routine antenatal visits.
- Obesity: 35% of all the women who died were obese.
- Domestic violence: 14% of all the women who died disclosed that they were subject to violence in the home.
- Substance abuse: 8% of women who died were substance misusers.

The 2007 CEMACH report concluded the following:

- 295 mothers died of pregnancy related conditions between 2003 and 2005. Direct causes were thromboembolism, sepsis, pre-eclampsia and amniotic fluid embolism.
- There were fewer deaths from haemorrhage, anaesthesia, and trauma to the uterus.
- Risk factors for maternal deaths were linked with social exclusion as previously.

The CEMACH report[1,2] has provided an overview of the findings and recommendations specifically related to midwives and their practice. This is intended to stimulate debate on what lessons can be learned from the management of the women who died. There are detailed recommendations on antenatal care and specific guidance for developing ways to meet the needs of women in the above-named groups.

1 Confidential Enquiry into Maternal and Child Health (2004). *Why Mothers Die 2000–2002*. London: CEMACH. Available at: ℘ www.cemach.org.uk (accessed 25.2.11).

2 CEMACH (2007). *Saving Mothers' Lives Reviewing Maternal Deaths to Make Motherhood Safer 2003–2005*. London: CEMACH. Available at: ℘ www.cemach.org.uk (accessed 25.2.11).

Blood tests results during pregnancy, detecting deviations from the norm

Table 19.3 Haematalogical values during pregnancy: detecting deviations from normal

Test	Non-pregnant	Pregnancy	PIH/PET	DIC	Notes	Causes of abnormal result
Full blood count						
Haemoglobin (g/dL⁻¹)	11.5–16.5	(↓) 11.0	–	–	Normal reduction in pregnancy (physiological).	Anaemia due to any cause Haemolysis in HELLP. Also decreased in some haemoglobinopathies
Packed cell volume (PCV)	0.35–0.47	(↓) 0.34–0.36	–	–	Decrease PCV represents increased plasma to red cell ratio seen in pregnancy	
White cell count (×10⁹/L⁻¹)	6(4–11)	(↑) 9–11	–	–	Normal increase through pregnancy. Polymorphonuclear cells	Labour can (↑) levels to 13–15. infection causes (↑ levels).
Platelet count (×10⁹/L⁻¹)	150 000–350 000	140 000–440 000	(↓) to (↓ ↓)	<50 000	Decreased platelet count affects blood clotting efficiency.	Idiopathic (ITP), PIH, HELLP

Test	Non-pregnant	Pregnancy	PIH/PET	DIC	Notes	Causes of abnormal result
Coagulation						
Prothrombin time (seconds)	10–12	10–12	May (↑)	>100	Measures II, V, VII, and X	Increased with liver problems or anticoagulant use (warfarin).
Partial thromboplastin time (seconds)	35–45	35–50	May (↑)	>100	Measures II, V, VIII, IX, X, and XI	Increased in factor VII, IX and X deficiency and heparin use.
Thrombin time (seconds)	16–20	15–20	May (↑)	>100		
Fibrinogen (mg/dL⁻¹)	150–400	450	May (↓)	(↓) to (↓↓)	Normally increased in pregnancy. Hepatic dysfunction affects production.	PIH/HELLP, major haemorrhage and DIC
FiDPs (micrograms/mL⁻¹)	<5	<16	May (↑)	>200	Raised levels are evidence of clot breakdown	(↑) levels are seen in thrombo-embolic disease (pulmonary embolism/DVT). Also (↑) in small APH and DIC.

Table 19.4 Blood chemistry values in pregnancy: detecting deviations from normal

Test	Non-pregnant	Pregnancy	PIH/PET	DIC	Notes	Causes of abnormal result
Biochemistry						
Sodium (mmol/L⁻¹)	132–144	132–144	–	–	Fall to lower end of non-pregnant range. Body sodium increases in pregnancy but levels unchanged due to water retention	Low sodium in hyperemesis
Potassium (mmol/L⁻¹)	3.6–5.1	3.6–5.1	May (↑)		Raised levels represent deterioration of renal function	PIH, HELLP, primary renal disease.
Urea (mmol/L⁻¹)	4.3 (2.5–6.6)	2.3–4.3	(↑)		Normally ↓ due to increased renal blood flow. Raised levels represent deterioration of renal function	PIH, HELLP, primary renal disease
Creatinine (μmol/L⁻¹)	73 (55–150)	50–73	(↑)			
Chloride (mmol/L⁻¹)	95–107	95–107	–	–		
Uric acid (mmol/L⁻¹)	0.2–0.35	0.15–0.35	(↑)		Raised levels represent deterioration of renal function	PIH, HELLP, primary renal disease.

Test	Non-pregnant	Pregnancy	PIH/PET	DIC	Notes	Causes of abnormal result
Liver function tests						
Total protein (g/L⁻¹)	78 (60–80)	70	(↓) to (↓↓)	–	Normally just below non-pregnant reference range. Increased loss of protein and decreased production due to liver dysfunction in PIH/HELLP	PIH, HELLP
Albumin (g/L⁻¹)	45 (36–47)	33	(↓) to (↓↓)	–		
ALT (U/L⁻¹)	10–40	10–40	May (↑)	–	Raised levels indicate hepatic cellular damage.	PIH, HELLP, primary liver disease
AST (U/L⁻¹)	10–35	10–35	May (↑)	–		Levels slightly ↑ post partum
γ-glutamyl transpeptidase (U/L⁻¹)	7–50	7–50	–	–	No significant change	Alcohol abuse, enzyme-inducing drugs such as barbiturates and warfarin

Table 19.5 Blood chemistry values in pregnancy induced hypertension and o/e

Test	Non-pregnant	Pregnancy	PIH/PET	DIC	Notes	Causes of abnormal result
Bilirubin (mmol/L⁻¹)	2–17	2–17	May (↑)	–	Product of red cell breakdown.	PIH/HELLP
Lactic dehydrogenase (LDH) (U/L⁻¹)	100–300	100–300	May (↑)	–	Levels may (↑) in last few weeks of pregnancy. Significant increases in PIH/HELLP.	Significant increases in PIH
ALP (U/L⁻¹)	40–125	(↑) 2–4 times	–	–	Normal increase (2–4 times) due to placental production	
Calcium (mmol/L⁻¹)	2.12–2.62	2.12–2.62	–	–	Fall to lower end of reference interval due to reduction in serum albumin. No change in ionized calcium	
Bile acids (µmol/L⁻¹)	0–6	0–14	–	–	Measured in pruritus	(↑ to ↑↑) in cholestasis of pregnancy

Test	Non-pregnant	Pregnancy	PIH/PET	DIC	Notes	Causes of abnormal result
Blood gas results						
P$_a$O$_2$ (kPa)	13 (12–15)	13.7	May (↓)	–	May be lower in the supine position	Fall in PIH/HELLP due to fluid overload. Blood gas results may deteriorate due to respiratory disease as well as pregnancy-induced disease
PaCO$_2$ (kPa)	5.3 (4.4–6.1)	4	–	–	Hyperventilation associated with pregnancy	
HCO$_3^-$ (mmol/L^{-1})	24 (21–27.5)	20	–	–	Metabolic compensation for the respiratory alkalosis—incomplete	
PH	7.4 (36–44)	7.44	–	–	Reflects incomplete compensation of alkalosis	
Base excess (mmol/L^{-1})	–4 to +4	–4 to +4	–	–	Little change in pregnancy. Lower end of reference range	
Other						
Glucose (mmol/L^{-1})	3.6–5.8	3.6–5.8	May (↓)	–		Severe hepatic dysfunction in PIH/HELLP

In utero transfer

The midwife may be asked to transfer a woman in preterm labour to a unit with a vacant cot at specialist neonatal facilities. The ambulance service will provide transport. The decision to transfer lies with the senior obstetrician but the midwife involved should feel confident about transfer.

She or he should have the time and opportunity to assess the woman's progress in labour, and should discuss alternative arrangements if, for example:

• The woman is experiencing, or has recently experienced, fresh bleeding
• The woman is experiencing frequent strong contractions regularly and is distressed
• The woman is severely pre-eclamptic.
  The midwife dealing with the transfer must:
• Ensure that the obstetric team which will be receiving the woman is identified and agree to the transfer
• Liaise with the ward or unit that will accommodate the woman
• Establish IV access
• Ensure that all medications have been given as prescribed
• Ensure that all information, including the receiving consultant's name, is recorded in the notes
• Ensure that a photocopy of the woman's hospital notes and summary is available for the receiving hospital
• Ensure that facilities are available to monitor and care for the woman during transit
• Arrange an ambulance and arrange for support by trained paramedical staff during the transfer
• Ensure that the woman, the woman's partner and family understand the rationale for transfer and that the family are able to visit
• Arrange transport for the midwife's return to base since the ambulance service will not routinely do this.

The midwife should travel with the woman and give care and support as appropriate on the journey ensuring that the woman is comfortable at her destination before returning home.

Hypoxia and asphyxia

The fetus has increased oxygen-carrying capacity because it has a high fetal haemoglobin and relatively high cardiac output. However, fetal oxygen supply can be reduced as a result of changes in:

- Maternal oxygenation and blood flow (cardiac or respiratory disease or maternal hypotension as a result of supine position, epidural, haemorrhage, or shock)
- Uterine blood flow (during labour, each strong uterine contraction temporarily restricts the blood/oxygen supply to the placenta; this may be more severe if oxytocin is used and contractions are hypertonic)
- Placental sufficiency (PIH)
- Fetal circulation (cord compression, abnormal fetal cardiac function). In hypoxia, oxygen supply is insufficient for tissue energy requirements.

Fetal responses to hypoxia

- Heart rate increases to increase cardiac output.
- Blood flow is directed to main organs (heart, brain).
- Reduced fetal activity/movement and, in chronic situations, IUGR.
- Eventually glucose and liver glycogen are metabolized (anaerobic metabolism—without oxygen) to provide energy to maintain organ function. This results in the production/accumulation of lactic acid, and metabolic acidosis occurs with a fall in blood pH and rise in base deficit.
- As the fetus becomes acidotic with depleted glycogen reserves, bradycardia develops.
- The fetus may pass meconium into the liquor.

Glycogen stores are used up quickly and the length of time the fetus can withstand hypoxia depends on reserves. Asphyxia will occur if hypoxia continues. Finally, energy balance cannot be maintained and tissue damage then organ failure will ensue. A growth-retarded fetus (IUGR) with low glycogen stores will be particularly susceptible to asphyxia.

Detecting hypoxia in labour

- The normal fetus is well able to withstand normal labour stress, but if the fetus has already been compromised during pregnancy it may be even more vulnerable during labour. Fetal surveillance during labour therefore depends on an assessment of risk (📖 see The partogram, p. 234) and, if indicated, institute continuous monitoring (CTG).
- Abnormal FHR patterns may indicate fetal hypoxia and asphyxia. The most frequently noted abnormalities include loss of baseline variability, a baseline tachycardia, and decelerations.
- A deceleration is a transient fall (>15 beats) in the baseline rate for >15s, classified as:
  - *Early:* deceleration occurs at the beginning and returns to baseline at the end of the contraction, and is usually a repeating pattern of similar decelerations.

- *Variable:* decelerations that do not necessarily occur with the contraction. They may occur in isolation. They vary in depth with quick onset/recovery.
- *Late:* deceleration may occur partway through the contraction or following it, with the lowest point more than 20s after the height of the contraction.
- *Isolated prolonged:* a deceleration that lasts 60–90s.
- NICE guidelines[1] suggest analysis of the CTG to facilitate early detection of fetal compromise. They suggest that abnormal patterns are *suspicious* if one of the following features is present but otherwise the trace is reassuring:
  - Abnormal baseline rate
  - Reduced baseline variability
  - Decelerations present
  - Accelerations absent (though the significance of this in an otherwise normal trace is uncertain).[1]

Abnormal patterns may be regarded as *pathological* if two or more non-reassuring features are found or one or more abnormal features are present (Table 19.6).

Table 19.6 Fetal heart rate patterns

	Baseline bpm	Variability	Decelerations	Accelerations
Reassuring	110–160	+ 5	None	Present
Non-reassuring	100–109; 161–180	<5 for >40 to <90min	Early deceleration, variable deceleration, single prolonged deceleration	Absent
Abnormal	<100, >180 sinusoidal pattern for +10min	<5 for +90min	Atypical variable decelerations, late decelerations, single prolonged deceleration >3min	Absent

- A CTG recording with loss of baseline variability and accompanied by shallow late decelerations is particularly pathological and should be reported.
- A rare occurrence in labour is a sinusoidal trace—a regular, smooth, sine wave-like baseline with loss of variability but with normal baseline. It is associated with hypoxia as a result of severe fetal anaemia, feto-maternal haemorrhage, diabetes, prolonged pregnancy, or cord compression.

A non-reassuring fetal heart

It is important to recognize that management of care should be holistic and not simply related to CTG patterns. Factors other than hypoxia may make the fetal heart appear abnormal. You should ask:

- Is the pattern precipitated by care procedures, maternal position, or temperature/pulse?
- Is this client high risk?
- What is the rate of progress in labour?
- What is the current cervical dilatation?
- Is the liquor meconium stained?

Initial intervention

- Monitor and record the maternal pulse and blood pressure on the CTG tracing.
- Discontinue IV oxytocin if in use, since this may cause hyperstimulation of the uterus and subsequent decelerations on CTG tracing.
- Help the woman to change position to left/right lateral, to avoid supine hypotension.
- Always ensure adequate IV fluids are available before 'topping up' an epidural. Measure blood pressure regularly and correct hypotension.
- If the FHR remains non-reassuring after 5min, inform the labour ward coordinator or registrar.

  If delivery is not imminent, the obstetric registrar may wish to assess fetal condition by performing FBS.

Fetal blood sampling

A sample of blood is obtained from the fetal scalp and tested for a low-ering of blood pH, which is indicative of metabolic acidosis. Indications include:

- An FHR pattern which is assessed to be suspicious or pathological.
- Meconium-stained liquor noted during labour if the fetus is 34–37 weeks' gestation.

FBS is avoided if:

- There is HIV, hepatitis B or C, herpes simplex, or other viral bloodborne infection in the mother
- Gestation <34 weeks
- Clotting disorders in the fetus are suspected.

  Under these circumstances, inform the consultant obstetrician; delivery may be the best option.

Procedure

Be sensitive to the needs of the parents. Explain the procedure and obtain verbal consent. Preserve the woman's dignity and provide support and adequate pain relief.

- Encourage the woman into the left lateral position or the lithotomy position with a wedge support to prevent supine hypotension.
- The obstetrician uses an amnioscope to view the fetal scalp.
- The area in view is cleaned and ethyl chloride is sprayed on to the scalp to stimulate hyperaemia.
- Sterile grease is smeared on the scalp to facilitate collection of the fetal blood sample into a pre-heparinized capillary tube.

- A small incision is made and 0.4mL blood collected.
- The obstetrician ensures wound haemostasis.
- Sometimes obtaining an adequate sample is problematic. Repeated attempts should be avoided.
- Discuss the plan of management with the obstetric consultant.
- The pH measurement is done straight away using a pH meter
  - pH >7.25 is regarded as normal.
  - pH <7.20 is regarded as indicative of fetal acidosis. Urgent delivery is necessary.
  - pH between these readings suggests the fetus may be on the verge of acidosis and the sample should always be repeated in 30min to obtain an improved reading.
- Cord blood samples should be obtained at delivery.

Cord blood samples: fetal pH at delivery[2]

Oxygen from the maternal blood diffuses to the fetus via the placenta and cord vein. Deoxygenated blood returns via the cord arteries to the placenta and carbon dioxide diffuses to the maternal blood.

- Thus cord arterial blood should give an indication of fetal acid–base balance.
- Venous blood should reflect maternal acid–base status and placental function.
  Cord blood samples should be considered if:
- An emergency caesarean section is performed
- A forceps delivery is performed
- FBS is taken during labour
- The Apgar score at 5min after delivery is 7 or less.

Double clamping

When there has been active management of the third stage, it may be recommended that the cord be double clamped at delivery:

- Clamp the cord as usual near the baby's umbilicus
- Clamp a second time to allow for cutting of the cord
- Leave 10–15cm between the second and a third clamp, which preserves blood in a segment of the cord.

Obtaining the samples

- Arterial and venous samples are obtained from the cord in a pre-heparinized syringe.
- The result should remain accurate for up to 10min at room temperature.
- Ensure that there is no air in the syringes, that they are capped, and that the heparin is mixed with the sample by rolling the syringe between the fingers.

Measurements

The following measurements are obtained (Tables 19.7 and 19.8):

- pH: measure of acidity or alkalinity.
- pO_2: oxygen tension in the blood (units kilopascals, kPa).
- pCO_2 carbon dioxide measure (units kilopascals, kPa).
- Base deficit: an indirect measure of anaerobic metabolism. It allows distinction between a low pH caused by a build-up of CO_2 (respiratory

acidosis) and that caused by a build up of metabolic acids as a result of anaerobic metabolism (metabolic acidosis). The former is resolved quickly at birth when the lungs are inflated, the latter indicates that a significant period of hypoxia has occurred which may affect the baby in the neonatal period.
- Cord blood results are influenced by mode of delivery, gestational age, and analgesia during labour.

Table 19.7 Normal arterial blood gas values[2]

	Artery	**Vein**
pH	7.26 (7.05–7.38)	7.35 (7.17–7.48)
pCO$_2$ (kPa)	7.3 (4.9–10.7)	5.3 (3.5–7.9)
Base deficit	2.4 (2.5–9.7)	3.0 (–1.0–8.9)

Table 19.8 Criteria for diagnosis of acidosis—analysis of blood gases results

	Respiratory	**Metabolic**	**Mixed**
pCO$_2$	High	Normal	High
pO$_2$	Normal	Low	Low
HCO$_3$ (bicarbonate)	Normal	Low	Low
Base deficit	Normal	High	High

What should you expect to find in a baby who has intrapartum asphyxia?
- Metabolic acidosis in cord sample.
- Need for resuscitation at birth.
- Evidence of organ dysfunction in the neonatal period: convulsions due to CNS malfunction.
- Hypotension, poor cardiac function, hypoxia.
- Blood and oxygen redistributed from peripheral organs results in respiratory distress, renal failure, hepatic damage.
- Neonatal hypoglycaemia resulting from depletion of liver glycogen.

---

1 National Institute for Health and Clinical Excellence (2007). *Intrapartum care. Clinical Guideline 55.* London: NICE. Available at: ℜ www.nice.org.uk/nicemedia/live/11837/36275/36275.pdf (accessed 25.2.11).

2 The Practice Development Team (2010). *Jessop Wing, Labour Ward Guidelines 2010.* Sheffield: Sheffield Teaching Hospitals NHS Trust (quoted from Plymouth Perinatal Research Group, 1994).

Cord presentation and cord prolapse

Cord presentation and cord prolapse occur in any situation where the presenting part is poorly applied to the lower segment of the uterus or high in the pelvic cavity, making it possible for a loop of cord to slip down in front of the presenting part.

Definitions

- *Cord presentation*: the umbilical cord lies in front of the presenting part with the membranes intact (Fig. 19.1).
- *Cord prolapse*: the umbilical cord lies in front of the presenting part and the membranes have ruptured (Fig. 19.2).
- *Occult cord prolapse*: the cord lies alongside, but not in front of the presenting part.

Predisposing conditions

- High or ill-fitting presenting part.
- High parity: due to a weakened lower uterine segment or loss of abdominal muscle tone, there is an increased incidence of non-engagement of the presenting part until labour is well established.
- Prematurity: the size of the fetus in relation to the uterus constitutes a high risk of cord prolapse, hence there is a high mortality rate associated with prematurity.
- Multiple pregnancy: especially malpresentation of the second twin.
- Malpresentation: breech presentation is particularly vulnerable, especially complete or footling breech. The close proximity of the umbilicus to the buttocks is an added risk. Other malpresentations such as shoulder presentation or transverse lie carry a high risk of cord prolapse.
- Polyhydramnios: the cord may be swept down with a gush of liquor if the membranes rupture spontaneously.
- Obstetric practices and interventions may possibly make a difference to the incidence of cord prolapse, dependent on the intrapartum practices of individual hospitals, such as ARM in early labour; displacement of the presenting part during a vaginal examination.
- Long umbilical cord: usually associated with one of the above.

Cord prolapse

Where there are factors that predispose to cord prolapse, a vaginal exam should be undertaken following spontaneous rupture of the membranes. An abnormal heart rate, such as bradycardia, may indicate cord prolapse. The risks to the fetus are hypoxia or death.

Diagnosis

- The cord is felt below or beside the presenting part on vaginal examination.
- A loop of cord may be felt in the vagina or the cord may be visible at the vulva.
- There may be bradycardia.

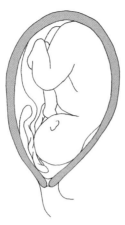

Fig. 19.1 Cord presentation.

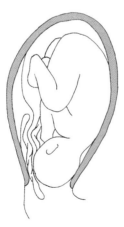

Fig. 19.2 Cord prolapse.

Management
- Call medical aid.
- Explain the situation to the mother.
- Carry out a vaginal examination.
- If an oxytocic infusion is running, this should be stopped immediately.
- Relieve pressure on the umbilical cord by keeping your fingers in the vagina to push the presenting part away from the umbilical cord.
- Assist the woman to move into the knee-chest position, which helps to relieve compression of the umbilical cord (Fig. 19.3). Alternatively, the exaggerated Sim's position (Fig. 19.4) may be adopted, by lying her on her side with a wedge or pillow to raise her hips. The foot of the bed can be elevated.
- Monitor the FHR.
- Urgent delivery.
- In some units alternative management may involve displacing the presenting part by filling the bladder with 500mL of normal saline. The catheter is then clamped and the fingers may then be withdrawn from the vagina. The clamp is released when the incision for LSCS is being made and therefore delivery is imminent.

Cord presentation
- Will usually have been diagnosed on vaginal examination.
- May be associated with deceleration of the FHR.
- Do *not* rupture the membranes.
- Discontinue the vaginal examination.
- Call for medical assistance.
- Monitor the FHR.
- Encourage the woman to adopt a position as above that will reduce the occurrence of cord compression.
- Expedite delivery as soon as possible—LSCS is the most likely outcome.

Cord presentation and cord prolapse constitute a serious threat to fetal well-being. In order to reduce mortality and morbidity, it is important that urgent delivery is initiated. This will usually be by caesarean section if the fetus is alive and delivery is not imminent. In some instances, with a multiparous woman, a second-stage vaginal delivery may be possible. In the community, where the fetus is alive, arrange urgent transfer to hospital.

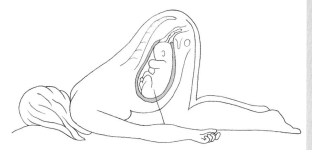

Fig. 19.3 Knee chest position (relieves compression on prolapsed cord).

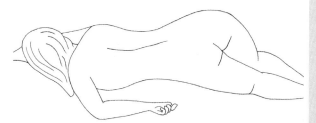

Fig. 19.4 Sim's position.

Vasa praevia

- This is a rare occurrence when a fetal blood vessel is situated over the cervical os and therefore is in front of the presenting part.
- There may be a velamentous insertion of the cord (or possibly a succenturiate lobe) resulting in a fetal vessel running through the membranes.

Diagnosis

- The presence of the vessel might be suspected during vaginal examination while the membranes are still intact.
- If a careful speculum examination were performed with a good light it might be possible to see the vessel.

Rupture of the vessel

- This may occur if the membranes rupture.
- The fetus may die unless quickly delivered.

Signs and symptoms

- Minimal fresh red loss occurring typically at the rupture of the membranes.
- On monitoring the fetal heart there are signs of fetal compromise which are disproportionate to the amount of blood loss.
- There may be a sinusoidal fetal heart pattern sometimes seen when the fetus is severely anaemic. This is characterized by increased variability of >15 beats and resembles a sine wave with 2–6 cycles per min.

Immediate care

The midwife should:

- Recognize the risk of fetal asphyxia (see Hypoxia and asphyxia, p. 434).
- Call for help speedily from the obstetric registrar and team.
- Continue to record a CTG.
- If the fetal compromise is apparent prepare the woman for very urgent caesarean section (see Emergency LSCS, p. 379) if this is the first stage of labour.
- If delivery is imminent or the woman is multiparous in the second stage of labour encourage pushing or/and if requested prepare for forceps/ventouse delivery.
- The paediatrician should be called to the delivery.
- The cord should be double clamped and blood should be obtained for blood gases and also for haemoglobin estimation in the baby.
- The paediatric team will transfer the baby to SCBU for observation and treatment. S/he may require a blood transfusion.

Shoulder dystocia

Definition
Impaction of the anterior shoulder behind the symphysis pubis, which impedes the spontaneous delivery of the baby.

Incidence
- 0.15–2% of all vaginal deliveries.
- Although this is a relatively rare event, the perinatal mortality can be between 2.6% and 29%, with surviving babies at risk of long-term morbidity.
- The Confidential Enquiry into Stillbirths and Deaths in Infancy (CESDI) (1996)[1] report recommended that all professionals involved with delivery of a baby must be trained to deal with this emergency.
- This is one of the most frightening emergencies experienced, as it is difficult to predict and the midwife facilitating the birth may be working alone.

Predisposing factors
- Maternal obesity
- Maternal diabetes
- Post dates, >41 weeks
- Previous shoulder dystocia or big baby
- Macrosomia in present pregnancy
- Prolonged first and/or second stage of labour
- Operative delivery, especially mid-cavity instrumental delivery for delay.

The predisposing factors may not be present in every case, so the first sign is often failure of the baby's chin to escape the perineum, or failure of the baby's head to undergo restitution or rotation. This is sometimes referred to as the 'turtle' sign. The baby's head is pressing so tightly against the perineum that it is impossible to insert a finger into the vagina, and the baby's face becomes suffused and discoloured.

The following mnemonic, HELPER, is adapted from the Advanced Life Support in Obstetrics:
- **H = HELP**, call for help: obstetrician, anaesthetist, midwives, paediatric team, and support workers.
- NOTE THE TIME OF THE DELIVERY OF THE HEAD
- **E = EVALUATE for EPISIOTOMY**, episiotomy scissors open, symphysiotomy tray available.
- **L = LEGS**, lay the bed flat, remove pillows, lift the woman's knees to her shoulders (McRobert's position, see Fig. 19.5).
- **P = PRESSURE: SUPRAPUBIC**, constant for 30s, direct the baby's shoulder towards his or her chest, rocking pressure for 30s (see Fig. 19.6).
- **E = ENTER PELVIS**
  - Episiotomy.
  - Pressure on posterior aspect of the baby's anterior shoulder, try to get baby's shoulders into oblique diameter.

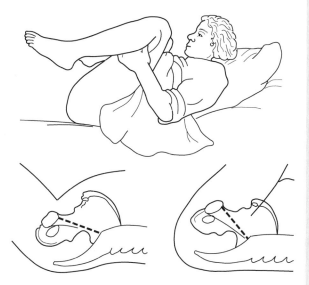

Fig. 19.5 McRobert's manoeuvre.

Reprinted by permission of Henry Lerner M.D. from 🖰 www.shoulderdystociainfo.com

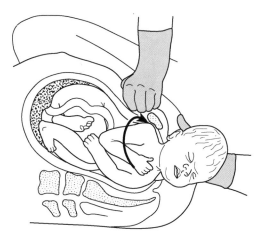

Fig. 19.6 Suprapubic pressure, divert the baby's shoulder towards his chest.

Reprinted by permission of Henry Lerner M.D. from 🖰 www.shoulderdystociainfo.com.

- Continue pressure and rotate the baby by 180° (the baby's anterior shoulder now be posterior) (Fig. 19.7).
- Pressure on the posterior aspect of the baby's posterior shoulder, try to get baby's shoulders into oblique diameter.
- Continue pressure and rotate the baby by 180° (the baby's posterior shoulder becomes anterior) (Fig. 19.8).
- **R = REMOVE POSTERIOR ARM**, midwife's hand enters posteriorly along arm, flexes arm and grasps hand, sweeping the baby's arm across his chest and face to deliver.

Consider other options;

- Place mother in all fours position: change of position may dislodge the anterior shoulder, may facilitate access for internal manoeuvres.
- Fracture clavicle, symphysiotomy (division of symphysis), and Zavanelli manoeuvre (cephalic replacement and delivery by caesarean). (The last three options would need to be performed by an obstetrician. They are last resort measures.)

Document the head to body delivery interval, order of manoeuvres, and cord pH.

Debrief—full and clear explanations should be given to the parents. The professionals involved should be offered the chance to discuss the case in a supportive environment.

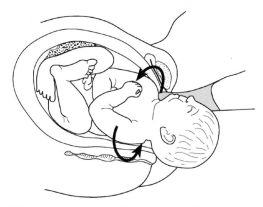

Fig. 19.7 Wood's screw manoeuvre. Rotate anterior shoulder.

Reprinted by permission of Henry Lerner M.D. from www.shoulderdystociainfo.com.

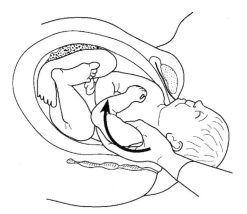

Fig. 19.8 Rubin's manoeuvre. Rotate posterior shoulder.
Reprinted by permission of Henry Lerner M.D. from ℬ www.shoulderdystociainfo.com.

1 The Confidential Enquiry into Stillbirths and Neonatal Deaths. 5th Annual Report. London: CESDI, pp. 73–9. Available at: ℬ www.cesdi.org.uk (accessed 25.2.11).

Guidelines for admission to neonatal ICU

'Provision for sick neonates has developed rapidly over the last two decades from a small area on a maternity ward to a giant, technical, scientifically based system of care. Advances in technology and an increased understanding of the problems and needs of premature and low birth weight babies have increased the survival rates of babies who would have died a few years ago.'[1]

In 1992 the WHO[2] clarified the definitions for premature and small for date babies:

- A **premature baby** is any baby born before 37 completed weeks of gestation.
- A **small for date baby** is a baby whose weight falls below the 10th percentile for its gestational age.

These definitions indicate that a baby can be both premature and small for dates, or term and small for dates.

- About 6.7% of babies born in the UK will weigh <2.5kg.
- One-third will be small for dates; 70% will weigh between 2kg and 2.5kg.
- About 50% of those weighing 1.5–2kg will have minimal or no illness in the neonatal period.
- A **term baby** is one born between 37 and 42 weeks' gestation, with an average weight of 3.5kg on the 50th percentile.
- A baby can be **large for dates**, with a weight of 4.5kg or more at birth, which is on the 90th percentile. This can be normal, but is also associated with maternal diabetes.

In 1990 the Human Fertilization and Embryology Act stated that a baby is capable of surviving from 24 weeks of pregnancy. Viable gestational age is considered by law to be 24 weeks, whatever the baby's weight.[1,3]

The current structure of neonatal care in the UK

Regional units

Full intensive expert care is provided for the smallest, sickest babies. There is also provision for neonatal surgery. Mothers are referred to these centres for delivery if problems are indicated, or retrieval teams will collect the baby following delivery and stabilization. It is preferable to transfer the baby *in utero* as, once born, its survival depends on provision of a stable thermal environment and effective management of oxygenation. Transferring a small, sick baby in the back of an ambulance can prove to be very hazardous. The baby returns to the referring unit once he or she is well enough.

Subregional units

These are subsidiary to the regional units. They provide full expert intensive care. The only difference being that they do not provide surgery, and will transfer any baby requiring surgery to the nearest surgical unit.

Special care baby units

These are based in all maternity hospitals, for the care of small babies from 32 weeks' gestation. They can also provide emergency treatment and stabilization for the smaller, sicker babies, until transfer to the regional unit can be arranged. They usually have two or three intensive cots and may keep the baby if it can be managed within that context.

Transitional care units

These are usually based on a maternity ward away from the intensive and high-dependency care contexts, thus keeping the baby with or near to its mother, and cared for by midwives or neonatal nurses. Babies needing this level of care usually require treatment for jaundice or infections, or they may be small but are otherwise well.

Criteria for admission to the NICU[4]

- Any baby weighing <1700g from 23–34 weeks' gestation.
- Any baby who is ill at birth; for example, extremely small for dates.
- Any baby who has severe congenital abnormalities requiring emergency management and/or surgery.
- Term babies who have birth asphyxia, meconium aspiration, or respiratory difficulties requiring extensive resuscitation at birth.

Babies with congenital abnormalities who are not seriously ill, for example, babies with Down's syndrome who are otherwise well, stay with their mothers on the maternity ward or in the transitional care unit (📖 see Guidelines for admission to transitional care, p. 452).

1 Yeo H (ed.) (2000). *Nursing the Neonate*, 2nd edn. Oxford: Churchill Livingstone, pp. 1–16.

2 World Health Organization (1992). *International Statistical Classification of Diseases and Related Health Problems*, 10th revision. Geneva: WHO.

3 Roberton NRC (1993). Should we look after babies less than 800 grams? *Archives of Diseases of Childhood* 68, 326–9.

4 Rennie JM, Roberton NRC (eds) (1999). *Textbook of Neonatology*, 3rd edn. London: Churchill Livingstone, pp. 389–99.

Guidelines for admission to transitional care

A transitional care ward is an environment where infants requiring specific nursing and medical management can be cared for without being separated from their mothers. The typical length of stay varies between 2 and 3 days and 3 weeks.

Transitional care is instrumental in the development of attachment between the mother and infant, as it allows 24h parenting. Moderately compromised babies (see below) gain weight more quickly and are discharged earlier with less chance of readmission than if they were cared for in a standard neonatal unit.

In a busy obstetric unit, over a 6-month period approximately 150 babies weighing >1.5kg will be admitted to the neonatal unit, for an average of 3.7 special care days each. It is likely that most of these infants could be cared for on a transitional care ward, reserving neonatal care facilities for sicker infants.

Admission criteria

- Gestational age 34 weeks to term
- Birth weight >1.5kg
- Babies requiring nasogastric tube feeding
- Babies requiring calculated feeding regimens
- Persistently hypoglycaemic babies
- Hypothermic babies
- Dehydrated babies
- Babies requiring increased observation, e.g. traumatic delivery
- Babies with congenital abnormalities.

It may be possible to extend the admission criteria, if the ward is well established and adequately staffed, to include:
- Infants of unstable diabetic mothers
- Difficult to manage babies with neonatal abstinence syndrome (☐ see Neonatal abstinence syndrome, p. 648).
- Babies requiring palliative care.

Not for admission

- Sick babies requiring the care of a neonatal unit, e.g.:
  - Any baby requiring extensive resuscitation and/or ventilatory support
  - Any baby requiring oxygen therapy.
- Babies who can be cared for on a normal postnatal ward, e.g.:
  - Babies who only require IV cannulation and antibiotics
  - Babies who are slow to feed with no excessive clinical symptoms of hypoglycaemia/dehydration
  - Multiple births babies who are clinically well.
- Sick babies for foster care or adoption, are treated in a neonatal unit whether or not they meet admission criteria for a transitional care ward.

Neonatal resuscitation

Stimuli resulting in the initiation of respiration
- At birth, gas exchange changes from placental to alveolar.
- As the fetus is propelled down the birth canal, a negative intrathoracic pressure is exerted, so that on delivery air is sucked into the lungs.
- Clamping and cutting the cord.
- Physical stimuli: tactile, cold, and gravity.[1]

Changes from fetal to normal circulation
- The first breath increases paO_2 and closes the ductus arteriosus between the aorta and pulmonary artery, allowing more blood to flow to the lungs.
- There is a decrease in the pulmonary vascular resistance and an increase in blood flow from the lungs.
- The increased left atrial pressure and decreased right atrial pressure closes the foramen ovale.[1]

Prevent hypothermia
- The intrauterine environment is 1.5°C higher than maternal temperature.
- The temperature of a newborn is approximately 37.8°C. The core temperature of a wet, asphyxiated infant will decrease by 5°C in as many minutes.
- Surfactant production is decreased if body temperature goes <35°C.
- The baby will increase oxygen intake by breathing rapidly, using up glycogen stores to produce body heat, leading to hypoglycaemia.[1]

Preparation for delivery
Ensure that:
- Personnel capable of initiating resuscitation are always available
- A person capable of complete resuscitation is in attendance for all high-risk deliveries
- Resuscitaire and overhead heater, with dry and warmed towels are prepared
- Oxygen with a Neopuff® ventilation system is available. This system allows for the setting of an inspiration pressure which will not cause damage to the lungs. It also allows for the setting of a positive end expiratory pressure to help prevent the collapse of the alveoli at expiration thus allowing for more efficient oxygenation
- Suction and suction tubes (varying sizes) are available
- Laryngoscopes, endotracheal tubes, and connections are at hand
- Medications are readily available.[2]

Initial assessment at birth
- Start the clock.
- Dry and warm the baby.
- Assess:
  - Colour
  - Breathing

- Heart rate by listening with a stethoscope or palpate the base of the cord
- Tone
- Response to stimuli.

These observations form the basis of assessment and reassessment throughout the resuscitation.

Provided the airway is clear, most babies who are apnoeic at birth will resuscitate themselves.[2]

ABC of resuscitation

- **Airway**. To secure a clear airway:
  - Hold the head in a neutral position.
  - Do not flex or overextend the neck.
  - Apply gentle suction to the mouth and nose, but this is not always needed. Avoid deep pharyngeal suction as the vagal stimulation can cause bradycardia.
  - Jaw thrust will be needed if the baby is very floppy, with one or two fingers under each side of the angle of the jaw, push forwards and outwards.[2] These manoeuvres may be all that is required to initiate breathing.
- **Breathing**. If not breathing:
  - Administer 5 inflation breaths.
  - Inflation pressure 30cmH$_2$O for 2–3s.
  - This will sufficiently aerate the lungs.
  - As the first few inflations will be replacing lung fluid with air, chest movement will not be detected until the fourth or fifth inflation.
- **Circulation**. If the heart rate is less than 60bpm and not increasing despite adequate lung inflations:
  - Start chest compressions for 30s.
  - After 30s, check the heart rate. If there is still no response despite adequate inflations and chest compressions, emergency drugs may be needed.[2]

Chest compression

There are two methods:
- The two-thumb method
- The two-finger method.

The main principles for both are the same, using the lower third of the sternum one finger's breadth below the nipple line:
- Rate: 90/min
- Ratio: three compressions to one ventilation/inhalation
- Depth: one-third of the depth of the baby's chest (1–2cm)
- Action: well controlled, not jerky or erratic.

Allow for expansion after each compression to facilitate venous return.[2]

Emergency drugs are given if adequate ventilation and effective chest compressions have failed to increase the heart rate above 60bpm. They are given to increase cardiac output and improve cardiac and cerebral perfusion. They are usually administered through an umbilical venous catheter.

- *Adrenaline:* improves cerebral and cardiac perfusion.
  - Dose 10micrograms/kg; 0.1mL 1:10 000 solution can be given via an endotracheal tube but is less effective.
- *Sodium bicarbonate:* reverses acidosis, 'kick starts' the heart
  - Dose 1–2mmol/kg; 2–4mL 4.2% solution.
  If there is no response to adrenaline and sodium bicarbonate, use:
- *Glucose:* 2.5mL/kg 10% solution.
  Occasionally volume expansion may help. Use:
- Plasma, whole blood or normal saline, 10mL/kg.
  In addition:
- *Naloxone* 1.0mg/kg is given intramuscularly to reverse the effects of pethidine given during labour. Do not use this if the mother has been taking opiate drugs during pregnancy.
- *Calcium* 2mL/kg 10% solution. Give when the heart rate remains below 80bpm, despite a minimum of 30s, of adequate ventilation with 100% oxygen, chest compressions, and the administration of adrenaline or if the heart rate is 0 and there is no response to ventilation despite the administration of adrenaline and cardiac compressions.[2]

Tracheal intubation

Is indicated where there is:
- Ineffective face-mask ventilation
- The need for tracheal suction at the level or below the vocal cords due to thick meconium
- Extreme prematurity and surfactant administration (see Respiratory distress syndrome in the newborn, p. 640)
- Prolonged ventilation
- During transfer from the labour ward/theatre to the neonatal unit
- Some congenital abnormalities, where the baby has abnormalities of the face and neck, for example a cystic hygroma which is large enough to obstruct the airway
- Lung pathology due to diaphragmatic hernia, pneumothorax, hypoplastic lungs, and hydrops.[2]

Meconium-stained liquor

- Meconium aspiration syndrome (MAS) is a problem associated with term babies.
- If peristalsis is stimulated by hypoxia *in utero*, the anal sphincter relaxes and the fetus will pass meconium into the amniotic fluid.
- The asphyxia also causes the fetus to make gasping movements, taking the meconium into the lungs.
- Aspiration can occur at any time, but the risk is greatest with intrauterine asphyxia.[3]

Thin meconium

May be an 'innocent' finding due to fetal maturation processes. It is often associated with post-term deliveries.

Thick meconium

- Is a marker of fetal hypoxia.
- Must be cleared from the oropharynx prior to delivery of the shoulders.

- Normal respiration should not be initiated until it has been cleared, otherwise it will be driven into the lungs, causing MAS.

Management of meconium-stained liquor

Thin meconium

- A small amount of meconium with light staining and no particulate material presents minimal risk of aspiration.
- The baby will be lively, have cried and breathed spontaneously.
- Assess and treat as any other birth.
- Some gentle suction to the mouth may well be sufficient.

Thick particulate meconium

- Increases the risk of aspiration.
- The infant will be depressed and not making any respiratory effort.
- Attempt to remove the meconium before initiating normal respiration.
- Do not stimulate or ventilate.
- Place the infant under a radiant heater on the resuscitaire.
- Examine the upper airway for residual meconium.
- Suck out under direct vision using a large-sized catheter or a Yankauer® sucker.
- Dry the baby and keep warm.
- The trachea should be intubated and meconium suctioned from the lower airways.
- This may require several attempts.[3]

Post-resuscitation care

- Babies who receive minimal or no resuscitation can normally be handed straight to the parents. Routine observations will be made.
- Babies who receive prolonged resuscitation will need to be transferred to the neonatal intensive care unit. This will involve:
  - Stabilization
  - Safe transfer
  - Identification and treatment of problems.
- Babies with MAS will require antibiotics, physiotherapy, and suction to remove the meconium from the lungs. They are also at risk of a pneumothorax due to the meconium blocking the airways.[2]

Communication and record keeping

- An accurate written record detailing the resuscitation events is vital, as it can help to protect practitioners if defence of their actions is required.
- All documentation should be legible, signed, dated, and timed.
- Parents need a clear, detailed account of the baby's problems and further treatments should the baby require specialized care and transfer to the NICU.[2]

When to stop

Hospitals will have their own policies in place regarding when to stop resuscitation, usually based on the following factors:

- No cardiac output after 15min.
- No respiratory effort after 30min, despite effective ventilation and chest compressions.

When all reversible factors have been eliminated, the decision to stop is made by the most senior clinician available.[2]

1 Roberton NRC (1999). Resuscitation of the newborn. In: Rennie JM, Roberton NRC (eds) *Textbook of Neonatology*, 3rd edn. London: Churchill Livingstone, pp. 241–62.

2 Resuscitation Council (UK) (2001). *Resuscitation at Birth. The Newborn Life Support Provider Course Manual*. London: Resuscitation Council.

3 Greenhough A (1995). Meconium aspiration syndrome: prevention and treatment. *Early Human Development* **41**, 183–92.

Perinatal mortality

Perinatal mortality is defined as the sum of all stillbirths and neonatal deaths in the first week of life. The rate is expressed as numbers of deaths per thousand births.

CEMACH (2004)[1] produced a report on stillbirth, neonatal, and post-neonatal mortality from 2000 to 2002.

- The report shows a rise in the rate of stillbirths from 4.83 to 5.20.
- The perinatal death rate for 2002 was 7.87.
- The stillbirth rate for multiple pregnancies is 3.5 times higher than for single pregnancies.

Under one type of classification, 70% of the deaths were unexplained antepartum deaths. For those where a diagnosis had been made, the leading causes were:

- Congenital malformation (15.7%)
- Intrapartum-related events (6.9%).

Unexplained antepartum deaths were then described using the obstetric classification, with the largest identifiable causes being:

- APH (13.9%)
- Maternal disorders (6.7%)
- Pre-eclampsia (4.7%).

Half of all the stillbirths reported remained unexplained.

Neonatal deaths are those occurring during the first month of life. CEMACH (2004)[1] reported that the leading causes of neonatal death were:

- Immaturity (47.7%)
- Congenital malformation (23.6%)
- Infection (9.1%).

The leading causes of post-neonatal death were:

- Congenital malformation (29.7%)
- Sudden infant death, cause unknown (22.9%)
- Infection (16%).

The CEMACH report (2009) that reviewed perinatal mortality noted some positive key findings:[2]

- An improvement in neonatal mortality 3.3 per 1000 livebirths in 2007
- A stillbirth rate of 5.2 per 1000 in 2007
- A reducing stillbirth rate among twins 12.2 per 1000 livebirths and neonatal mortality rate of 18:1000 livebirths.

The report showed that neonatal mortality was highest amongst teenage mothers: 4.4:1000 compared with other age groups. Extremes of maternal age, non-white ethnicity, and maternal deprivation continue to be risk factors. Maternal obesity could be associated with adverse outcomes.

1 CEMACH (2004). *Why Mothers Die 2000–2002*. Available at: www.cemach.org.uk (accessed 25.2.11).

2 CEMACH (2009). *Perinatal Mortality 2007*. Available at: www.cemach.org.uk (accessed 25.2.11).

Intrauterine death and stillbirth

Definition

- Intrauterine death refers to death of the fetus at any stage in the pregnancy after the first trimester and before the onset of labour.
- A stillbirth is a baby born after 24 weeks' gestation which shows no signs of life. A baby born before 24 weeks is defined (from a medical viewpoint) as a spontaneous abortion.
- The fetus may be retained in the uterus for weeks or be born a few days following intrauterine death.

Factors associated with intrauterine death

Maternal

- Social factors, e.g. low socio-economic status
- Maternal age (teenagers and >35 years)
- Smoking, alcohol, and drug misuse
- Viruses/infection: rubella, cytomegalovirus, toxoplasmosis, listeriosis
- Exposure to environmental hazards:
  - Lead, cadmium, mercury
  - Air pollution
- Direct trauma to abdomen
- Placental dysfunction: abruption, placenta praevia
- PIH, cholestasis of pregnancy
- Poor previous obstetric history: abortions, preterm labour, stillbirth
- Maternal illness: diabetes, renal disease, severe anaemia, epilepsy, antiphospholipid syndrome.

Fetal

- Fetal malformation (e.g. associated with diabetes)
- Fetal anoxia
- Severe IUGR
- Rh incompatibility
- Multiple pregnancy (especially monozygotic twins)
- Cord accidents, compression, entanglement, true knot
  The cause of intrauterine death and stillbirth is often unknown.

Complications of intrauterine death

- DIC may occur if the fetus is retained 3–4 weeks.
- Induction of labour may be prolonged or difficult.
- The woman and her partner are at risk of psychological trauma.

Signs

Signs will depend on the time lapse since intrauterine death:
- No fetal movements will be felt by the woman
- No fetal heart heard with abdominal transducer
- The uterus may be smaller than expected for dates
- The woman may experience full breasts and may produce milk
- Any hypertension may settle
- There may be a brownish discharge PV.

Diagnosis
- Ultrasound scan will confirm no heart beat.
- Spalding's sign: overlap and misalignment of fetal skull bones.
- Robert's sign: gas in the great vessels and heart of the fetus (1–2 days).
- Fetal curl: there is arching of the fetal spine.

Management of care
- The woman who presents with anxieties about reduced or no fetal movements should be seen urgently.
- Be sensitive to her anxiety. You may be able to reassure the woman quickly by hearing the fetal heart using the CTG or Sonicaid®. When doing this, it is important to differentiate the fetal and the maternal pulse.
- If the fetal heart is not heard (or the pregnancy is <20 weeks and the FHR is not easily audible), explain the findings and contact an experienced ultrasonographer and a registrar to assess by ultrasound whether or not the FHR is present.
- The diagnosis of intrauterine death should be confirmed by two experts.
- Women booked under midwifery-led care should be transferred to consultant-led care. However, continuity of midwifery care should still be given high priority in order to facilitate adequate support and co-ordination of information throughout the episode. A midwife specializing in bereavement care may be available.
  When giving bad news note that:
- Support for the woman should be sought from her partner/family/ friend
- Information should be clear and honest, given in a way sensitive to individual needs and feelings. Parents will always remember the way the news is delivered and the attitudes of staff
- The parents may react with shock or 'numbness' or disbelief. Some may experience physical symptoms
- Parents need time to receive the information
- Any information given may need to be repeated, and distressed clients may need the information to be written down so that they can review it later
- Support for staff is also important
- The supervisor of midwives, community midwife, health visitor liaison, and GP should be informed of the intrauterine death as soon as possible after diagnosis.

Induction of labour
- An obstetric consultant should discuss a plan for care and delivery with the parents.
- Once the diagnosis is made, some women will want to wait a day or two, others will request induction of labour as soon as practical.
- If the death of the fetus is thought to be related to maternal complications such as placental abruption, PIH, or infection, urgent delivery is indicated.

- A full explanation should be given of the procedures, a possible time scale, and how the baby may look at delivery. Obtain consent for treatment. Those close to the couple should be encouraged to stay and give support.
- Ensure that the room for induction of labour is comfortable, and remove any inappropriate items (e.g. fetal monitor).
- Take IV samples of blood to test for FBC/platelets and G&S. Obtain a clotting screen if the intrauterine death occurred more than 3 weeks previously. Other samples may be requested, depending on the clinical picture.

Induction regimen
- Mifepristone 200mg is given orally and the woman may go home and return in 36–48h.
- On re-admission: misoprostol 800micrograms is given PV.
- Misoprostol 400micrograms is given PV 3h later.
- This is repeated 3h up to five doses. The regimen should be continued even when the cervix dilates, to maintain uterine activity.
- If delivery does not occur, the senior obstetrician should be informed. After 24h it is safe to repeat the five doses of misoprostol.
- ARM should be avoided until delivery is imminent because:
  - There is a risk of infection
  - The fetal skull is cushioned by the waters.
- Choice in analgesia is important. Opiates may be given or an epidural if there is no coagulopathy.
- Syntometrine® is indicated at delivery. Be aware that PPH may occur.

Care immediately after delivery
- Support the parents, and, if they are willing, encourage them to look at and hold the baby. They should be left alone with the baby for a period of time if they so wish.
- Acknowledge the parents' feelings of loss. A few kind words, a clasped hand or hug, or a small posy of flowers from staff can enrich the few memories the couple take away.
- The obstetric registrar or consultant should see the baby and complete a stillbirth certificate. It is important that this is obtained early in the proceedings because the parents will need it to make arrangements for registration and burial.
- Weigh the baby and measure his or her length. The parents may want to help with bathing and dressing the baby. They will wish to give the baby a name. Photographs, a lock of hair, handprints, and footprints are taken and transferred to a card as a keepsake.
- Carefully label the baby with the mother's identification details.
- Enquire whether the parents would like to see the hospital chaplain or other person who may provide spiritual support.

Administration
It is good practice to complete a bereavement checklist and to have a communication book to ensure that all administration is recorded efficiently (see Table 19.9).

Investigations into cause of fetal loss

- To complete the process of grieving for their baby the parents often need to know the cause of death.
- Certain blood, tissue samples and swabs may be requested from mother, fetus, and placenta, and are important for obtaining accurate information for counselling the parents at a later date (Table 19.10).
- The placenta may be sent to histology for examination.
- A postmortem may be indicated. A senior obstetrician or midwife should obtain consent after a full but sensitive explanation of the procedure. The parents should be given written information about the examination and have an opportunity to read it before consent.
- Photographs of the baby may be required and can be requested from medical photography.
- An appointment with the consultant should be arranged 4–6 weeks after the stillbirth to discuss any findings.

Transfer to the community

- If the woman is physically well after the delivery, the parents may want to go home and return, as they wish, to see the baby and discuss further arrangements. The baby will be kept in the hospital until decisions have been made about postmortem and funeral.
- If the fetal death occurred unexpectedly in labour, it is especially important that the parents be given plenty of time to talk through the incident with staff involved at the earliest opportunity.
- The parents need to know what might have been the cause; otherwise some in their grief may irrationally blame themselves or others. A mutually convenient appointment should be arranged.
- Anti-D may be given prophylactically to Rh-negative women.
- If the woman's pregnancy was more than 20 weeks' gestation and she has no history of PIH, she may be given a prescription for cabergoline 1mg, to be taken on the first postpartum day. This will help to suppress lactation.
- Give the woman and her partner literature that puts them in touch with other parents who have been bereaved; for example the Stillbirth and Neonatal Death Society (SANDS). The Child Bereavement Trust provides support for parents and siblings.
- Mark the hospital notes with the SANDS teardrop logo, indicating a perinatal bereavement.
- Where possible, postal advertising for pregnancy is cancelled.
- Some units keep a remembrance book and hold yearly memorial services for parents and families who have experienced the loss of a baby.

Registration and funeral arrangements

- If the gestation is <24 weeks, no registration is required.
- All stillborn babies after 24 weeks' gestation require a stillbirth certificate.
- This certificate is taken by the parents to the registrar of births and deaths at the registry so that the registration of the stillbirth can take place.

- The registration should be completed within 42 days.
- Unless legally married, the woman and her partner should attend together if the father's name is to be registered on the certificate.
- The parents should ask for a copy of the certificate for themselves.

Table 19.9 Example of bereavement checklist for labour ward

	Signature	Date
Name of doctor examining baby after delivery		
Mother informed or death by		
Father informed of death by		
New page in bereavement diary		
Notes marked with SANDS logo		
Cancellation card Bounty advertising		
Community midwife informed ASAP Name: Phone: Is a visit wanted at home?		
GP informed. Name: Phone: Is a visit wanted at home?		
Cancel antenatal clinic appointment		
Health visitor (HV) referral form: HV notified by phone		
Inform chaplaincy		
Parents given time to handle baby		
4 Polaroid photographs taken		
Medical illustration card completed		
Hand- and footprints/hair taken		
Computer details completed		
Congenital anomalies register		
Mortuary identification labels attached ×2		
SANDS booklet and other literature given		

- The registrar will issue a certificate of disposal following a stillbirth.
- This, when given to the funeral directors, allows them to proceed with arrangements for the funeral.
- The hospital may arrange the funeral, or parents may arrange a private cremation or burial if they wish.

For further information 📖 see Bereavement care, p. 516.

Table 19.10 Example of checklist for maternal, placenta, and fetal investigations

Maternal investigations	Bloods	Signature	Date	Required
Viral studies: toxoplasmosis, CMV, herpes, rubella	Virology			(Yes/no)
Blood group, antibodies, Kleihauer	BTS			Regardless of blood group
Haemoglobin	Haematology			
Listeriosis	Microbiology			

Fetal and placental	Bloods	Signature	Date	Required
Viral PCR studies: toxoplasmosis, CMV, herpes, rubella	Virology			
Blood group and Coomb's test	BTS			
Haemoglobin	Paediatric vial, haematology			
Chromosome analysis	Paediatric vial, cytogenetics; + sample of membrane, placenta, and cord. Sent in culture solution to Cytogenetics (consent required)			
Placental swabs	From maternal surface and from fetal surface; bacteriology			
Placenta to histology	Send as soon as possible regardless of whether a postmortem is required			

CMV, cytomegalovirus; BTS Blood Transfusion Service; PCR, polymerase chain reaction.
Adapted from Bereavement guidelines (2004). Jessop Wing Sheffield Teaching Hospitals Trust.

Part 4

Postnatal care

Postnatal care

Principles of postnatal care

The principles of postnatal care are mother and family centred, to meet her physical, psychological and emotional needs, in recovering from the birth experience and caring for her baby. In providing effective postnatal care, the midwife must ensure:

• The mother and her family are treated with kindness, respect and dignity
• Excellent communication that respects the views, values and beliefs of the woman, partner and her family
• A documented, individualized care plan developed in partnership with the mother and reviewed at each contact
• Timely and relevant information to enable her to promote her own and her baby's health and well-being and recognize and respond to any problems arising
• The mother is encouraged to make informed decisions about her care and any treatment needed
• The mother's emotional well-being is monitored and what family and social support she has in the postnatal period. Encourage the mother and her partner and family to tell the midwife about any changes in mood, emotional state, and behaviour that are outside of her normal pattern
• Contact details of all healthcare professionals involved in her care
• The mother knows the signs and symptoms of potentially life threatening conditions and how to summon help from the midwife or doctor or emergency services, if required
• Contemporaneous and accurate records about maternal and neonatal health and well-being, information, and advice given, agreed in partnership with the mother, and readily available to all healthcare professionals involved in her care.

The midwife must ensure that postnatal care complies with the following:

• Department of Health (2007). *Maternity Matters*. London: Department of Health.
• National Institute for Health and Clinical Excellence (2006). *Routine Postnatal Care of Women and their Babies*. Clinical guideline 37. London: NICE.
• National Institute for Health and Clinical Excellence (2007). *Antenatal and Postnatal Mental Health*. Clinical guideline 45. London: NICE.

Physiological aspects of postnatal care

Aim

- To ensure optimal physical health and to detect deviations from normal.
- A methodical top-to-toe examination, accompanied by a discussion about her health.
- Exact interpretation of the findings will depend on:
  - Whether the woman had a normal pregnancy and a spontaneous vaginal birth
  - Pre-existing health or obstetric problems
  - Problems occurring in labour.

Physiological changes

- Involution of the uterus and other parts of the genital tract.
- Initiation of lactation.
- Physiological changes in other body systems.

Vital signs

- Temperature: normal range 36–37°C. Once returned to the normal range after birth, it is unnecessary to check it routinely, unless the mother complains of, or shows, signs that suggest infection: feeling unwell, flu-like symptoms, or actual signs of infection.
- Pulse: normal range 65–80bpm. A rapid pulse rate may also indicate infection.
- Respiratory rate: normal range 12–16 per min at rest.
- Blood pressure: should return to normal within 24h of birth. Unless the blood pressure was raised pre-pregnancy, during pregnancy, and/or labour, there is no need to monitor routinely postnatally.

Involution of the uterus

Definition
The return of the uterus to its pre-pregnant size, tone, and position.

Process
- Ischaemia: the uterine muscle contracts and retracts, restricting the blood flow within the uterus.
- Phagocytosis: redundant fibrous and elastic tissue is broken down.
- Autolysis: muscle fibres are digested by proteolytic enzymes (lysozymes).
- All the waste products pass into the bloodstream and are eliminated via the kidneys.
- The decidual lining of the uterus is shed in the vaginal blood loss, and the new endometrium begins to develop from about 10 days after birth and is completed by 6 weeks.
- Uterine size decreases from 15cm × 11cm × 7.5cm to 7.5cm × 5cm × 2.5cm by 6 weeks.
- Uterine weight decreases from 1000g immediately after birth to 60g by 6 weeks. At the end of the first week it weighs about 500g.
- Rate of involution: there is a steady decrease by 1cm/day. On the first day it is 12cm above the symphysis pubis and by the 7th day is approximately 5cm above the symphysis pubis. By day 10 it is barely palpable, if at all.
- Involution will be slower after caesarean section.
- Involution will be delayed if there is retention of placental tissue or blood clot, particularly if associated with infection.

Assessment of postnatal uterine involution
- Discuss the need for uterine assessment with the mother.
- Obtain verbal consent.
- Ask her to empty her bladder if she has not done so in the last half hour.
- Ensure privacy.
- Ask her to lie on her back, with her head well supported.
- Cover her legs and abdomen.
- Wash your hands thoroughly.
- Ask the mother to expose her abdomen.
- Talk to the mother throughout the examination, explain what you are doing and why, and answer her questions.
- Face the mother and place the lower edge of the examining hand on the abdomen at the level of the umbilicus.
- Palpate gently inwards towards the spine and gently move downwards until the uterine fundus is located.
- Note the level of the uterine fundus and the degree of uterine contraction and retraction.
- Note any pain, tenderness, or bulkiness.
- Ask her about her vaginal loss: odour, amount, abnormal colour, or any concerns at all about her loss.
- Discuss the findings with the mother.

- Document the findings in the mother's records.
- Report any abnormalities to the doctor without delay.

Practice points

▶ It is important that:

- Wherever possible, the same midwife carries out the regular postnatal examination, to monitor normal involution and detect early deviations from normal.
- The uterus remains contracted and retracted and centrally positioned in the lower abdomen.

Daily uterine palpation is unnecessary after the first 3 days, unless there is any reason for concern or deviations from normal are apparent. The midwife should use her discretion.

Vaginal blood loss

- Blood is the major component of vaginal loss in the first few days.
- As uterine involution progresses, the vaginal loss changes to stale blood products, lanugo, vernix and other debris from the products of conception, leucocytes, and organisms.
- Towards the end of the second week the discharge is yellowish white, consisting of cervical mucus, leucocytes, and organisms.
- This process may take as long as 3 weeks, and research has shown that there is a wide variation in the amount, colour, and duration of vaginal loss in the first 12 weeks postpartum.

Practice point

▶ It is important that the midwife asks focused questions about the nature of the vaginal loss, to determine whether it is normal or not.

The perineum

- Even if the perineum remains intact at the time of birth, women experience bruising of the vaginal and perineal tissues for the first few days.
- Women may be embarrassed about exposing the perineum after birth, so, unless there is a clinical indication, i.e. pain or evidence of infection, routine daily observation by the midwife is unnecessary, and may actually serve to introduce infection, when strict hand washing before and after the procedure and the wearing of disposable gloves is not carried out.
- Ask her specific questions about perineal pain and soreness.
- Dependent on the suturing technique used, and on the suture material, sutures may have to be removed approximately 1 week after birth. However, absorbable, non-irritant suture material is now increasingly used.

Practice points

- The first few days after birth can be difficult physically, emotionally, and psychologically for a woman with perineal trauma, restricting her mobility, her rest and sleep, the enjoyment of her baby, and the ability to find a comfortable position for feeding, particularly if breastfeeding.
- Long-term physical and psychological trauma may be the result, and the midwife must be sensitive and supportive of the mother at this time.

Perineal pain

- If the mother has sustained perineal trauma, the midwife may wish to inspect the perineum daily for the first few days, to ascertain the comfort of any sutures, wound healing, and cleanliness.
- If she has interrupted sutures, removal of a particularly tight suture may be all that is required to ease perineal pain and tension.
- Advice should be given, as appropriate, about cleansing and changing the sanitary pad regularly, to avoid infection.
- Vaginal blood loss can also be assessed, as can the presence of haemorrhoids.
  Pain relief may be achieved in a number of ways:
- Try the simple remedies first, such as a bath, bidet, or cool water poured over the perineum.
- Bath additives, such as salt or Savlon®, have been shown in research to be of no added value, neither have treatments such as ultrasound, infrared heat, or pulsed electromagnetic energy in promoting healing or reducing pain.
- Keeping the area clean and dry, with pain relief, as above, allows healing.
- Oral analgesia such as paracetamol may be administered 4–6h.
- Lavender oil or tea tree essential oils, five drops added to bath water or applied as a topical compress. Homeopathic remedies, such as arnica, calendula and Bellis perennis may be applied topically or taken orally (📖 see Homoeopathy, p. 120 for detailed information).

Practice points

- If administering any of the above treatments, ensure personal knowledge and competence with regard to the current research evidence, and the use of complementary therapies, or refer the mother to an appropriately trained complementary therapist
- Document all examination, findings, and treatments clearly in the mother's and/or your notes.

Circulation

- The increased blood volume of pregnancy is gradually reabsorbed and excreted in the diuresis of the first few days after birth.
- Oedema of the feet and ankles may be experienced, even if not experienced in pregnancy.
- Check that the woman's blood pressure is not abnormally raised, and advise her to mobilize, avoid long periods of standing, and elevate the feet and legs when sitting.
- The swelling should be bilateral and without pain. Swelling in one leg, accompanied by pain in the calf or femoral area may indicate deep vein thrombosis (☐ see Deep vein thrombosis, p. 502 and Principles of thromboprophylaxis, p. 190, for further details).

Legs

- ► It is important to observe for swelling, oedema, inflammation, colour, and pain, particularly in a woman confined to bed or mobilizing in a limited way, particularly after operative delivery.
- ►► Any abnormality may be due to a DVT and medical aid should be sought immediately.

Haemoglobin level

- In some maternity units it is routine to check the maternal haemoglobin level on the 2nd or 3rd postnatal day.
- This practice is now occurring much less, as women are transferred home from hospital much earlier, often 6h after birth.
- It should not be necessary in fit, healthy women, where blood loss at birth has had no detrimental effect.
- In a mother who has had a traumatic birth and/or sustained a heavy blood loss, a FBC may be undertaken on the third postnatal day.
- Generally it is not now done unless clinically indicated.

General health

General observations
- Overall body temperature.
- Abnormal body odour that may suggest infection.
- Overall colour and complexion, e.g. flushed or pale.

Skin
- Skin texture and tone will return to normal soon after birth.
- Any skin irritation caused by obstetric cholestasis or skin stretching will soon resolve. A moisturizing lotion is all that is normally required to ease irritation and any dry feeling.

Nutrition
- Encourage the mother to maintain a balanced diet as much as possible and to include as much fresh food as possible.
- Adequate water intake is important, at least 2L a day.
- Adequate fluid and nutrition are essential for lactation, to encourage normal gastrointestinal activity, and resume normal bowel action as soon as possible.

Bowel action
- This should return to normal in 2–3 days after birth.
- Fresh fruit, vegetables, and a good fluid intake will encourage this.
- After caesarean section it may take a day or so longer, particularly if diet and fluids have been restricted in the first few hours after operation.

Practice point
The mother may be afraid of rupturing any perineal sutures, so supporting the perineum with a pad may help during the first bowel action.

Urinary output

- A marked diuresis will occur in the first 2–3 days after birth, but there should be no dysuria (pain on micturition).
- There may be some soreness from perineal trauma.
- Ask the mother whether she is passing urine normally and whether there is any discomfort or any stress incontinence.
- The bladder neck and urethra may have been damaged during labour and birth, which could result in a lack of sensation to pass urine in the first couple of days. This can lead to retention with overflow, causing intense pain and discomfort, urinary tract infection, and sub-involution of the uterus, a cause of primary or secondary postpartum haemorrhage.

Practice points

- ► Passing very small amounts of urine is often a sign of retention with overflow. Palpate the bladder after she has been to the toilet. If a portable ultrasound bladder scanner is available, the midwife may scan the bladder to estimate the amount of urine retained.
- If the mother has difficulty in passing urine, try the simple remedies first, such as running water, asking her to sit on the bidet or in a bath of warm water, in an attempt to stimulate micturition.
- Oral fluids should not be restricted, but encouraged.
- If a mother has difficulty with micturition, burning sensation, or pain with micturition, obtain a midstream specimen of urine in a sterile container and send for laboratory culture.
- Initial inspection of the urine for colour, clarity, and odour will yield useful information if infection is suspected.

Psychological and emotional aspects of postnatal care

- Psychological and emotional well-being and positive mental health are as important as the physical aspects of care.
- Postnatal emotional and psychological changes following childbirth are commonly experienced by women.
- Midwives have an important role in the early detection of psychological problems and have a responsibility as part of the multi-professional team, to ensure that women are referred appropriately and receive support and care.
- Psychological conditions in the postnatal period cover a spectrum of conditions that vary from mild to severe.
- At each postnatal contact the mother should be asked about her emotional well-being, what family and social support she has, and her usual coping strategies with day-to-day matters.[1]
- Good communication, listening to what the mother is telling you and responding appropriately, will do much to alleviate situations causing the mother anxiety, most commonly concerning baby care and feeding.
- The mother and her partner should be offered the opportunity to talk about their birth experiences and ask questions about the care they received and the events of labour. For further information (📖 see Postnatal afterthoughts for parents, p. 510).
- The mother and her partner/family should be encouraged to tell the midwife about any changes in mood, emotional state, and behaviour that are outside the woman's normal pattern.[1]
- The midwife must always be able to recognize the risks, signs, and symptoms of domestic abuse and whom to contact for advice and management.[2,3]

Temporary mood alteration (postpartum 'blues')

This is a transient, self-limiting condition, often referred to as 'baby blues'. It occurs between the third and tenth days, although it occurs most often around the fourth day. It is considered a normal reaction to childbirth and between 50% and 80% will experience the condition.[1]

Symptoms
These include:
- Tearfulness
- Mood swings
- Irritability.

The condition usually resolves spontaneously within a day or two, although women with postnatal depression have been shown to have higher occurrences of the baby blues. Provide emotional support and reassurance that it is a temporary condition that will resolve.

1 National Institute for Health and Clinical Excellence (2006). *Routine Postnatal Care of Women and Their Babies.* Clinical guideline 37. London: NICE.

2 Department of Health (2004). *National Service Framework for Children, Young People and Maternity Services. Standard 11: Maternity Services.* London: DH. Available at: ℘ www.dh.gov.uk (accessed 2.5.10).

3 Department of Health (2005). *Responding to Domestic Abuse: A Handbook for Health Professionals.* London: DH. Available at: ℘ www.dh.gov.uk (accessed 2.5.10).

Transfer home from hospital

- The exact timing of transfer home is normally negotiated between the mother and the midwife, and is dependent on her circumstances and needs.
- Care is transferred back to the community midwife, if the model of care operating locally has not involved the named community midwife in her care in hospital.
- Examine the mother, to ensure that she is physically fit to go home, and ensure that the baby has been fully examined by a paediatrician or a midwife appropriately trained and competent to undertake this first complete examination of the newborn. Community midwives now also undertake this examination in the UK, for mothers who have had a home birth, or they may carry out the examination on the first visit after transfer home.
- Explain to the mother about the continued visiting by her community midwife, give her her personal notes, duly completed to date, and letters for her family doctor and community midwife, containing the relevant details about the birth and progress of the mother and baby to date.
- This is accompanied by a range of leaflets and details of how to get advice and support night and day, e.g. the telephone number of the community midwife, postnatal ward, community midwifery office, and infant feeding adviser.
- The mother makes her own arrangements for transport home.
- The importance of car safety for mother and baby should be stressed, although it is the mother's/parents' responsibility to ensure that the baby is transported in a car seat, appropriately secured in the car.
- On no account must the midwife have any involvement in the process of putting the baby in the car seat or securing the seat in the car.
- It is important that the transfer home between hospital and community midwife is seamless, in that there is continuity of care, no conflicting advice, and records clearly show progress and problems to date and advice given.

Parent education

Aims
- To promote health improvement
- To give appropriate information and support
- To develop confidence in parenting skills
- To facilitate parental involvement in decision making
- To provide emotional and psychological support for the new parents
- To encourage peer support.

Practice points
- The social, emotional, and psychological needs of parents are as important as the physical skills of caring for the baby.
- Every mother/parent has differing needs.
- Certain groups have special needs, e.g. the young, single, women with disability, ethnic minorities, women whose first language is not English, women with learning difficulties, asylum seekers, refugees.
- Don't forget the men!
- Preparation for parenthood begins in childhood; in the home, in school, and the social environment, e.g. television, books, magazines.
- Continuity of care and carer, as far as possible, will enable the mother to express her concerns, fears, and anxieties more freely, and will enable the midwife to be more effective in education activities.
- Every meeting with new parents is an opportunity for health education, health promotion, parent education, or referral to other health or social care professionals or agencies that can more effectively address or meet their needs.
- Use each care setting as an educational opportunity.
- Small groups aid discussion and can encourage women/parents to air their problems, learn from each other, and aid peer support for new parents. With the development of local Children's Centres in the UK, the opportunity for networking and developing social networks of support for the mother, also offers the midwife and other health and social care professionals the ideal opportunity for health education and promotion.
- When offering group sessions, consider the target group and its needs carefully. You may need to offer a choice of groups and times.
- Be realistic about what can be achieved in a series of meetings.

Main educational activities
The mother:
- Adequate rest and sleep
- Well-balanced diet
- Personal hygiene, particularly of the vulval and perineal area
- Prevention of infection
- Healthy lifestyle, e.g. smoking cessation
- Postnatal exercises and encouragement to continue with them for at least 6 weeks
- Resuming normal exercise regimens, e.g. returning to the gym
- Continuing contact with healthcare professionals for personal support and infant care, e.g. immunizations and child development.

The baby:
- Provide a safe, child friendly environment
- Teach infant care skills
- Cord care
- Hygiene
- Room temperature—keep baby warm but not overheated
- Prevention of infection
- Breastfeeding (📖 see Chapter 24 for further information):
  - Establishing and maintaining lactation
  - Correct fixing technique
  - Hand expression technique
  - Safe storage of expressed breast milk
- Formula feeding:
  - Sterilization of feeding and other equipment
  - Making up feeds safely
  - Choosing the correct formula
  - Storage of made-up feeds
  - The dos and don'ts of formula feeding
- Responding to and interpreting baby's cry
- Getting to know the baby
- Sleep patterns
- General behaviour
- Car seats and safety
- Prevention of sudden infant death
- Risks of co-sleeping with parents.

Emotional:
- Effect of the new baby in the home
- Changing roles and responsibilities
- Relationship with partner and family
- Sibling jealousy
- Psychological adaptation to parenthood.

Father/partner:
- Increasing involvement in the care of the immediate family
- Important adjustments
- Aid his partner in adjusting to motherhood
- Jealousy of the baby
- Sharing his partner
- Supporting his partner
- Sharing baby care
- Helping with other children and care of the home
- Encourage him to be as involved as possible
- Paternity leave entitlement.

Sexual:
- Resumption of sexual relationships
- Dyspareunia
- Contraception
- Sexual health
- Cervical screening.

Postoperative care

- The most common reason for postoperative care is caesarean section, but reasons may include manual removal of the placenta or dealing with persistent post-birth bleeding from the genital tract.
- Immediate postoperative care is normally undertaken in the theatre recovery room by theatre staff, but in many cases the midwife will find herself undertaking this care.
- Clear and accurate documentation of all aspects of care is vital.
- Postoperative observations of the mother will consist of observation and management of:
  - Vital signs and level of consciousness, if she has had a general anaesthetic
  - Epidural site and degree of anaesthesia
  - Pain
  - Vaginal blood loss
  - Wound drain
  - IV fluids and the cannula area
  - Bladder drainage (if a urinary catheter is *in situ*).
- As soon as possible after the birth, the mother should have skin-to-skin contact with her baby, as would happen in a normal birth. If her condition/level of consciousness do not immediately allow this, then the father could undertake the initial skin-to-skin contact, until the mother is able to (☐ see Skin-to-skin, p. 310).
- Once the mother's condition is stable and she is fully conscious, she is transferred to the postnatal ward with her baby.
- A caesarean section is major abdominal surgery, and if it was undertaken following a complicated or traumatic labour, the mother has to recover from the physical and the mental stress of labour, as well as from the anaesthetic and the operation.

Immediate care

Position
- General anaesthetic: nurse her in the left lateral or 'recovery' position until fully conscious.
- Epidural or spinal anaesthesia: as directed by the anaesthetist, particularly noting her respiratory rate, because of the narcotic analgesia given.
- Gradually sit her up as soon as possible, provided her blood pressure is stable.

Observations
The frequency of the observations carried out will be according to local policy and practice guidelines, but generally will follow this pattern for the first 12h:
- Blood pressure and pulse rate: half hourly for the first 2h, hourly for 2h then 4h.
- Wound and wound drain inspection, as above.
- Vaginal blood loss, as above.
- Temperature: 2h for the first 4h then 4h.

Analgesia

Postoperative pain relief can be given in a number of ways:
- Epidural opioid (observe respiratory rate).
- Intravenous opioid: patient-controlled device.
- Subcutaneous opioid or other similar analgesia.
- Intramuscular opioid, never use in conjunction with an epidural opioid.
- Rectal, e.g. diclofenac.
- Oral drugs, e.g. dihydrocodeine or paracetamol.

An anti-emetic, such as cyclizine, may be prescribed and given intra-muscularly or subcutaneously, to counteract nausea or vomiting caused by opioid drugs.

Care in the postnatal ward

Unless the baby has been transferred to the neonatal unit, the mother and baby should be transferred together and stay together. Attachment should be encouraged and a clip-on cot, which fits on to the mother's bed, will make it easier for the mother to touch and handle her baby.

The midwife should employ a model of care that ensures a holistic and integrated approach to meeting the individual woman's needs and encouraging increasing self-care, but limiting over-exertion.

Observations

Continue the regimen begun in the theatre recovery room for the first 12h:
- Blood pressure and pulse rate: half hourly for the first 2h, hourly for 2h then 4h
- Wound and wound drain inspection, as above
- Vaginal blood loss, as above
- Temperature: 2h for the first 4h then 4h.

The IV infusion is usually removed 8–12h after operation, once the mother's blood pressure is stable and she is tolerating oral fluids.

Wound care

- Prophylactic antibiotics may be prescribed to reduce the incidence of wound infection; the regimen and route of administration are dependent on local policy and practice, e.g. IV, intramuscularly, or oral.
- The principle of wound care is to keep it dry and clean. The dressing is usually removed after 24h, if one has been applied initially.
- If the woman is obese and lower abdominal skin folds are present, allowing the wound to become warm and moist, the dressing may be left on.
- Offer advice about drying the wound thoroughly after a shower.
- Observe the wound for the following, reporting any occurrence to the doctor:
  - *Infection*: hot, tender, inflamed area, pyrexia; obtain a swab for laboratory culture.
  - *Haematoma*: pain, hard to touch, tender.
- Broad-spectrum antibiotics will usually be started at this point, if they are not being taken prophylactically. They may be given IV or subcutaneously or taken orally, depending on local policy.

Thromboprophylaxis

📖 See Principles of thromboprophylaxis, p. 190.

- Pulmonary embolism and thromboembolic disease are the main causes of direct maternal death in the UK.[1]
- Encourage the mother to move her legs, with leg stretching and ankle rotation exercises, at least every hour.
- Administer low-molecular-weight heparin, tinzaparin, subcutaneously, daily for 48–72h.
- Measure the woman for thromboembolic prevention stockings prior to operation and ensure they are put on prior to operation and worn until full mobility is regained.
- Encourage mobilization as soon as possible.

Urine output

- An indwelling catheter is usually *in situ* for the first 24–48h postoperatively, after which it is removed.
- Observe and record the urine output carefully and empty the catheter bag, measure and record the amount 6–8 hourly. Never let the drainage bag get too full, as this can be very uncomfortable, cumbersome, and embarrassing for the mother, as she begins to mobilize.
- The mother should be encouraged to use the bidet when she is able to get up, to keep the vulva and catheter area clean.
- It is good practice to obtain and send a catheter specimen of urine to the lab at the time of removal of the catheter, or any time before that if the mother is complaining of pain, which could be associated with urinary tract infection.
- After catheter removal it is important to ask the mother about her ability to pass urine and the amount passed.
- Observe and palpate the abdomen for evidence of retention of urine at least twice a day for the first day.
- At first the bladder may not be completely emptied and a bladder scan after passing urine will estimate the residual urine in the bladder. This should be <30mL as bladder tone gradually returns.
- Report any haematuria to the doctor.

Fluid and nutrition

- The mother is encouraged to drink plenty and to gradually introduce a light diet. Plain water is the fluid of choice if there are any problems with nausea or vomiting following general anaesthesia, until this has passed.
- If there has been trauma to any part of the pelvic structures or handling of the bowel, the surgeon will usually request water only by mouth until bowel sounds return, 24–48h after surgery, to avoid the risk of paralytic ileus.
- Appetite will vary from woman to woman, and those who have had a general anaesthetic will be less keen to eat initially.

Mood and feelings

- After a general anaesthetic some women feel very tired and have a sense of detachment for several days.
- She may not relate well to the baby immediately.
- She may feel guilty, disappointed, or a failure at not achieving a normal birth.
- Pain and the analgesia given may make her sleepy.
- She will need help with caring for and feeding her baby.

1 Lewis, G (ed.) (2007). *The Confidential Enquiry into Maternal and Child Health (CEMACH). Saving Mothers' Live; Reviewing Maternal Deaths to Make Motherhood Safer—2003–2005.* The 7th Report on Confidential Enquires into Maternal Deaths in the United Kingdom. London: CEMACH.

Postnatal care of the breasts

The advice that is given to the mother on the care of the breasts postnatally will depend upon her choice of infant feeding method.

Postnatal care for breastfeeding mothers

- Mothers are no longer advised to wash their breasts before each feed, as the use of soap may remove the natural oils that keep the nipples and areola supple.
- Advise mothers that adequate personal hygiene is sufficient.
- A supportive well-fitting maternity bra may add to the mother's comfort but care should be taken that it does not dig into the breast tissue.
- There is no evidence to support the use of creams, ointments, sprays, or tinctures to prevent nipple soreness and, in some cases; these have been shown to increase the incidence of soreness.
- Provide help and assistance to ensure correct positioning and attachment of the baby at the breast.
- The duration and frequency of feeds should not be restricted.
- For mothers with specific problems, 🕮 see Breastfeeding problems, p. 690).

Breast care for mothers who are bottle feeding

The mother should be informed that although she is not breastfeeding the milk will still 'come in' between 2 and 4 days postnatally. Advise the mother:

- To handle her breasts as little as possible
- To wear a good supporting bra
- Not to express the milk as this will encourage further milk production
- To use heat and cold, either via a shower or soaking in the bath, to help relieve discomfort
- Take mild analgesics, e.g. paracetamol to help relieve the discomfort.

Reassure the mother that this is a transient condition that will resolve within 24–48h.

Occasionally, pharmacological preparations (bromocriptine and cabergoline) may be used for the suppression of lactation. Bromocriptine has adverse side-effects and therefore cabergoline is usually the drug of choice.

Care of the mother with pre-existing medical conditions

Diabetes

Most diabetic women can return to normal management of their diabetes after the birth, as soon as the first meal is taken. In gestational diabetes there is a rapid return to normal and usually no further insulin is required.

If the mother is insulin dependent:

- The dosage of insulin should reflect the blood glucose measurement.
- Energy requirements vary considerably in the postnatal period, especially if the mother breastfeeds.
- Most women need extra carbohydrates if breastfeeding, 40–90g/day.
- The mother may experience more hypoglycaemic episodes and may need a snack when feeding her baby at night.
- Many breastfeeding diabetics find that their insulin requirements are lower because of the energy expenditure of lactation. This remains so while fully breastfeeding and needs adjustment when the baby starts weaning.

Epilepsy

Women are often concerned about how they will manage once their baby is born, and there may be safety issues for some women with epilepsy. Precautions aim to minimize any risk to the baby and mother and maximize opportunities for bonding. The mother should be advised to avoid extreme tiredness (this makes seizures more likely), which can be difficult with the demands of a new baby! The woman's partner helping to settle the baby after feeds at night or helping with formula feeds helps protect against exhaustion. Where the mother has sudden, frequent, or unpredictable seizures, the following safety measures are recommended:

- The mother can feed her baby while sitting on the floor, supported by cushions
- Changing the baby's nappy can take place at floor level on a changing mat
- Bathing the baby should take place when the mother is least likely to experience a seizure or when there is someone there to assist if necessary. Alternatively, washing the baby on a towel instead of immersion in water might be preferable.

❶ Antiepileptic drugs (AEDs) are excreted in breast milk, but breastfeeding is safe, and it should be recommended if this is the mother's preferred choice, as it may even help wean the baby from the higher levels of AEDs to which he or she was exposed *in utero*. Mothers should watch for drowsiness in their infants.

A postnatal epilepsy review should take place at 6 weeks and the mother should be seen by a specialist at 12 weeks.[1] If the dose of AEDs was increased during pregnancy, this may need to be gradually reduced under supervision.

Effective contraception must be discussed with a woman taking antiepileptic drugs and the contraceptive pill should be avoided if possible, because drug interactions reduce its effectiveness.

---

1 National Institute for Health and Clinical Excellence (2004). *Epilepsy in Adults and Children*. Clinical guideline No.20. London: NICE. Available at: ℘ www.nice.org.uk/nicemedia/pdf/CG020niceguidline.pdf.

Chapter 21

Disorders of the postnatal period

The uterus

- The uterus that is deviated to one side, usually to the right, is usually the result of a full bladder. If the woman cannot empty her bladder, or the bladder still palpates as full after voiding urine, catheterization of the bladder is required to remove the urine, allow the uterus to involute normally, and prevent urinary tract infection.
- As a precaution, an MSU should be sent to the laboratory for bacterial culture.
- Constipation may also inhibit the rate of uterine involution.

Sub-involution of the uterus

- The uterus fails to involute at the expected rate, feels wide and 'boggy' on palpation.
- The vaginal blood loss is markedly brighter red and heavier than normal.
- The mother may be passing clots of blood and/or her loss may smell offensive. This may indicate genital tract infection or retained products of conception.
- The mother may also feel unwell and have a raised temperature and pulse rate.
- Seek urgent medical aid to investigate and treat the cause.
- The usual treatment is a course of antibiotics and, if retained products are suspected, an evacuation of the uterus under general anaesthesia, to prevent infection and PPH.
- Thereafter undertake twice-daily monitoring of vital signs, palpation of the uterus and monitor vaginal blood loss, until the situation returns to normal.

Practice point

▶ It is so important that, at the birth, you check the placenta for completeness and note any apparent missing pieces of cotyledon or membrane in the birth records. This information must be passed to the midwife giving postnatal care.

Primary postpartum haemorrhage

Definition
Profuse bleeding from the genital tract from after completion of the third stage of labour until 24h after birth.

Signs and symptoms
- Sudden or excessive vaginal blood loss
- The uterus may fell enlarged, soft, and 'boggy' on palpation
- Pallor
- Rising pulse rate
- Falling blood pressure.

More serious
- Maternal collapse
- Altered level of consciousness: drowsy, restless
- Heavy blood loss.

Immediate action
- Summon medical aid.
- Summon other colleagues if able to.
- Stop the bleeding: if the uterus feels soft and relaxed:
  - Rub up a contraction by massaging the uterine fundus gently in a circular motion
  - When contracted, stop the massage.
- Administer a uterotonic drug:
  - Oxytocin 5–10 units intramuscularly (effective in 2–2.5min)
  - Oxytocin/ergometrine 1mL intramuscularly (effective in 2–2.5min)
  - Ergometrine 0.25–0.5mg IV (effective in 45s)
  - Consider further resuscitative measures according to maternal response.
- Put the baby to the breast.
- Empty the bladder by catheter.
- Empty the uterus: gentle pressure on the contracted uterus, in an attempt to expel any retained placental tissue, membranes, or blood clots.
- If the bleeding continues and the uterus is well contracted, consider other causes of bleeding:
  - Cervical tear
  - Deep vaginal wall tear
  - Perineal trauma
  - Uterine rupture (rare).
- Attempt to locate the source of the bleeding. Direct pressure can be applied to a lower vaginal or perineal tear.
- A vaginal pack can be inserted to attempt to arrest bleeding from higher up the genital tract, as a first-aid measure.
- Keep all pads and linen to assess blood loss.
- If possible, and if trained to do so, ask a colleague to cannulate a suitable vein in the arm or hand, with a cannula suitably large enough to administer blood, and commence IV fluids, sodium chloride 0.9%, or Hartmann's solution 1L.

- Record vital signs every 5–15min, according to the mother's condition.
  This emergency may occur in the home, when the mother may be
  alone, and the community midwife may be the first person to arrive.
- Tell the mother to leave the access door unlocked and lie down flat
  until you arrive.
- If severe or uncontrolled blood loss, summon urgent aid, as
  determined by local policy, either the emergency obstetric unit or a
  paramedic ambulance.
- Reassure the mother and others present, warn her of the possible
  need for theatre, for exploration and treating the cause of the bleeding
  under general anaesthesia.
- Accompany the mother to hospital with her baby.

Afterwards

- Continue IV therapy according to prescription.
- Monitor blood pressure, pulse rate, temperature, and respirations, as
  described above.
- Monitor vaginal blood loss.
- Administer antibiotics as prescribed, usually IV at first.
- Monitor the mother for signs of infection.
- Give psychological support and reassurance to the mother,
  partner, and others concerned, and explain what happened and the
  ongoing care.

Secondary postpartum haemorrhage

Definition
- Profuse bleeding from the genital tract, occurring after the first 24h until 6 weeks after birth.
- It most commonly occurs between 7 and 14 days after birth.

Signs and symptoms
- Often preceded by a heavy red loss, which may be offensive and accompanied by sub-involution of the uterus. Some clots or pieces of membrane may be seen.
- Tachycardia and low-grade pyrexia will indicate the presence of infection.

Management
- Massage the uterus, if palpable, to encourage uterine contraction.
- Summon medical aid, according to local policy.
- Ensure the bladder is empty; catheterize if necessary.
- To control bleeding:
  - If bleeding is severe, give 250–500micrograms of ergometrine maleate IV, or intramuscularly if you are unable/not trained and competent to administer IV drugs.
- Insert an IV cannula, if competent to do so, and start an IV infusion of sodium chloride 0.9%. Otherwise, get the equipment ready for the doctor or paramedic to carry out this procedure.

Practice point
▶▶This emergency normally occurs in the home 7–14 days after birth. Transfer the mother to hospital as quickly as possible via paramedic ambulance and accompany her, continuing to carry out emergency procedures, as required.

Maternal collapse within 24h without bleeding

Possible causes

- Inversion of the uterus
- Amniotic fluid embolism
- Pulmonary embolism
- Cerebrovascular accident
- Fitting: eclamptic fit, even with no previous signs of hypertension or pre-eclampsia.

Midwifery management

- Ensure a safe environment.
- Summon emergency medical aid and help from other midwives in the vicinity.
- Lay her down flat.
- Commence basic emergency care:
  - **A**irway—ensure it is patent
  - **B**reathing—ensure she is breathing. Monitor respiratory rate and depth of respirations
  - **C**irculation—check pulse rate.
- If trained and able, ask a colleague to insert an IV cannula and commence IV fluids, e.g. Hartmann's solution, 1L. This is best done as soon as possible, before her veins collapse as her blood pressure falls.
- If collapse is total and she has stopped breathing, and her pulse is weak or absent, initiate emergency resuscitation procedure drill until help arrives.

Hypertensive disorders

- All women who have pre-existing hypertension and hypertensive disorders of pregnancy can develop eclampsia in the hours and days following birth.
- Although postnatal eclampsia is rare, it is not unknown for a woman with a history of a normal blood pressure to develop postnatal pre-eclampsia or eclampsia.
- Continue monitoring the blood pressure, twice daily for at least 3 days after birth, until you are sure it is back within normal range and there are no other signs of pre-eclampsia.
- Keep accurate records of the recordings in the mother's records.
- If necessary, the doctor may prescribe antihypertensive treatment, in which case regular blood pressure recording must be continued until the blood pressure has been back within normal range and stable for at least 24h.

Essential hypertension

- This woman was hypertensive prior to pregnancy and has probably required an increase in her medication in pregnancy.
- Continue monitoring the blood pressure daily for 48h, then daily while the antihypertensive medication is satisfactorily readjusted and the blood pressure is stable within normal limits.
- If the mother is breastfeeding, check that the medication is not harmful to the baby. If the medication is contraindicated in breastfeeding, discuss it with the doctor, to find one that is suitable.

Practice point

- ▶ It is essential that the blood pressure is controlled within the normal range, to prevent eclampsia, cerebrovascular accident, and renal damage.
- Monitor urine output, as well as monitoring the blood pressure in the early postnatal period.

Circulatory disorders

Varicose veins
- Generally, these start in pregnancy and are due to hormonal relaxation of the veins, increased venous pressure, and increasing weight as pregnancy progresses.
- Most common in the legs, but may present as vulval or femoral varicosities.
- Generally they regress after birth.
- Some women have pre-existing varicose veins and for some women they become worse with successive pregnancies and increasing age.

Signs and symptoms
- They may become inflamed and painful, particularly in the early postnatal period.
- Vulval varicose veins may rupture during the second stage of labour, from pressure of the fetal head or from perineal tearing, and can be a cause of significant haemorrhage.
- May predispose to increased risk of DVT.

Treatment
- Early ambulation and walking out each day is encouraged.
- Rest with legs raised, whenever possible.
- Local anti-inflammatory treatment and oral analgesia.
- ► Support stockings should *not* be worn, as they restrict blood flow in the legs. Support tights are better.
- In subsequent years some women will require surgical treatment for varicose veins.

Superficial thrombophlebitis
Signs and symptoms
Localized inflammation and tenderness around the affected varicose vein, and, perhaps, a mild pyrexia.

Treatment
- Support, anti-embolic stockings.
- Early ambulation. Support when sitting, with leg raised on a footstool or, preferably, on the bed, in the acute stage.
- Anti-inflammatory drugs (care if breastfeeding).

Deep vein thrombosis
Signs and symptoms
- Unilateral oedema in the affected leg
- Calf pain and stiffness
- Difficulty in walking
- Positive Homan's sign.

Treatment
- Urgent referral to the doctor is required.
- If necessary, transfer the woman back to hospital medical services by ambulance.
- Anticoagulant therapy must be started as soon as possible, IV heparin initially for 24–48h, followed by daily subcutaneous tinzaparin injection of 3500 or 4500mg.

- Observe and monitor the woman for signs and symptoms of pulmonary embolism.
- Document all observations and treatment in her notes.

Pulmonary embolism

- Pulmonary embolism remains a major cause of maternal death worldwide and is the most common cause in the UK.[1]
- Early ambulation for all women is the most effective form of prevention.
- Women most at risk are those with:
  - Previous history of DVT or pulmonary embolism
  - Pre-existing or pregnancy-induced medical or obstetric complications resulting in prolonged immobility
  - Epidural anaesthesia
  - Operative birth
  - Prolonged labour
  - Anaemia.

Signs and symptoms

- Severe chest pain
- Breathlessness
- Gasping for breath
- Fear
- Tachycardia
- Shallow, gasping respirations
- Sweating, pallor
- Cyanosis, particularly at the peripheries and around the mouth.

Treatment

- Ensure a safe environment.
- Summon emergency medical aid and help from other midwives in the vicinity.
- Ask for emergency trolley and defibrillator.
- Lay her down flat.
- Commence basic emergency care:
  - **A**irway—ensure it is patent
  - **B**reathing—ensure she is breathing. Monitor respiratory rate and depth of respirations
  - **C**irculation—check pulse rate.
- If trained and able, ask a colleague to insert an IV cannula and commence IV fluids, e.g. Hartmann's solution, 1L. This is best done as soon as possible, before her veins collapse as her blood pressure falls.
- If collapse is total and she has stopped breathing, and her pulse is weak or absent, initiate emergency resuscitation procedure drill until help arrives.

Practice points

- ▶ Pulmonary embolism is the highest major cause of direct maternal death in the UK.[1]
- ▶ It is essential that all midwives know and practise the emergency drills regularly, in order that, should an emergency occur, the emergency procedure works well and all know what to do.

1 Lewis, G (ed.) (2007). *The Confidential Enquiry into Maternal and Child Health (CEMACH). Saving Mothers' Live; Reviewing Maternal Deaths to Make Motherhood Safer—2003–2005. The 7th Report on Confidential Enquires into Maternal Deaths in the United Kingdom.* London: CEMACH.

Postnatal pain

- *'After pains'*: the most common cause of postnatal pain, is experienced as the uterine involution and pelvic musculature return to normal. All women experience them to some degree, from mild discomfort to pain equivalent to moderate labour pains. It is caused by the release of oxytocin to cause uterine contraction and retraction and is exacerbated in a breastfeeding mother, in response to suckling and the 'let down' response. An appropriate analgesic, taken prior to breastfeeding, will usually help. The pain is intermittent in nature.
- *Abdominal or pelvic pain* may also be associated with a full bladder, constipation, flatus, intrauterine infection or, in rare cases, a pelvic vein thrombosis.
- *Pain in the uterus*, which is constant or present on abdominal palpation, is most likely due to infection. Other signs, such as a raised temperature and pulse rate, and heavy, offensive vaginal blood loss, may be present.
- *Symphysis pubis pain* occurs 8–60h after birth and may inhibit mobility. Whenever possible, the midwife should seek the support of the obstetric physiotherapist. Bed rest with hips adducted and analgesia may be supplemented by a pelvic binder, an elasticated support bandage, or trochanteric belt. Lying on her side in bed helps reduce symphysis pubis separation. Elbow crutches or a walking frame may be needed to support weight-bearing for several weeks. She will also need considerable help with the baby's care.

Headache

General headache

As with the general population, there are many causes of postnatal head-ache. The duration, severity, and frequency are important in the postnatal period.

- Tiredness, lack of sleep, the hot, dry environment of the postnatal ward, dehydration, worrying about her baby, her ability as a mother, infant feeding, particularly establishing breastfeeding, may all cause tension and anxiety leading to headache.
- Simple analgesia, such as paracetamol or ibuprofen, should be effective in these situations.
- Ensure that she drinks sufficient fluid, particularly water.
- ▶ A walk in the fresh air, in the cooler part of the day, will also often help, as will support and encouragement with baby care.

Epidural anaesthesia

- Headache arising from a dural tap once the mother is mobile again, and is worse when she is standing. The headache may be accompanied by neck stiffness, vomiting, and visual disturbances.
- The anaesthetist must be informed, to manage the leakage of CSF.
- She may already have returned home and will require readmission to hospital with her baby.

High blood pressure

- It is most important to monitor the blood pressure if there has been a pre-existing raised blood pressure.
- ▶ An untreated raised blood pressure will cause increasing headache and may lead to fits or a cerebrovascular accident.

Psychological stress

- It is important that issues pertinent to birth are explored sensitively in privacy, also other issues that may be worrying her.
- Take time to explore her feelings and ascertain whether there are problems at home; for example, domestic abuse.
- Deal sensitively and confidentially with any issues that arise, with the mother's permission; this may mean referral to other members of the multidisciplinary team.

Urinary tract disorders

The physiological changes that occurred in pregnancy and labour may take up to 6 weeks to resolve after birth, hence the potential for urinary problems and infection is considerable.

Problems are relatively common in the immediate postnatal period and usually resolve as the pelvic floor regains its muscle tone and the pelvic structures return to the pre-pregnant state. However, for a small number of women, the problem persists for weeks or months.

Common disorders
- Difficulty in voiding urine
- Frequency of micturition
- Acute retention of urine
- Cystitis
- Urinary tract infection.
  Most at risk are those with:
- Antenatal asymptomatic bacteriuria
- Antenatal urinary tract infection or pyelonephritis
- Catheterization in labour
- Epidural or spinal anaesthetic
- Long second stage with slow progress
- Vaginal delivery of a large baby
- Instrumental delivery, particularly forceps, causing trauma to the bladder and urethra
- Perineal trauma, particularly vulval grazes and tears
- Lax abdominal wall.

Management
- Determine the cause.
- Catheterize if retention of urine is present.
- Reassure the mother.
- Give analgesia if required.
- Exclude urinary tract infection through laboratory culture of an MSU.
- Postnatal pelvic floor exercises.

Acute retention of urine
- Usually caused by trauma to the bladder and urethra during labour.
- Bladder feels hard and distended abdominally.
- Lower abdominal severe discomfort and pain, if sensation is present.
- After an epidural or spinal anaesthetic, the sensation to pass urine may be lost for a number of hours.
- The uterus is higher in the abdomen than it should be and is displaced to one side.

Management
- Catheterize to remove the urine, and withdraw the catheter.
- Advise the mother to drink plenty of fluid, and keep an accurate fluid balance chart until you are sure the crisis period is over.
- An indwelling catheter must not be left in at this stage.

- Encourage her to void urine at regular intervals, to regain bladder tone.
- If retention reoccurs, an indwelling catheter may be inserted for 24–48h, to help the bladder regain its tone.

Urinary tract infection

Signs and symptoms

- Frequency of urine
- Dysuria
- Urine may be cloudy in appearance and have an offensive odour
- Rise in temperature
- Feeling unwell.

Treatment

- Obtain an MSU and send to the laboratory for microscopy.
- Report to the doctor.
- Commence broad-spectrum antibiotics, and change, if necessary, once the results of laboratory microscopy are known.
- Ask the mother to drink at least 3L of fluid a day.
- Maintain an accurate fluid balance chart.
- Repeat the MSU once the antibiotic course is completed to ensure the infection is successfully treated.

Pyelonephritis

Signs and symptoms

- As above, but more severe.
- The woman looks and feels very unwell, and has flu-like symptoms.
- Pain radiating from the loin to the groin, usually unilaterally.
- Pyrexia.
- Rigors.
- Vomiting.
- Lack of any appetite.
- Urine smells offensive, has an acid reaction, and is 'cloudy' in appearance.
- On laboratory microscopy pus cells are seen in the urine.

Treatment

- Notify the doctor.
- Give antipyretic drugs.
- Commence a broad-spectrum antibiotic immediately and change, if necessary, according to the result of the microscopy.
- IV fluids for the duration of the period of vomiting.
- She should drink at least 3L of fluid a day.
- Maintain an accurate fluid balance chart.
- Repeat MSU after the antibiotic treatment is completed.
- Help with baby care.

Stress incontinence

The precise role of pregnancy and birth in the immediate and long-term problem is unclear, but stress incontinence is usually linked to pelvic floor stretching and nerve damage during childbirth. Twenty per cent of women complain of stress incontinence at 3 months postpartum,[1,2] and many of these women are still symptomatic several years later.[3]

Most at risk:
- The older mother
- Long second stage of labour
- Vaginal birth of a large baby.

Management
- Encourage postnatal pelvic floor exercises, as these have longer term benefits.
- Refer the woman to a specialist physiotherapist.
- Encourage regular exercise.

Vesico-vaginal fistula

A rare complication, when a fistula (hole) develops between the bladder or the urethra and the vagina, through the anterior vaginal wall. There are two main causes:
- Damage during labour, caused by prolonged pressure of the fetal head against the symphysis pubis:
  - The damaged tissue takes 1–2 weeks to break down, after which the mother becomes incontinent of urine
  - Surgical repair and antibiotics are required
  - This should never be seen where there are professionally skilled attendants present during labour and birth. Prolonged labour and/or obstructed labour should be quickly diagnosed and immediate delivery by caesarean section carried out. It is more common in situations where this skilled help is not available.
- Direct trauma to the bladder during difficult instrumental delivery, notably with forceps:
  - Incontinence occurs almost immediately
  - Initial treatment is antibiotics and continuous bladder drainage for 2–3 weeks, to encourage spontaneous healing
  - If this fails, surgical repair is required.

1 Wilson PD, Herbison PW, Herbison GP (1996). Obstetric practice and the prevalence of urinary incontinence three months after delivery. *British Journal of Obstetrics and Gynaecology* **103**, 154–61.

2 Sleep J, Grant A, Garcia J, Elbourne D, Spencer J, Chalmers I (1984). West Berkshire perineal management trial. *British Medical Journal* **289**, 587–90.

3 Sleep J, Grace A (1987). West Berkshire perineal management trial. Three year follow up. *British Medical Journal* **295**, 749–51.

Bowel disorders

- Difficulties in regaining normal bowel function are common in the first few postnatal days and are a common problem for the midwife to deal with.
- Most women are embarrassed to talk about bowel problems, but it is important to ascertain her normal pre-pregnancy bowel habits, to determine what is normal for her.
- Bowel problems are common in the latter stage of the pregnancy, due to the relaxing effects of progesterone on the smooth muscle of the bowel, diminishing peristaltic movement. The relative dehydration and lack of dietary intake in labour exacerbate this, along with pelvic pressure and pushing in the second stage of labour.
- Inform the mother about the importance of drinking plenty of water and eating a diet high in fibre, fruit, and vegetables, to regain normal bowel action.

Haemorrhoids

- These are swollen varicose veins of the lower rectum and anal margin.
- They may be present in pregnancy and exacerbated by pelvic pressure and pushing in the second stage of labour.
- Perineal trauma may exacerbate the pain and discomfort of haemorrhoids.
- They may occur for the first time in the early postnatal period.
- Instrumental delivery, particularly forceps, is twice as likely to cause haemorrhoids.

Management

- Dietary advice: high fibre, plenty of fruit, vegetables, and fluids.
- Avoidance of constipation.
- Proprietary treatments in the form of creams or suppositories may be bought or prescribed by the doctor.
- Compress of cypress and lavender essential oils in a 1% dilution of grapeseed or vegetable oil. This may also be added to the bath water. (lavender oil used alone: three drops on a pad may be applied directly to the perineal skin).
- Oral analgesia, such as paracetamol. Codeine should be avoided, as it can cause constipation.

Constipation

- A common problem of the early postnatal period.
- It is usually 2–3 days after birth when the mother has a bowel movement, especially if perineal sutures are painful or after operative birth.
- A mild aperient may be offered 24–48h after birth, but research has shown that laxatives are generally unnecessary.
- Irritant laxatives, such as senna, bisacodyl, or other herbal remedies may cause maternal discomfort and diarrhoea in breastfed infants.
- A balanced diet, with plenty of fruit and vegetables, and plenty of fluids is all that is required.

Postnatal afterthoughts for parents

This is often referred to as debriefing, but the use of this term is contentious.

- Postnatal afterthoughts discussion is the responsibility of every midwife.
- ▶ Offer every mother, and others present at the birth, such as partner, friend, or grandparents, the opportunity to discuss the events.
- Appropriate and effective communication is vital to this process and should be handled with empathy and understanding.
- Honesty is essential and euphemisms should be avoided.
- Even if you consider the birth to have been normal, with no complications, there still needs to be an opportunity for the parents to ask any questions and for you to ensure that explanations have been understood.
- As the midwife present at the birth, you should set aside time for discussion with the parents before you leave the labour ward or home, and definitely within 24h of the birth.
- It is particularly important to offer a clear explanation of events and the reasons for a particular course of action to those who have experienced traumatic events or complications in labour, as soon as possible. Appropriate documentation is essential to this process.
- The effects of intense pain, use of technological or operative intervention, and insensitive and/or disrespectful care from one or more carers in labour can cause intense distress.
- ❶ One discussion may be insufficient; more questions may arise as the parents contemplate on events and possible/actual long-term consequences. Providing an opportunity to discuss these, together with good support from the midwife and, where appropriate, the doctor involved, will, in the majority of cases, prevent further long-term consequences, such as postnatal depression or post-traumatic stress disorder.
- Women (and their partners) will react differently. Experiences that some will understand as necessary and normal and will eventually overcome, will be intensely distressing to others, and may become ingrained in their psyche, adversely affecting their relationship with their partner and baby.
- In some cases parents may need more specialist help, such as professional counselling, psychological or psychiatric care.
- Women who experience nightmares and flashbacks need specialized help. The sensitive support of a midwife will be essential should they ever embark on a future pregnancy.
- ▶ In the increasing litigious world, provision of a postnatal afterthoughts service could prove cost-effective in reducing complaints and legal action. The majority of complaints and threats of legal action arise from the fact that parents want someone to listen to them, to give them a clear explanation, and to say 'sorry', where appropriate.
- Increasingly, maternity units are identifying and training specialist midwives to lead this service, provide specialist discussion and counselling for the parents, and advise midwifery managers on professional development and risk management issues that may arise.

Postnatal afterthoughts for midwives

- Midwives also need the opportunity to reflect and discuss events after caring for a woman who has experienced traumatic complications during childbirth.
- Reflection with senior midwifery colleagues or a supervisor of midwives can put the events in perspective and help the midwife learn from the experience.
- It is also important to reflect on the midwife's actions and records and, where appropriate, praise their actions and assure them that they have done nothing wrong.
- All those present at the birth must be given the opportunity to work through their feelings and obtain support.
- In the UK, the supervisor of midwives should provide the confidential support required, identify any professional development required for the midwife, and draw up an action plan to meet any identified need.

Psychological and mental health disorders

- Mental health disorders in the antenatal and postnatal period can have serious consequences for the mother, her baby and other family members. They may be pre-existing or occur for the first time in pregnancy or the postnatal period.[1]
- There should be clearly specified care pathways in each NHS trust, to enable the midwife to make an appropriate referral.[1]
- Women who require inpatient care for a mental disorder within 12 months of childbirth should be admitted to a specialist mother and baby unit, wherever possible.[1]

Postnatal psychosis

This condition is at the other end of the spectrum to baby blues and is the most severe form of psychiatric morbidity. It is the least common of the postnatal psychological conditions but different studies report varying levels of incidence from 1:500 to 1:1500.[2,3] It is usually sudden and dramatic in onset and usually occurs very early, within the first week, the majority presenting before the 16th day postnatally.

Symptoms

These may be variable but can include:

- Changes in mood state
- Irrational behaviour
- Restlessness and agitation
- Fear
- Perplexity, as the woman loses touch with reality
- Suspicion
- Insomnia
- Episodes of mania, where the mother becomes hyperactive
- Neglect of basic needs
- Hallucinations and morbid delusional thoughts
- Profound depression.

Twenty five per cent of women admitted for postnatal psychosis within 3 months of birth will have consulted for psychological symptoms in pregnancy; 50% will have had symptoms of anxiety or depression in pregnancy; 50% will have non-puerperal episodes of psychosis and/or a family history of mental illness.[2]

►► There should be immediate referral to the mental health team, as the condition will usually warrant admission to hospital. Prognosis is good, but there is a high risk of recurrence in subsequent pregnancy.

The psychotropic drugs often used in the treatment of postnatal psychosis and for other long-term mental health conditions make it imperative that the woman understands the need for effective contraception and the risks of severe damage to the fetus in a subsequent unplanned pregnancy. The midwife should encourage her to attend the contraception and sexual health clinic for effective contraceptive management.

1 National Institute for Health and Clinical Excellence (2007). *Antenatal and Postnatal Mental Health*. Clinical guideline 45. London: NICE.

2 Kendell RE, Chalmers L, Platz C (1984). The epidemiology of postnatal psychosis. *British Journal Psychiatry* **150**, 662–73.

3 Cox J (1986). *Postnatal Depression: A Guide for Health Professionals*. Edinburgh: Churchill Livingstone.

Postnatal depression

Postnatal depression refers to depression with its onset during the first postnatal year. It is a non-psychotic depressive disorder that varies in severity and is not fundamentally different from depression occurring at other points in a woman's life. The incidence varies according to different reports, but is thought that around 10–15% of women suffer postnatal depression following childbirth.[1] However, this may only be the tip of the iceberg, as many incidences go unreported and untreated.

Symptoms

There is a wide range of symptoms that the mother may exhibit, including:

• Anxiety
• Panic attacks
• Tension and irritability
• Feelings of despair and emptiness
• Exhaustion
• Lack of concentration
• Rejection of partner or baby
• Inappropriate or obsessional thoughts
• Loss of libido
• Physical symptoms
• Desire for sleep
• Feels better in the morning
• Guilt and anxiety about the baby
• Preoccupied with baby's health.

Aetiology

There has been wide research into the causes of postnatal depression, but no one single cause is apparent. It has been linked with both physiological and psychosocial factors.

Physiological factors

• Genetic background
• Hormonal changes
• Oestrogen is seen as being more significant than progesterone
• Thyroid dysfunction.

Psychosocial factors

• Events surrounding the birth
• Difficult to care for baby
• Previous history of depression
• Age of the mother
• Prior experience with babies
• Stressful life events
• Marital stress
• Inadequate postnatal sexual relations
• Mother's own childhood experiences
• Social condition
• Personality
• Linked with parenthood rather than pregnancy or birth experiences.

Effects of postnatal depression on the family

A review of research[2] revealed that postnatal depression had profound and long-lasting effects on both the children and the families of women. It can have adverse effects on the children's emotional and intellectual development, and boys appear to be affected more than girls.

Detection

Early diagnosis and treatment is important not only for the woman but also her family. The midwife has an important role in recognizing women at high risk of postnatal depression, and the early signs of postnatal depression.

- Assess the mother's emotional state as part of the routine postnatal care.
- The Edinburgh Postnatal Depression Scale, or other validated assessment tool, is useful in assisting the diagnosis of the condition.
- If you suspect that the mother may be affected, be sensitive and reassuring and refer to appropriate resources.

Treatment

A wide range of treatments have been suggested for postnatal depression. The treatment required will depend upon the severity of the illness and the support available for the woman. For some women the condition will resolve spontaneously, but for many the condition will become chronic and may last for the first year or longer following the birth. The *Saving Mothers' Lives* report into maternal death[3] has shown suicide to be the leading cause of maternal death in the first year after birth.

Treatments may include:

- Social and emotional support
- Self-help groups
- Prophylactic progesterone
- Oestrogen treatment
- Placentophagy
- Psychotropic drugs
- Electro-convulsive therapy.

1 Cox J (1986). *Postnatal Depression: A Guide for Health Professionals*. Edinburgh: Churchill Livingstone.

2 Cooper PJ, Murray L (1998). Postnatal depression. *British Medical Journal* **316,** 1884–6.

3 Lewis G (ed.) (2007) Confidential Enquiry into Maternal Deaths (2007). *Saving Mothers' Lives 2003–2005: Seventh Report of the Confidential Enquiries Into Maternal Death in the United Kingdom*. London: CEMACH. Available from: ℞ www.cemach.org.uk (accessed 25.2.11).

4 Cox JL, Holder J (eds) (1994). *Perinatal Psychiatry: Use and Misuse of the Edinburgh Postnatal Depression Scale*. London: Gaskell.

Bereavement care

- This section refers to loss of a non-viable fetus, stillbirth, or neonatal death.
- Legal definitions and requirements stated are those currently required in the UK.
- Please check your own local policies and procedures.
- ▶ The disposal of a baby's body is of immense importance and therapeutic value to the parents. It can be the means towards the healing of the inner hurt sustained in the death of their child. Poorly managed, it can be the foundation of severe psychological damage.
- ▶ Respect and facilitate religious customs and rituals. Time spent in getting everything right will save many years of heartache.

Aims for the midwife[1]

- To achieve optimal communication with families when their baby dies before, during, or soon after birth
- To ensure parents are fully aware of, and understand, all the choices open to them
- To help parents to face the reality of the situation as they grieve for their baby
- To act as an advocate for the family, demonstrating sensitivity while maintaining professional boundaries
- To ensure that the family's cultural and religious traditions are respected
- To provide families with a choice of appropriate follow-up support and counselling arrangements.

Post-mortem examination

- This may be legally required, in certain circumstances particularly for a neonatal death. It may also be requested by the parents.
- Explain sensitively the reason for the post-mortem examination.
- One of the parents will be required to sign the consent form.
- If the parents refuse consent, their wishes must be respected, unless the death has been reported to the coroner (in Scotland the Procurator Fiscal), in which case the coroner will order the post-mortem. Try to avoid this if at all possible, as it will cause unnecessary distress.

Practice point

❶ If the baby is to have a post-mortem, the body must be kept dry and not bathed after birth.

The non-viable fetus

- *Definition*: a fetus born dead before the legal age of viability, i.e. before 24 weeks' gestation.
- After 16 weeks', but before 24 weeks', gestation the parents may be given the opportunity to have their baby buried, either by the hospital making the arrangements or by the parents making their own funeral arrangements.
- The law requires that the funeral director undertaking such a burial is given a letter signed by the qualified health care professional present at the birth.

- It is also possible to arrange for the hospital chaplain or a minister of the parents' own choice to officiate. This applies to all religious faiths.

Stillbirth

- *Definition:* a baby who neither breathes nor shows any other sign of life after being completely expelled from its mother after 24 completed weeks' gestation.
- The Certificate of Stillbirth must be completed by the midwife present at the birth. This is given to the parents to register the stillbirth with the local Registrar of Births and Deaths, which must be done within 42 days and before the baby can be buried or cremated.
- Encourage the parents to give the baby a name, as forenames cannot be added to the certificate retrospectively.
- Inform your supervisor of midwives of the stillbirth.

Neonatal death

- *Definition:* a baby born alive, but who dies within 28 days of birth.
- You will have completed the notification of birth in the normal way and the doctor certifying the baby's death will issue the death certificate.
- Both the birth and the death must be registered by the parents within 5 days. This often occurs simultaneously.
- Encourage the parents to give the baby a name, as forenames cannot be added to the certificate retrospectively.

Baby's body

- Handle the baby sensitively and respectfully at all times.
- Wash or bathe the baby to remove traces of blood, unless a post-mortem examination is to be carried out. Wear gloves for this procedure.
- The mother or father can bathe the baby if they wish. Allow sufficient time for this to be done properly.
- Dress the baby in its own clothes, disposable nappy, and bonnet, if possible.
- Apply small waterproof dressings to any wounds.

Photographs

- Take at least two photographs of the baby after consent gained and give one to the parents.
- If they do not wish to keep the photo, seal it in an envelope and save in the mother's notes. She may ask for it at a later date.
- Encourage the parents and family to take as many photos as they wish. Have a camera and film ready for their use, if required.
- Offer a professional photograph taken by the hospital photographer.

Mementos

- Foot and handprints, a lock of hair, cot card, and name bracelets need to be collected for the memento folder.
- Parental permission *must* be obtained before obtaining a lock of hair.
- Small toys or other mementos may be kept with the baby.

Religious customs and ceremonies

- Ask the parents, at the outset, about any religious customs or ceremonies they wish to be observed. They may wish to make their own arrangements or the hospital chaplain will facilitate this for them.
- The parents may appreciate a simple blessing and naming ceremony.

Parent information booklet

- It is important that all information for parents, including helpful leaflets, booklets, support group and website addresses, and telephone numbers, should be made available in each maternity unit.
- Go through this page by page to help the parents understand the help and support available.

The environment

- This is so important and should be as homely and non-clinical as possible.
- Each maternity unit should have a 'quiet room' to ensure the family is not disturbed.
- A door notice asking others to respect their privacy should be available for them to use at their discretion when they feel the need for privacy.
- Encourage the parents to see and cuddle the baby.
- Allow the family to be alone with the baby for as long as they wish.
- Have a Moses basket or a cot available to put the baby in when they are ready.
- Have a telephone in the room for the parents to use. The hospital switchboard may need to be informed, so that they can connect calls sensitively.
- After the baby has been taken to the mortuary, the parents may ask for it to be brought back to the ward, while the mother is in hospital, or to visit it in the mortuary viewing room.

Transport of the baby's body

- Inform the mortuary technician when the baby is to be collected and whether or not a post-mortem is required.
- Inform the porter when the baby is ready to be collected.
- Refer to local guidelines as the arrangements may differ slightly depending on location.

Arranging the funeral

- In the cases of both stillbirth and neonatal death, the Registrar of Births and Deaths will issue the Certificate for Burial or Cremation once the death has been officially registered.
- The parents may wish the burial or cremation arrangements to be made by the hospital, or they may make their own arrangements. The hospital chaplain or a minister/religious leader of their own choice may officiate.
- Occasionally, parents may ask to take the baby home. This can be arranged and the undertaker will collect the baby from home for the funeral. This usually requires additional paperwork and the police may need to be informed.

Memorial book

- This may be kept in the hospital chapel and should be on view at all times.
- Invite the parents to place the baby's name and date of birth in the book. There should also be a space for a short verse.
- If the parents cannot do this themselves, the hospital chaplain may do it for them.

Memorial service

- A memorial service, which may be multi-faith, may be held annually, to which all families and staff are invited, to remember newborn babies who have died.
- Parents and families will decide for themselves how many years they wish to attend. They should never be excluded by time limit or other obstacles.

Counselling

- Encourage parents to talk to staff about how they feel. Set aside time to do this.
- It is helpful if the maternity unit has one or two midwives, trained in counselling skills and experienced in dealing with families in this situation, to lead this work.
- Home visits can be arranged, if the parents do not wish to return to the maternity unit for counselling.
- Some parents may need longer counselling and psychological support than you are able to offer; in which case, establish appropriate referral mechanisms.

1 Child Bereavement Trust (2003). Available at: ℘ www.childbereavement.org.uk/professionals (accessed 27.2.11).

Part 5

Family planning

Contraception

Contraception

▶ Important points for the midwife to remember:

- Any discussion about contraception is both sensitive and highly personal to individual women and their partners
- You need to be knowledgeable both about the range of contraceptive methods available and the local services available to best meet the woman's needs
- Ensure that you have up-to-date information on the full range of contraceptive methods available in the locality, access to relevant appropriate websites, NICE guidelines, and useful books that might help (📖 see Contraceptive methods, p. 525)
- Allow enough time for discussion, and ensure an appropriate environment to maintain confidentiality and allow a relaxed discussion, ideally in the woman's home
- Encourage discussion
- Offer any leaflets and suitable websites available to support information given
- Remember that to be effective the chosen contraception must be used properly and therefore acceptable to the woman and, ideally, to her partner
- As with any other form of treatment, informed decision making and consent is required
- Brand names of contraceptives apply to the UK, but these will vary throughout the world.

Contraception following abortion/miscarriage

- First trimester: hormonal contraception can be commenced or recommenced immediately.
- Second trimester: hormonal contraception should not be commenced or recommenced until at least 21 days after abortion or miscarriage until uterine changes have reverted to the pre-pregnant state.
- However, there will be exceptions to consider in individual cases, when effective contraception is paramount.

Contraception after giving birth

- Normally, hormonal contraceptive methods are not commenced until at least 21 days after birth.
- However, should the need for contraception be the paramount concern, it may be started sooner.

Important points to remember

- **Never recommend the combined oral contraceptive pill to a breastfeeding woman**. Oestrogen will inhibit the release of prolactin and suppress her lactation within 24h.
- Giving progesterone while the postnatal vaginal loss is still present may cause an increase in the amount of blood loss and prolong the bleeding time.
- Progesterone-only methods, if started too soon in a breastfeeding mother, may also cause suppression of lactation.

Contraceptive methods

Table 22.1 lists the methods that will be discussed in this chapter.

Table 22.1 Contraceptive methods

Hormonal	
Combined oestrogen and progesterone	Combined pill
	Skin patch
	Vaginal ring
Progesterone only	Oral progesterone-only pill
	Injectables
	Implant
	Intrauterine system (IUS)
Emergency contraception	**Oral pills**
Non-hormonal	**Intrauterine device**
IUD	
Barrier	Male condom
	Female condom
	Diaphragm and cervical cap
Natural	Breastfeeding
Sterilization	Fertility awareness
	Male sterilization
	Female sterilization

Useful websites

British Association of Sexual Health and HIV: www.bashh.org.uk.

Faculty of Sexual and Reproductive Health: www.fsh.org.uk.

Faculty of Sexual and Reproductive Healthcare; UK medical eligibility criteria for contraceptive use (2009). Available at: http://www.ffprhc.org.uk.org/admin/uploads/UKMEC2009.pdf (accessed 10.4.10).

International Planned Parenthood Federation: www.ippf.org.

Journal of Family Planning and Reproductive Health Care: www.pmn.uk.com/healthcare/familyplan/home.htm.

The Family Planning Association: www.fpa.org.

World Health Organization: www.who.int/topics/familyplanning/en/.

Recommended reading

Everett S (2004). *Handbook of Contraception and Reproductive Sexual Health*, 2nd edn. London: Balliere Tindall.

Guillebaud J (2008). *Contraception Today*, 6th edn. London: Taylor and Francis.

Guillebaud J (2009). *Contraception: Your Questions Answered*, 5th edn. Edinburgh: Churchill Livingstone.

National Institute for Health and Clinical Excellence (2006). Routine postnatal care of women and their babies. Clinical guideline 37. London: NICE.

National Institute for Health and Clinical Excellence (2007). Long acting methods of contraception. Clinical guideline 30. London: NICE.

Lactational amenorrhoea method

How does it work?

The lactational amenorrhoea method (LAM; Fig. 22.1) will inhibit ovulation if the following criteria are all met:

- *Amenorrhoea* since the postnatal vaginal blood loss ceased
- *Full lactation*: the mother is fully supplying the baby's nutritional needs day and night
- *Baby is <6 months old*.

In these circumstances the operating prolactin levels inhibit gonadotrophin release from the anterior pituitary gland, thus inhibiting ovulation, and the risk of pregnancy occurring is only approximately 2% (i.e. 98% effective as contraception).

Efficacy

- A WHO multicentre study[1] supports this, with a reported pregnancy rate in the first 6 months after childbirth of 0.9–1.2%.
- Prolactin levels are highest during the night, and to ensure that LAM works, it is essential to continue night-time feeding as long as possible.
- The failure rate will increase if the mother is not fully breastfeeding, and in the Western world women are encouraged and motivated to stop night feeding as soon as possible, and the baby encouraged to sleep the night through, by giving supplementary solids in the evening.
- Before modern times, LAM was the only contraceptive method available, and is still the only method available to women in many parts of the world.

Additional contraception

- Many women choose to rely on an additional method, such as the condom or the progesterone-only pill (POP).
- If the mother is using the a POP while fully breastfeeding, it is unnecessary to give emergency contraception if a pill is missed.
- If a breastfeeding mother chooses a POP, the amount passed to the baby in the breast milk is the equivalent of one POP in 2 years, considerably less progesterone than in formula milk.[2]
- As soon as the baby begins to be weaned or the mother has a period, it is important that, if she wants effective oral hormonal contraception, she is switched to desogestrel 75micrograms or the combined contraceptive pill.

Return of ovulation

- The time taken for return of ovulation depends on the frequency, intensity, and duration of feeding, maintenance of night feeds, and introduction of supplementary feeding.
- Midwives should be confident in recommending this method to mothers, *provided the criteria are met*.

Ask the mother:

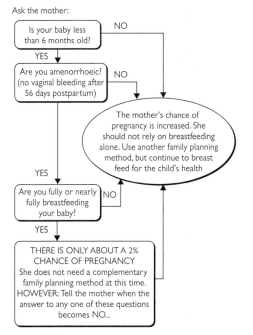

Fig. 22.1 Lactational amenorrhoea method of contraception.
Reprinted by permission of Fertility UK from www.fertility.uk.org.

1 World Health Organization (1999). Multinational study of breast feeding and lactational amenorrhoea method. III Pregnancy during breastfeeding. *Fertility and Sterility* **72**(3), 431–40.

2 Guillebaud J (2008). *Contraception Today*, 6th edn. London: Taylor and Francis.

Combined oral contraceptive: 'the pill'

Contents
Each tablet contains a combination of oestrogen and progesterone. Most brands contain 30–35micrograms of ethinylestradiol and a progestogen.

In the UK, the combined oral contraceptive pill is the most commonly used form of contraception:
- It is highly effective
- It is convenient
- It is not related to intercourse
- It is reversible
- It reduces the incidence of ectopic pregnancy
- It results in lighter and less painful periods
- It possibly helps to reduce premenstrual symptoms
- It protects against ovarian and endometrial cancer.

When is it taken?
- Ideally, the woman should start the first pack on the first full day of menstrual bleeding and definitely within the first 5 days of the cycle. If this is done, then follicle stimulating hormone (FSH) inhibition will be complete for that cycle, and no additional contraception will be necessary.
- If the pill is started later than the 5th day of the cycle, she should use a condom every time sexual intercourse occurs in the next 7 days. After that the hormonal control will be established.
- It is not started in the latter half of the menstrual cycle, because of the risk of pregnancy.
- Tell the woman to take one pill daily, at approximately the same time every day, choosing a time of day that is most convenient and best remembered. She should follow the arrows on the pack until all 21 pills have been taken. Then she will have a 7-day break, during which a withdrawal bleed, 'period', will occur. The next pack should be commenced 7 days later.

Follow-up
- Normally, the first prescription is for 3 months, with an appointment to return to clinic in 8–10 weeks for review.
- Unless there any menstrual irregularities or other side-effects are evident, follow-up and repeat prescription is then 6–12 months, depending on local policy.

Points to remember
- A useful tip for an effective pill-taking regimen is to ask the woman to make a note of the day she started the pill for the first time: that is the day she will always start a new pack.
- She should make a note of the new pack start date. Again, a paper diary, electronic diary, or mobile phone calendar and alarm can be used.

- Missed pill: there is a 'window' of 12h, during which a pill may be taken later than normal and still be within the normal regimen. If more than 12h late, then advise her to follow the regimen given in 📖 When the pill may not be effective, p. 532.
- If the woman smokes, she must be warned of the increased risk of coronary heart disease and venous thromboembolism.
- After giving birth:
  - Ideally the combined pill should not be started until at least 21 days after birth, to allow the body to recover physiologically from birth and to avoid increasing the thrombo-embolic risk.
  - However, there are some women for whom the risk of further pregnancy is high and who need highly effective contraception. In this case, refer the woman to the contraception and sexual health clinic for appropriate management.
  - The combined pill should never be given to a breastfeeding mother, as the oestrogen component will suppress her lactation within 24–48h.
  - If a breastfeeding mother requires hormonal contraception, then advise a progesterone-only method.
  - If the combined pill is started while the mother still has a vaginal blood loss, the progesterone component will cause bleeding to become heavier and more prolonged. Be aware of this and also warn the mother.
  - The combined pill should be avoided, wherever possible, in a mother who has reduced mobility following birth, e.g. after caesarean section, because of the increased thrombo-embolic risk.
- Blood pressure and personal and family medical history are checked annually for any significant changes that may signal caution or discontinuation of this method of contraception, notably cardiovascular issues such as hypertension, heart attacks, and stroke or thrombo-embolic disorders.

When the pill may not be effective

Missed pill(s)

The WHO[1] issued new missed pill guidance in 2004, which was adapted for UK use in 2005[2] (see Fig. 21.2):

- If the pill for that day is taken more than 12h late, advise the woman to take the missed pill as soon as it is remembered and take the next scheduled pill at its normal time. In practice, what often happens is that two pills are taken together.
- Up to two pills can be missed anywhere in the pack (only one if taking Loestrin® 20, Mercilon®, or Femodette®). No additional contraception is needed.
- If three or more pills are missed (two if taking Loestrin® 20, Mercilon®, or Femodette®). Take the last pill missed as soon as it is remembered. Leave any earlier missed pills in the pack. Use an extra method of contraception for the next 7 days (the male condom is the easiest).
- If three or more pills have been missed and the woman has had unprotected sex in the last few days, advise her to consider emergency contraception, as she may be at risk of pregnancy.
- If seven or more pills are left from now until the end of this cycle: she should continue taking the pill in the normal way to the end of the pack and have the normal 7-day break. The normal period should occur.
- If fewer than seven pills are left from now until the end of this cycle: she should continue to the end of the pack, but not have the 7-day break. Tell her to start the new pack immediately and follow the normal daily regimen to complete the pack in the normal way. In this case there will be no period between the two packs, but there should be a normal period at the end of the second pack.

Points to remember

- She should only take one missed pill. If more than one pill has been missed, advise her to leave the other missed pills in the pack. If this happens, it is important that a condom is used for every act of sexual intercourse for the next 7 days.
- ▶ When a pill has been missed for more than 12h in a cycle, the risk of pregnancy is increased. Any disturbance in menstrual cycle as a result should be followed up with a pregnancy test.

Antibiotic therapy

The well-established guidance that the use of additional precautions must be used when taking any broad spectrum antibiotic has changed, in the light of worldwide research evidence, and is no longer the case.[4] This also applies to fluconazole, used in the treatment of *Candida* ('thrush').

Antiretroviral therapy

Drug interactions between the antiretroviral drugs and the combined hormonal contraceptive may alter the effectiveness of the combined hormonal contraceptive and consistent additional use of the condom should be recommended.[3]

Nausea and vomiting

If the woman vomits within 3h of taking the pill, she may not have absorbed sufficient amounts of the oestrogen component to suppress ovulation effectively. In this case a condom should also be used for every act of sexual intercourse for the duration of the episode of illness involving vomiting and for the next 7 days, to allow the contraceptive effect to return.

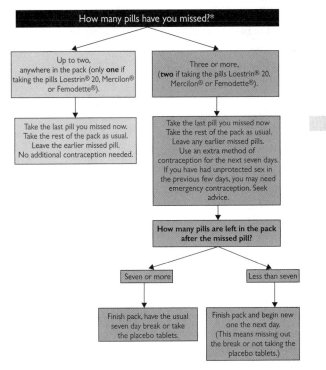

* If you miss pills and have also missed pills in your previous packet, speak to your doctor or nurse as you may need emergency contraception.

Fig. 22.2 Missed pill guidance.

Copyright © fpa 2007, reprinted by permission of the publisher.

Drug interactions

Certain drugs may inhibit absorption/reduce the effectiveness of the pill, so it is imperative that you check whether or not the woman is taking any other medication when discussing possible use of the pill.[4]

The main interacting drugs are:

• Enzyme-inducing anticonvulsants used in the treatment of epilepsy, tuberculosis, and HIV.
• Drugs used in the treatment of TB.
• Coumarin anticoagulants (e.g. warfarin).
• St John's wort (a herbal complementary medicine often taken by women).

Refer the woman to the contraception and sexual health clinic or general practitioner for review of the drug regimen. Advise her that St John's wort must not be taken when using combined hormonal contraception.

1 World Health Organization (2004). *Selected Practice Recommendations for Contraceptive Use.* Geneva: WHO.

2 Faculty of Family Planning and Reproductive Health Care (2005). *Faculty Statement: Missed Pills: New Recommendations.* London: FFPRHC.

3 Faculty of Sexual and Reproductive Health Care (2009). *UK Medical Eligibility for Contraceptive Use.* London: Faculty of Sexual and Reproductive Health Care. Available at: ℜ www.ffprhc.org.uk/admin/uploads/UKMEC2009.pdf (accessed 10.4.10).

4 Faculty of Sexual and Reproductive Health Care (2011). *Drug Interactions with Hormonal Contraception.* London: FSRSH. Available at: ℜ www.ffprhc.org.uk/admin/uploads/CEUGuidanceDrugInteractionsHormonal.pdf

Contraceptive patch

The 'pill in a patch' first became available in the UK in 2003. It is a combination oestrogen and progesterone drug and can be given to any woman who is suitable for the combined pill. Each pack contains 3 months' supply.

Using the patch

The woman should:

- Start using the patch on the first day of the next period or no sooner than day 21 after giving birth or having a second trimester abortion. After a first trimester abortion she can start immediately. Ask her to note the start day. This is most easily done using the calendar wheel on the underside of the box lid provided to store the patches.
- Place the patch on any part of the body, *except the breasts*, where it is unseen and where clothes are unlikely to rub excessively. The adhesive will allow normal activity, bathing, sport, and swimming.
- Leave the patch in position for 7 days and then change the patch weekly for the next 3 weeks. After the 3 completed weeks, tell her to then have a 7-day break, during which withdrawal bleeding will occur.

Points to remember

- Remind her not to place the patch on the breasts.
- Remind her to check daily that the patch is firmly in place.
- If the patch comes off, she must replace it with a new one within 24h for continuous contraception. If left off for over 24h, the 7-day rule applies and should intercourse occur in the following 7 days, condoms should be used. Lack of condom use warrants use of emergency contraception if the patch was off for more than 24h.
- She should restart the next cycle with a new patch.
- She should report any side-effects to the doctor or contraception and sexual health clinic supplying the patch.
- This method is expensive.
- Contraindications to its use are as for the combined pill.
- ❶ Care should be taken when prescribing this form of contraceptive for any woman who has a sensitive skin or allergy. Monitor her for evidence of skin irritation or allergy, even though the patch is hypoallergenic, and ask her to return immediately if skin irritation should occur, but to continue to wear the patch until an alternative method of contraception is organized.
- Additional support is available from the company making the patch in the form of:
  - A 24h telephone helpline
  - Online support
  - Text message reminder on patch change day.

Contraceptive vaginal ring

- The 'pill in a ring' (Fig. 22.3) became available in the UK in 2009 and is designed as an alternative to taking a pill daily. Known as Nuvaring® in the UK.
- It is a combination oestrogen and progesterone drug and can be given to any woman who is suitable for the combined pill.
- Each ring lasts for 3 weeks, i.e. one ring per menstrual cycle, with a ring free week in the fourth week, during which a withdrawal bleed 'period' will occur.
- The daily release of hormone is 15micrograms ethinylestradiol and 120micrograms etonorgestrel. Hormone release occurs continuously and the body does not store the drug. It is designed to inhibit ovulation.

Using the ring

She should:
- Insert the vaginal ring on the first day of the next period or no sooner than day 21 after giving birth or having a second trimester abortion. After a first trimester abortion she can start immediately. Ask her to note the start day. This is the day that she will always insert a new ring.
- Place the ring as high in the vagina as she can; a similar technique to inserting a tampon.
- Leave the ring in position for 21 days. After the three completed weeks, tell her to then have a 7 day break, during which withdrawal bleeding will occur.
- Remove the ring 3 weeks after insertion on the same day of the week at about the same time of day that it was inserted. Hook the index finger under the forward rim or hold the rim between the index and middle finger and pull it out.

Points to remember

- Remind her to check regularly that the ring is firmly in place.
- If the ring is accidentally expelled and is left outside of the vagina for less than 3h, contraceptive efficacy is not reduced. Replace the ring in the vagina.
- If the ring is out of the vagina for more than 3 continuous hours during weeks 1 and 2, contraceptive efficacy may be reduced. She should insert the ring as soon as she can. Additional contraception, usually in the form of the male condom, should be used for the next 7 days.
- If the ring is out of the vagina for more than 3 continuous hours in week 3 she should discard that ring. She can at that point either:
  - Insert a new ring immediately for another 3 weeks

or

  - Have a withdrawal bleed and insert a new ring no later than 7 days from the time the previous ring was removed or expelled. Additional contraception, usually in the form of the male condom, should be used for the next 7 days.

- She should report any side-effects to the doctor or contraception and sexual health clinic supplying the ring.
- This method is expensive.
- Contraindications to its use are as for the combined pill.
- ❶ Care should be taken when prescribing this form of contraceptive for any woman who has lax pelvic floor tone.

Storage
- The Nuvaring® can be stored for up to 4 months at 25°C.
- Avoid storing in direct sunlight or at temperatures above 30°C.

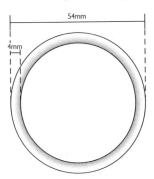

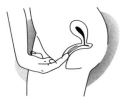

Insert in an upwards and backwards motion into the posterior fornix

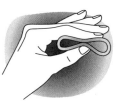

Squeeze the ring between thumb and forefinger ready for insertion into vagina

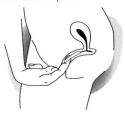

To remove, place the forefinger over the lower edge and pull gently

Fig. 22.3 Vaginal ring.

Copyright © fpa 2009 and reproduced by permission of the publisher.

Progesterone-only pill

Contents
- Tablets containing progesterone only.
- Dispensed in packs containing either 28 or 35 days' pills, depending on brand.
- Designed to prevent implantation of the fertilized ovum, which, depending on personal beliefs about when life begins, may not be acceptable to all women. However, in long-term users of the POP, ovulation does become inhibited.

The desogestrel pill, Cerazette®, licensed in the UK in 2002, has a different mode of action from standard POPs and is the first choice POP in women <40, who need highly effective contraception. It is designed to inhibit ovulation: in clinical trials ovulation was inhibited in 99% of cycles at 7 and 12 months after initiation and has been shown to be as effective as the combined pill.

Indications
There are a number of indications for the POP:
- The woman's choice
- Breastfeeding: all POPs secrete a very small amount of progestogen to the infant, the equivalent of one POP in 2 years, which is much less than the progesterone level found in dried cow's milk.[1] POPs do not interfere with lactation
- Hypertension
- Migraine (particularly focal migraine)
- Diabetes
- Obesity
- Older women, particularly smokers >35
- Side-effects of the combined pill
- Sickle-cell disease.

When is it taken?
- Advise the woman to choose a time of day that is most convenient and best remembered. A useful tip to help her remember is to set an alarm on her mobile phone if she has one. Her partner or other close relative could be of help in reminding her, if she is liable to forget.
- Ideally, the woman should start the first pack on the first full day of menstrual bleeding. If this is done, there is no need for additional contraception in the first cycle.
- However, if the pill is started later than the second day of the cycle it is advisable to use condoms every time sexual intercourse occurs in the next 7 days. After that, the hormonal control will be established. This advice also applies when started postnatally in a non-breastfeeding woman who has not yet had her first period following birth.
- It is not started in the latter half of the menstrual cycle, because of the risk of pregnancy, even if full sexual intercourse has not occurred.

Missed pill

- When a pill has been missed for more than the 3h window (12h with Cerazette®) advise the woman to take the missed pill as soon as she remembers it and to continue with her normal pill-taking routine.
- Only the *last* missed pill should be taken, if she has missed more than one.
- Additional barrier protection should be used if any sexual contact occurs in the next 48h, e.g. male condom.
- Additional emergency contraception may be used, particularly if more than one pill has been missed (📖 see Emergency contraception, p. 572).

Follow-up

- Normally, the first prescription is for 3 months, with an appointment to return to clinic in 8–10 weeks for review.
- Unless there any menstrual irregularities or other side-effects are evident, follow-up and repeat prescription is then 6–12 months, dependent on local policy.
- Check blood pressure and personal and family medical history annually, to check for any significant changes that may signal caution or discontinuation of this method of contraception, which is rare.

Points to remember

- ▶ There is only a 3h 'window' during which a pill may be taken late, but still be 'safe'. If more than 3h late, this must be classed as a missed pill. The exception to this rule is Cerazette®, which has a 12h window.
- If a breastfeeding mother requires hormonal contraception, the POP is ideal.
- The POP is highly effective if taken regularly each day, without any missed pills or breaks.
- In women >30 it is almost as effective as the combined pill.
- A useful tip for an effective pill-taking regimen is to ask the woman to make a note of the day she started the pill for the first time: that is the day she will always start a new pack.
- ▶ There are no pill-free days. The next pack must be started immediately.
- She should make a note of the new pack start date. Again, a paper diary, electronic diary, or mobile phone calendar and alarm can be used.

Following birth

- Ideally the POP should not be started until at least 21 days after birth, to allow the body to recover physiologically from birth. However, there are some women for whom the risk of further pregnancy is high and who need highly effective contraception. In this case, refer the woman to the Contraception and Sexual Health Clinic for appropriate management.
- If the POP is started while the mother still has a vaginal blood loss, it will cause bleeding to become heavier and more prolonged. Be aware of this and also warn the mother.

- The POP is a better choice than a combined oral contraceptive in a mother who has reduced mobility following birth, e.g. after caesarean section, because of the increased thrombo-embolic risk.

Antibiotic therapy

Any period of antibiotic therapy will not affect the uptake of this pill and the woman should continue to take it as normal. No additional barrier protection is required.

Antiretroviral therapy

HIV positive women on antiretroviral therapy should be advised to use consistent additional barrier contraception.

Nausea and vomiting

If the woman vomits within 3h of taking the pill, she may not have absorbed a sufficient amount of the pill for it to be effective. In this case, a condom should also be used for every act of sexual intercourse for the duration of the episode of illness involving vomiting and for the next 7 days, to allow the contraceptive effect to return. If she does not follow this advice, additional emergency contraception may be required (📖 see Emergency contraception, p. 572).

Drug interactions and the pill

Certain drugs *may* inhibit absorption or reduce the effectiveness of the POP, so it is imperative to check whether or not the woman is taking any other medication when discussing possible use of the pill. However, it is very unusual to find a drug that will inhibit the POP uptake and effectiveness.

1 Guillebaud J (2008). *Contraception Today*, 6th edn. London: Taylor and Francis.

Implant

Known as Nexplanon® in the UK (Implanon® previously available). The contraceptive implant offers 3 years' contraception, being most effective in the first 2 years.

Content

The implant is a single rate-limiting polymer capsule, 4cm long and 2mm in diameter, containing 68mg etonogestrel, which is released at over 30micrograms/day to inhibit ovulation.

Benefits

- Long-term effective contraception. Zero failure rate in initial clinical trials.
- One insertion.
- No daily pill-taking regime.
- Non-intercourse related.

Mode of action

- The subdermal implant is inserted into the under side of the upper arm by a doctor, midwife, or nurse trained and competent in the technique (Fig. 22.4).
- The hormone is released directly into the surrounding interstitial tissue and absorbed by capillaries into the bloodstream.
- Ovulation is suppressed at the level of the hypothalamus, therefore the luteal phase of the menstrual cycle is deficient, preventing implantation, should ovulation and fertilization occur.

Insertion

- Insertion is a minor surgical procedure under local anaesthesia.
- The preloaded single-capsule system is contained within a sterile, disposable applicator and is an easy and rapid subdermal injection technique.
- The implant should be inserted at the beginning of the menstrual cycle, ideally on day 1. If inserted on day 1, the serum etonogestrel levels will be sufficient for ovulation inhibition within the first day and no further contraception will be required in that cycle.
- If inserted on the 2nd day or later, then it is important to recommend 7 days extra barrier contraception, if sexual intercourse occurs within this period.

Points to remember

- Following first trimester abortion, the implant can be inserted immediately.
- Following second trimester abortion, it is wise to wait 21 days before insertion, because of the side-effect of prolonged or heavy bleeding.
- After giving birth, again it is wise to wait 21 days, for the above reason.
- At any time, it is important to remember that for some women the risk of repeated pregnancy is greater than the risk of early insertion.

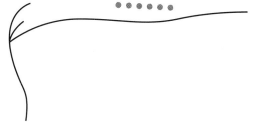

Fig. 22.4 Implanon® capsule showing position in arm. © Family Planning Association 2009, reprinted by permission of the publisher.

- When changing from another form of hormonal contraception to another it is important that there is planned change. Remind the woman to use condoms as additional protection for the first 7 days following insertion.

Follow-up
- Apart from a check of the insertion site to ensure there is no infection, it is not necessary to make a follow-up appointment.
- Give the woman the card that comes in the implant packaging which tells her the date of insertion and the date for removal.
- It is only necessary for her to return if there are any problems.

Suitable for
- Most women across the age range.
- Women who cannot take oestrogen or who have oestrogen-related side-effects.
- Diabetics, although possible adjustment of insulin dose may be required.
- Women weighing more than 70kg, but it may have reduced efficacy, particularly in the third year. In this case, the implant may be changed sooner than 3 years.
- Breastfeeding women, although a tiny amount of hormone may get into breast milk.
- Hypertensive women, as there is no adverse effect on blood pressure.
- Older women and smokers, who are at risk of cardiovascular incidents with oestrogen.
- Blood levels of hormone are steady, rather than fluctuating, as with injectable or oral POP.
- Absence of high-dose progesterone effects, as occur with Depo-Provera®.

Side-effects

- Disturbance of menstrual bleeding pattern:
  - 25% of women experience some change, with irregular cycles, inter menstrual bleeding, spotting, or prolonged bleeding in the first 6 months
  - 80% of problems settle without further management
  - 35% have normal cycles and no problems in the first 6 months
  - 20% become amenorrhoeic
  - Bleeding problems are the most common reason for early removal.
- Other possible effects:
  - Acne
  - Headaches
  - Abdominal pain
  - Weight gain
  - Breast pain
  - Dizziness
  - Mood swings
  - Hair loss.
- Functional ovarian cysts:
  - These are usually asymptomatic and managed conservatively
  - They will resolve on removal of the implant.
- Ectopic pregnancy: rare in implant users.

Return of fertility

- Plasma levels of etonogestrel are too low to measure 48h after removal and normal ovulatory cycles return within the first month after removal.
- The subsequent conception rate is comparable with that of women not using contraception, and you can, therefore, reassure women that the implant alone will not adversely affect their future fertility.

Drug interactions

- Antibiotics, except rifampicin and griseofulvin, do not affect effectiveness.
- Anti-epileptic treatment may reduce efficacy slightly. Advise additional consistent condom use.

Metabolic effects

- Minimal effects on carbohydrate metabolism, LFTs, blood coagulation, immunoglobulins, and serum cortisol levels have been reported.
- Lipoprotein levels: there should be a small fall in total triglycerides and cholesterol. High-density lipoprotein (HDL)/cholesterol ratio is unchanged or improved.
- These minimal metabolic effects make this a very suitable form of contraception for almost all women.

Injectables

Content

- The most common injectable contraceptive in use is Depo-Provera® (depot medroxyprogesterone acetate) 150mg, given every 12 weeks, but the interval may be extended up to 14 weeks.[1]
- Noristerat® (norethisterone oenanthate) 200mg, given by intramuscular injection every 8 weeks. Noristerat® is oily and must be warmed to near body temperature prior to administration. Normally, only used for those women who have persistent vaginal bleeding problems with Depo-Provera® and who wish to continue to use an injectable method.

Method of administration

- For both drugs the first dose should be given in the first 5 days of the menstrual cycle.
- For maximum effect injection should be on day 1.
- If given later than day 2, it is important to advise the woman to use extra barrier precautions for the next 7 days, if sexual intercourse occurs.
- Depo-Provera® is given by deep intramuscular injection into the gluteus muscle of the buttock, in the upper outer quadrant. It is important that the injection site is not rubbed afterwards, as this will accelerate breakdown of the drug and make it less effective.

After giving birth

- Normally given no sooner than 21 days after childbirth, to avoid prolonged or heavy bleeding, but can be given within 5 days of birth if not breastfeeding.
- Ideally wait 6 weeks before injection in a breastfeeding mother, if she chooses additional hormonal contraception. By this time the infant's enzyme system will be more fully developed and able to effectively metabolize any of the drug transmitted in the breast milk.

After abortion

- First trimester: can be given immediately.
- Second trimester: ideally wait 2 weeks.

Return of fertility

- ▶ After the last dose, return of fertility is commonly delayed (median 9 months) and the woman should be told this clearly.
- There is no evidence that injectable contraceptives cause permanent infertility.
- Over 80% of women are expected to conceive within 15 months of their last injection.

Benefits

The injectable progesterone-only method offers effective short- or long-term contraception.

- 0–1 failure per 100 woman years.
- Non-intercourse related.

- May be used in spite of a previous history of thrombosis.
- Ideal for women awaiting surgery, including sterilization.
- ▶ Women whose partners are awaiting vasectomy and postoperative confirmation of clear sperm count. It is important to stress the need to continue with effective contraception until the sperm count is clear or for 6 months after vasectomy.
- Studies show no adverse effect on blood pressure.
- Positively beneficial in women with endometriosis, epilepsy, sickle-cell anaemia, and pelvic inflammatory disease.
- Women being immunized against rubella.
- Minimal metabolic effects.

Effects
- Suppression of ovulation.
- Amenorrhoea usual within 6 months.
- Not reversible for duration of the injection.
- Injectables are safer than combined oral contraceptives.
- Delay in return of fertility (median 9 months).

Side-effects
Irregular bleeding
- This is the most common side-effect, usually in the first 3-month cycle.
- It usually resolves with second injection, which may be given early (not less than 4 weeks after the previous dose).
- May require added oestrogen, for example ethinylestradiol 20–30micrograms (usually given in combined oral contraception form) up to 21 days (i.e. one menstrual cycle). If the woman has a past history of thrombosis or focal migraine, this may be given as a natural oestrogen, for example Premarin® 1.25mg for up to 21 days.
- A withdrawal bleed may occur after oestrogen therapy.
- The treatment may be repeated if an acceptable bleeding pattern does not occur subsequently.

Amenorrhoea
- At least 90% of users have ceased having periods by 6 months.
- Prolonged amenorrhoea may cause hypo-oestrogenism, adverse lipid effects, and osteoporosis.
- When this form of contraception is administered over a long period of time, the woman should be reviewed at least once every 2 years by a doctor specializing in contraception. A bone mineral density scan may be undertaken.

Weight gain
- This may be slow and insidious or rapid and marked. Most women gain 0.5–2.0kg in the first year, and 10–12kg after 4–6 years of use.
- Progesterone use may increase the appetite, a similar effect to that of high progesterone levels in pregnancy. Weigh the woman regularly if weight gain is apparent or suspected.
- The evidence is that this weight gain is as a result of increased fat and not secondary to anabolic effect or fluid retention.

Mood
- Some women on Depo-Provera® complain of premenstrual-type depression.
- Others have reported marked mood swings, which were not there before they started to use Depo-Provera®.
- For postnatal mothers, these progestogenic side-effects may exacerbate postnatal depression.
- Women with history of endogenous depression should not be given Depo-Provera® if there is a suitable alternative.
- Hormone replacement therapy (HRT) on reaching menopause is advisable for women with a history of prolonged use of Depo-Provera®.

Bone mineral density changes
- Large, well-controlled studies are currently in progress.
- The evidence is that structure and bone mass return to normal once the drug is no longer taken.

1 World Health Organization (2004). *Selected Practice Recommendations for Contraceptive Use*, 2nd edn. Geneva: WHO.

Mirena® intrauterine system

Content

The IUS is a long-acting reversible contraceptive inserted into the uterus, mounted on a Nova T® IUD frame. It contains a Silastic capsule along its shaft, which secretes levonorgestrel 20micrograms daily.

It is licensed for 5 years' duration. If left longer than this the contraceptive effect of the IUD will continue, but the progestogenic effects will cease.

Indications for use

There are two main uses:
- Contraception, particularly in women who have heavy menstrual periods. After pregnancy a woman may experience notable and debilitating increase in menstrual flow and the IUS is ideal in these cases.
- Menorrhagia: the use of an IUS may prevent the need for hysterectomy.
- Other conditions: endometriosis, chronic pelvic pain, dysmenorrhoea and anaemia, associated with heavy menstrual bleeding, where there is no pathological cause.

It is *not* used for post-coital emergency contraception.

How does the IUS work?

In addition to the foreign body effect of the IUD there is the progestogenic effect:
- Frequency of ovulation is reduced
- Cervical mucus thickens to inhibit the passage of sperm through the cervix
- The foreign body reaction within the uterus causes the release of leucocytes and prostaglandins from the endometrium, making the environment hostile to the blastocyst
- The endometrium is thinned
- Menstrual bleeding becomes much lighter—this is in direct contrast to the copper IUD, which may cause heavier menstrual bleeding
- Irregular spotting or bleeding may occur in the first few months after insertion, but diminishes after the first 3 months.

The IUS and breastfeeding

The IUS and other progesterone-only contraceptives are not shown to affect milk supply or infant growth.[1] The risk of intrauterine perforation is increased in a lactating mother and fitting should ideally be delayed until at least 12 weeks post birth.

Fitting

For infection screen, when it is fitted and insertion notes, and other information, 📖 see Intrauterine devices, p. 550. As with other IUDs it *must* be fitted by a doctor or nurse trained and competent in the technique, assessing suitability and dealing with possible immediate complications. It is not usually fitted in a nullipara.

---

1 Truitt S, Fraser A, Grimes D, Gallo M, Schulz K (2003). Combined hormonal versus nonhormonal versus progestin-only contraception in lactation. *Cochrane Database Systematic Review* **2**, CD003988.

Intrauterine devices

- These are small polyethylene and copper devices, which come in a variety of shapes and sizes (Fig. 22.5), and are inserted into the uterus.
- IUDs provide excellent contraception, have the benefit of no 'user failures', and are the most popular form of contraception in some parts of the world, e.g. China.
- It is a myth that a nulliparous woman cannot be fitted with an IUD. Developments in IUDs now make this possible, particularly the frameless Gynefix®, which is ideal for nulliparae.
- In some parts of the world the IUD had received a negative press, but is now increasing in popularity again, as the newer IUDs are able to offer up to 10 years' contraceptive protection, and longer in the older woman, whose fertility is declining towards menopause.
- It is unsuitable for a woman who has a true copper allergy and for certain other women with uterine abnormalities, previous or current pelvic inflammatory disease or bacterial endocarditis, or those whose lifestyle puts them at high risk of pelvic infection. Other contraindications include past ectopic pregnancy, established immunosuppression, menorrhagia, unexplained vaginal or uterine bleeding, and heart valve replacement.
- It is important that the midwife knows the woman's medical, obstetric, gynaecological, and sexual history before advising her about an IUD.

How does the IUD work?

- The mode of action is not exactly known, but it is thought that the main mechanism of the copper is in preventing fertilization, by altering the composition of tubal and uterine fluids. In this way the IUD does not cause abortion. Within the uterus the IUD causes a foreign body reaction within the endometrium, with increased numbers of leucocytes.
- If fertilization does occur, then the IUD will stop implantation in the uterus, but this would only usually occur only if the woman keeps the device *in situ* longer than the recommended number of years for the copper content of the individual device to be effective. For the different IUDs this period ranges from 5 to 10 years.
- ▶ The IUD provides excellent post-coital emergency contraception, for the above reason, and may be removed after the next normal period or left *in situ* for long-term contraception.
- As the woman gets older, her fertility declines, so the IUD is more effective in women over 30. If an IUD is fitted in a woman over 40, it need not be changed and is removed at the time of the menopause.

When is it inserted?

- *After 1st trimester abortion*: it can be inserted immediately.
- *After 2nd trimester abortion*: wait 2–4 weeks, to allow uterine involution, and avoid the risk of expulsion.
- *After vaginal birth*: wait at least 6 weeks, to allow full uterine involution. If breastfeeding, the mother may be at increased risk of uterine perforation, and, if fully breastfeeding day and night, she could wait

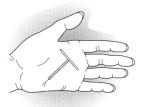

The actual size of the IUD

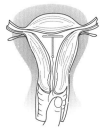

Palpating the threads after insertion

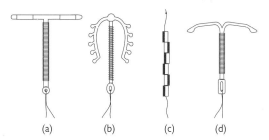

(a)   (b)   (c)   (d)

Fig. 22.5 The IUD. (a) Gyne T280; (b) Multiload Cu375; (c) Gynefix®; and (d) Nova T380.

up to 12 weeks to have her IUD inserted, because breastfeeding will prevent ovulation.
- *After caesarean section*: wait at least 8 weeks to allow uterine muscle healing. If breastfeeding, the above applies.
- The IUD will be inserted by a doctor or nurse trained in the technique.
- Ideally insertion takes place at the end of a period, when the cervix is more receptive to facilitate insertion.

▶ Pre-insertion infection screen
- Prior to insertion it is good practice to check for any current evidence of infection that could be extended into the uterine cavity with insertion. Explain this to the woman.
- The vagina and cervix are inspected and endocervical swabs taken for *Chlamydia* and gonorrhoea and a high vaginal swab for other infections such as bacterial vaginosis. Ideally this is done, and results are known, so that any infection can be treated before the IUD is inserted.
- In the case of emergency post-coital contraception, the swabs are taken at the time of insertion and infection subsequently treated, if necessary.

Insertion
- This is an aseptic procedure throughout.
- It is normal practice to apply lidocaine 2% gel around the cervix prior to the procedure. This not only reduces any discomfort felt, but also helps to relax the cervix during uterine sounding and IUD insertion.
- It also helps to advise the woman to take some simple analgesic, such as paracetamol or ibuprofen, about 1h prior to her appointment.
- ▶ The woman's colour and pulse rate are monitored to detect any evidence of shock.
- Once inserted, the monofilament threads are trimmed to approximately 3cm outside the cervix.
- At follow-up, 4–6 weeks later, the threads are further trimmed to 1cm. outside the cervix.

Teach the woman to feel for the threads after every period, to ensure that the device remains *in situ*. If she cannot feel them she should return to the clinic where the IUD was inserted.

Advantages
- Provides long-term, highly effective, reversible contraception.
- It is immediately effective.
- It is not related to intercourse.
- There are no tablets to remember.
- Very low morbidity.
- Once removed, the woman's fertility immediately returns to normal.

Disadvantages
- Periods may be longer, heavier and more painful, particularly the first couple of days.
- The woman may experience inter menstrual bleeding or spotting, particularly in the first 3 months.
- Infection: a small percentage of women may develop a pelvic infection, particularly in the first few weeks after insertion, which should be treated promptly with appropriate antibiotics. Pelvic infection is more likely in younger and nulliparous women and in those who are at risk of sexually transmitted infections.

Follow-up
- Usually the first appointment is at least 1 week after the next expected period, or up to 3 months, depending on local policy.
- This is to ensure that the IUD is comfortable, with no pain or discomfort; that there is no evidence of infection, that no part of the IUD can be felt or seen in the cervical canal; and to trim the threads once the IUD is settled in position.
- It is important to advise the woman to keep her follow-up appointments, even though she may not be experiencing any problems with her IUD.

Removal
The IUD is usually removed during a period. If removed later in the menstrual cycle, advise the woman to use an additional contraceptive method for 7 days prior to removal, to avoid possible pregnancy.

Problems with the IUD

Most problems occurring after IUD insertion can be attributed to faulty insertion technique:

- Failure to check the position and length of the uterine body, and obstructions in the uterus, such as submucous fibroids or septate or bicornuate uterus.
- The actual insertion technique was faulty.

Infection

Symptoms of infection may include pain during or after intercourse, unusual vaginal discharge, irregular bleeding, and lower abdominal or back pain.

Actinomyces-like organisms may be found in the genital tract of women with an IUD inserted. These potentially threaten future fertility and may be life-threatening if untreated.

❶ If any signs or symptoms of infection, such as abnormal vaginal discharge, pain, dyspareunia, tenderness, the woman must be immediately referred to a doctor for investigation and treatment. Ideally, this should be at a contraception and sexual health clinic. The IUD may have to be removed.

Bleeding

- Intermittent bleeding and spotting may occur for the first two or three cycles after insertion, after which it normally settles down.
- Warn the woman that this might occur.
- Periods may be heavier with an IUD fitted.

Ectopic pregnancy

It is a myth that an IUD will cause ectopic pregnancy. The main cause is infection of the fallopian tubes, with one or both tubes being affected. The IUD is highly effective at preventing uterine pregnancy and very few sperm actually penetrate the copper containing uterine fluid to reach the egg in the fallopian tube to be able to cause fertilization.[1]

Points to remember

- A modern copper-bearing IUD is a highly effective form of short- or long-term contraception, with an efficacy rate of over 99%. IUDs now on the market can have a copper efficiency of up to 10 years.
- Know her history for contraindications before advising a woman about an IUD.
- It does not cause abortion.
- Advise her about insertion after abortion or birth, particularly if breastfeeding.
- It is more effective than the oral form of emergency contraception, particularly between 3 and 5 days after intercourse in the fertile period of the woman's menstrual cycle.
- More effective in women <30.
- An infection screen is good practice, wherever possible, prior to IUD insertion.

- Advise her to take a simple analgesic about an hour before planned insertion, which will help with discomfort during insertion and any lower abdominal cramps in the hours after insertion.
- Advise the woman of the importance of checking for her threads after every period. If she cannot feel them, the doctor will check and an ultrasound scan will be advised to locate the IUD, if necessary.
- Advise her of the importance of attending follow-up appointments.
- Advise her to report any signs and symptoms of infection promptly, to prevent any possible long-term damage to her reproductive tract.

1 Guillebaud J (2008). *Contraception Today*, 6th edn. London: Taylor and Francis.

Female condom

- The female condom (Fig. 22.6) is a well-lubricated, loose-fitting polyurethane sheath, with an outer rim, designed to keep the condom outside the vagina in use, and a loose inner ring, with a retaining action similar to the diaphragm, designed to fit behind the suprapubic bone and over the cervix.
- It is easy to obtain over the counter, as well as at contraception and sexual health clinics, and does not need medical supervision. It is made in one size only and full instructions are contained in the packet. Each condom is individually packaged; they come in packs of three and each condom is single use only.

How is it used?

- For effective use it must be used before there is any genital contact. Remind the woman that, before opening the packet, she should push the condom well away from the edge of the packet that is to be torn to release the condom.
- The condom is inserted into the vagina, using the inner ring as a guide, as far as possible along the posterior vaginal wall towards the posterior cervical fornix. The outer ring lies flat against the body, outside the vulva, which helps prevent the condom being drawn up into the vagina during intercourse. It can be inserted any time before sexual intercourse and when correctly in place it will feel loose and comfortable. The man needs to be careful that the penis is not inserted between the condom and the vaginal wall. After use it should be carefully disposed of and *not* flushed down the toilet.
- Additional spermicides or lubricants of any kind can be used, although this should not be necessary, as the condom is very well lubricated.

Advantages

- The condom, when used carefully and consistently, is extremely effective in preventing pregnancy.
- Similarly, it is effective in preventing sexually transmitted infections and HIV.
- It is easy to obtain and use and requires no medical supervision.
- It does not require additional spermicide.
- It can be used with oil-based products.
- Polyurethane is stronger than latex. It is much less likely to split or break in use than the male condom.
- It does not require male erection before use.
- It may protect the woman against cancer of the cervix, by preventing transmission of HPV.
- The woman can take responsibility for contraception and STI prevention.

Disadvantages

- It needs forward planning each time.
- It needs to be used carefully to be effective.
- It can interrupt sex.
- It can get pushed into the vagina during intercourse.

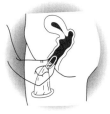

Insert the condom into the vagina holding and guiding the inner ring in an upwards and backwards direction following the posterior vaginal wall

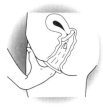

Ensure the condom is inserted high into the vagina and the inner ring covers the cervix and the lower edge remains outside the vagina at all times

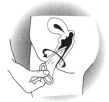

Twist the condom two to three times prior to removal to ensure semen does not escape

Fig. 22.6 The female condom.

Copyright © fpa 2007 and reproduced by permission of the publisher.

- It needs to be carefully disposed of.
- For women unable to touch their genital area with comfort it is not a good method to recommend.

Points to remember
- In the first few weeks after birth, intercourse may be uncomfortable or sore. Advise her to use an additional lubricant, if necessary.
- Advise the woman about the availability of emergency contraception, in case of failure to use or failure in use.

- If a mother is not breastfeeding or is post-abortion, her risk of pregnancy, even in the first menstrual cycle, is real. We have all seen the woman who comes for her postnatal examination and is pregnant again!
- For the mother who is fully breastfeeding, day and night, the risk of pregnancy is minimal. If this woman chooses to use a female condom, although it is very well lubricated, she may need additional lubrication because of the very low oestrogen levels while breastfeeding.
- If one or more partners are sensitive or allergic to latex, this is a useful alternative.
- She may use additional spermicides to increase efficacy of the condom.
- Emphasize that the condom is a 'once only' use and should never be re-used.
- In the UK all contraception is free of charge and the midwife can offer the woman a supply of female condoms. Make sure you know where the local contraception and sexual health clinics are located, to be able to advise her on further supplies.
- Remind her to check that the condom she is purchasing has the nationally agreed quality mark, e.g. the British Kite mark or the European Community CE mark.

Diaphragms and cervical caps

Diaphragms (Fig. 22.7) and cervical caps fit into the vagina and cover the cervix, providing a barrier to sperm, thus preventing fertilization.

Fitting and teaching of the method must be done by a doctor, nurse, or midwife trained and competent to do so. Accurate fitting is essential to their success in use.

How are they used?
- Diaphragms, in particular, are simple to use, once taught by a doctor or nurse experienced in fitting and teaching use of this method.
- The diaphragm comes in sizes from 55mm to 100mm and careful measuring and fitting is important.
- It can be inserted well ahead of intercourse and need not affect spontaneity.
- If more than 3h have elapsed since spermicide was applied, it must be reapplied before intercourse, usually in the form of a spermicidal pessary.
- The spermicide should be reapplied before repeated acts of intercourse.
- ▶ *It must be left in place for at least 6h after intercourse.*

Efficacy
- When used carefully and consistently, with spermicide, they have a 92–96% success rate.
- Typically the efficacy rate is 82–90%, with a spermicide.
- The failure rate depends on how effectively the woman uses the diaphragm or cervical cap.
- Age is relevant, as the woman aged 25 is generally more fertile than a woman aged 40+.

Disadvantages
- Requires motivation and needs to be used carefully and consistently.
- Needs to be used with a spermicide cream or gel for maximum effectiveness. Some women find the additional spermicide messy and unacceptable.
- No protection against HIV.
- May increase the incidence of cystitis and urinary tract infection (particularly if the diaphragm is too big).
- The woman must be comfortable with handling and exploring her body.
- Psychosexual problems may become apparent during discussion and teaching diaphragm or cervical cap fitting.

Advantages
- There is little reduction in sexual sensitivity.
- It may give some protection against cervical cancer and sexually transmitted diseases, if the cervix is covered.
- No hormones to take.
- It is under the control of the woman.

Contraindications
- Poor vaginal muscle tone, bladder, or uterine prolapse

Ensure the diaphragm completely covers the cervix

To remove the diaphragm place the forefinger over the power edge and gently pull downwards

Fig. 22.7 The diaphragm.

Copyright © fpa 2008 and reproduced by permission of the publisher.

- Allergy to spermicide or latex
- Undiagnosed genital tract bleeding
- Congenital abnormality, such as two cervices or septal wall defects in the vagina
- Current vaginal, cervical, or pelvic infection
- Recurrent urinary tract infections
- Past history of toxic shock syndrome
- Women unable to touch their genital area.

Side-effects

- Urinary tract infection
- Vaginal irritation
- Toxic shock syndrome if left in longer than 30h.

Points to remember

- ▶ After any pregnancy the diaphragm or cap should be refitted. This is particularly important after a full-term pregnancy.
- Fitting should be delayed until at least 6 weeks after birth, to allow for return of pelvic tone.
- Advise the woman to have a diaphragm or cap properly fitted by a competent nurse, doctor, or midwife.
- If her weight varies by more than 7lb (3kg) the fitting should be professionally reassessed.
- The diaphragm must be checked regularly for deterioration or holes.
- A new diaphragm should be fitted following any episode of treated vaginal infection.
- Only water-based lubricants should be used, as any other preparations damage the latex rubber.

Fertility awareness (natural family planning)

- Fertility awareness methods are natural, requiring no medical intervention, but do require competent education in their use.
- Natural methods of family planning are widely and successfully used, particularly in certain religious groups.
- Natural fertility awareness methods involve observation of female body changes within the woman's menstrual cycle, in order to detect ovulation, either to use as contraception or to achieve pregnancy in the fertile period.
- Many women/couples now want to utilize non-hormonal methods of contraception.
- There are four main methods of natural family planning and fertility awareness:
  - Temperature method
  - Calendar method
  - Cervical mucus method (Billing's method)
  - A combination of the above, known as the sympothermal method, which is the most effective and preferable method (see Fig. 22.8).

After pregnancy

▶ Because of the hormonal changes in pregnancy, it is important to remind the woman that this method should not be relied on until she has had at least three normal periods after abortion or birth. This is to ensure that her natural hormonal levels are back to normal.

Changing from a hormonal method of contraception

▶ As above, she should wait until at least three normal periods after discontinuing the hormonal method.

Breastfeeding

- ▶ This method cannot be used while a mother is breastfeeding, because of altered hormone levels (for further details, 📖 see Lactational amenorrhoea method, p. 528).
- She should wait until she has ceased breastfeeding and had at least three normal periods.
- She may need additional contraception in the intervening period.

Efficacy

- This depends on consistency and conscientiousness of method use.
- The efficacy rate varies from 80–90%.

Disadvantages

- Cannot be used immediately after pregnancy.
- Requires motivation and conscientiousness in use.
- Requires observation and recording of daily body changes.
- Requires specialist teaching.
- Takes time to learn (typically 3–6 months).

- Basal body temperature is affected by illness, alcohol, disturbed sleep, anxiety, and stress.
- Some cold and flu remedies can inhibit cervical mucus production.
- A vaginal infection will make it difficult to detect changes in cervical mucus.

Advantages

- It is under the control of the couple, once learned.
- No side-effects.
- Can be used to avoid or achieve pregnancy.
- Detects the beginning and end of the fertile period.
- Helps couples learn about their fertility and recognize body changes.
- Acceptable to a number of religious beliefs and cultures.

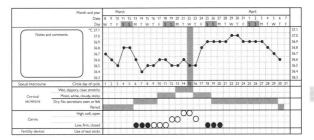

Fig. 22.8 Fertility indicator chart.

Copyright © J Knight and C Pyper. Adapted with permission of Fertility UK (2005) from ✋ www.fertilityuk.org.

Coitus interruptus

- The oldest known form of contraception, referred to in the Bible and in the Koran, and widely acceptable on religious grounds.
- The male withdraws his penis from the woman prior to ejaculation.
- Commonly called 'withdrawal' or 'being careful'.

Efficacy
- Variable.
- With careful and consistent use it may be up to 96% effective as contraception.
- Less careful use will result in it being 80% effective, at best.

Disadvantages
- Low efficacy.
- May inhibit enjoyment during sexual intercourse.
- May lead to erectile problems.
- The woman may experience anxiety that it will work.
- No protection against STIs or HIV.
- Efficacy is markedly reduced in men with erectile problems, such as premature ejaculation.

Advantages
- Easily used.
- No clinic appointments.
- Religious acceptability.
- It is under the control of the couple, when consciously used as a method of contraception.

Point to remember
▶ In discussing this method, it is important to remember to emphasize that sperm are present in the pre-ejaculate and, therefore, capable of fertilizing the female, even when full intercourse with ejaculation has not occurred.

Male condom

- This is the easiest form of contraception to obtain and use, and second only in popularity of use to the oral contraceptive pill in the under-30 age group, and to sterilization in the over-30s, in the UK.
- For a large proportion of the population it is a completely acceptable method.
- For those who have become used to alternative methods not related to intercourse, it may be completely unacceptable, even on a temporary basis.
- Male condoms come in various sizes, shapes, colours, and flavours, and are now produced from hypoallergenic latex.
- A non-latex polyurethane condom, Avanti® is available if either partner is allergic to latex.
- The main reason that men do not like to use them is the lack of sensitivity during sexual activity, but manufacturers are continually making attempts to overcome this problem.

How is it used?

- ▶ For effective use it must be used before there is any genital contact.
- Remind the woman that before opening the packet she should ensure that the condom is well away from the edge that is to be torn to release the condom.
- The closed end of the condom, the 'teat', is squeezed to expel any air and to leave about 1cm to receive the ejaculated semen.
- It is then gently rolled down the full length of the erect penis.
- After ejaculation, hold the condom firmly at the rim, to avoid any semen being spilt as the penis is withdrawn.
- It is then carefully and hygienically disposed of, *but not down the toilet.*

Advantages

- The condom, when used carefully and consistently, is extremely effective in preventing pregnancy.
- Similarly, it is effective in preventing sexually transmitted infections and HIV.
- It is easy to obtain and use, and requires no medical supervision.
- It may protect the woman against cancer of the cervix, by preventing transmission of HPV.
- The man can take responsibility for contraception and share prevention of transmission of STIs

Disadvantages

- It needs forward planning each time.
- It needs to be used carefully to be effective.
- It may interrupt sex, although putting and it on can be part of the enjoyment of foreplay.
- There may be possible loss of sensitivity during intercourse or loss of erection.
- It can slip off or split.
- It needs to be disposed of carefully.

Points to remember

- In the first few weeks after birth, intercourse may be uncomfortable or sore. Advise the woman to use a water-based lubricant, if necessary.
- ▶ Oil-based lubricants will interact with the latex and encourage the condom to split and should not be used. Baby oil will destroy up to 95% of the strength of condoms within 15min. Avoid *ad hoc* use of products from the kitchen or bathroom cupboards!
- Advise the woman about the availability of emergency contraception, in case of failure to use or failure in use.
- If a mother is not breastfeeding or is post-abortion, her risk of pregnancy, even in the first menstrual cycle, is real. We have all seen the woman who comes for her postnatal examination and is pregnant again!
- For the mother who is fully breastfeeding, day and night, the risk of pregnancy is minimal. If this woman chooses to use a condom, she may need additional water-based lubrication, because of the very low oestrogen levels while breastfeeding.
- If one or more partners is sensitive or allergic to latex, a hypoallergenic non-latex condom, Avanti®, is available.
- Because of allergic reactions, most manufacturers do not now coat the condom with Nonoxynol® 9 spermicide. For added protection, a spermicidal pessary or cream may be used.
- Emphasize that the condom is a 'once only' use and should never be re-used.
- In the UK, all contraception is free of charge and the midwife can offer the woman a supply of condoms.
- Make sure you know where the local contraception and sexual health clinics are located, to be able to advise her on further supplies.
- Remind the woman to check that any condom supplied or purchased has a recognized quality mark, e.g. the British Kite Mark or the European Community CE mark.
- Condom use is the only method proven to be effective against the transmission of HIV.

Male sterilization

Vasectomy

- Vasectomy has become a popular method of permanent contraception in the UK.
- It is simpler to carry out than female sterilization and is commonly done under local anaesthesia as an outpatient, in the contraception and sexual health clinic, or doctor's surgery.
- Vasectomy is a minor surgical procedure, involving incision, location and excising the vas deferens, preventing sperm from the epididymis reaching the seminal vesicles (Fig. 22.9). Sperm cannot then be ejaculated and the man becomes infertile, once the vas deferens has been cleared of sperm, which takes approximately 3 months.

Efficacy

- Highly effective.
- The immediate failure rate is 1:1000, with a later failure rate of 1:3000 to 1:7000.

Disadvantages

- Not easily reversible and must be regarded as permanent.
- Requires a surgical procedure.
- Requires local or general anaesthesia.
- ❶ Because vasectomy is not immediately effective, alternative contraception is required until two consecutive clear sperm counts are obtained.
- ❶ If a man does not produce the required two sperm specimens after surgery, the couple must be warned to wait at least 3 months before discontinuing the additional contraception.

Advantages

- Permanent
- Highly effective
- Safe and simple procedure
- Anxiety of unplanned pregnancy removed.

Contraindications

- Urological problems
- Relationship problems
- Indecision by either partner.

Side-effects

- Possibility of infection
- Haematoma
- Sperm granulation.

Counselling prior to vasectomy

- This is extremely important, because of the permanency of the method.
- Consider issues of regret and grief for loss of fertility.

- Ensure that the couple considers all the possible different scenarios that may affect their decision, particularly in respect of current children or future relationship breakdown.
- A particular worry in a lot of men is about their ability to maintain erections and have sexual intercourse following vasectomy. Vasectomy does not affect libido or erections, and they will ejaculate normally, but ejaculate will not contain sperm.
- Contraception is required for at least 3 months following vasectomy.
- There is no proven link between vasectomy and the incidence of testicular or prostatic cancer.
- Ensure that the decision that is made is without influence or coercion from healthcare professionals.

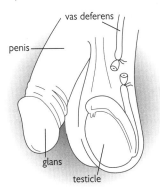

Fig. 22.9 Male sterilization.

Copyright © fpa 2008 and reproduced with permission of the publisher.

Female sterilization

- This is the only permanent form of female contraception.
- Usually a daycare procedure under regional or general anaesthesia.
- Involves incising and dissecting or blocking the fallopian tubes, preventing fertilization (Fig. 22.10).
- It is performed either by laparoscopy, mini-laparotomy, or vaginally.

Efficacy

Highly effective, with an efficacy rate of 99.4–99.8 per 100 woman years.

Disadvantages

- Involves a surgical procedure and anaesthesia.
- Not easily reversed and must be regarded as permanent.
- If it fails, there is a greater risk of ectopic pregnancy.

Advantages

- Permanent.
- Effective immediately.
- The anxiety of unplanned pregnancy is removed.
- The ultimate decision is the woman's.

Contraindications

- Indecision by either partner (if a partner is involved).
- Relationship problems.
- Psychiatric illness.
- A health problem or disability that may increase the risk of the surgical procedure.

Relative contraindications

- Obesity may be a contraindication for laparoscopy.
- Request for sterilization for a young woman <25.

Counselling prior to sterilization

- This is extremely important, because of the permanency of the method.
- ▶ Postoperative regret and grief for lost fertility happens in at least 10% of sterilized women and this must be discussed and the procedure considered thoroughly.
- Whenever possible, discussion should be undertaken with the couple together, to get each partner's perspective.

Practice points

- When discussing sterilization, it is important to emphasize that sterilization is not normally carried out at the time of termination of pregnancy, vaginal birth, or caesarean section, due to the increased vascularity of the tissue involved. This will increase the failure rate.
- In the UK, sterilization reversal is not carried out on the NHS, except in very exceptional circumstances.

- Termination of pregnancy or birth is an emotive time and a decision for sterilization made at this time is fraught with potential future psychological and psychosexual problems.
- It is normal to wait at least 6 weeks following termination of pregnancy or birth.
- Unless the mother is fully breastfeeding, effective contraception in the interim period is essential to prevent pregnancy.

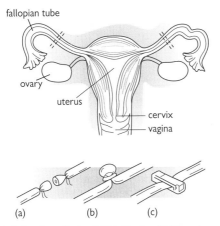

Fig. 22.10 Female sterilization. (a) Tubal ligation; (b) Falope ring; and (c) Filschie clip.

Copyright © fpa 2008 and reproduced with permission of the publisher.

Emergency contraception

There are three forms of emergency post-coital contraception:
- The levonorgestrel-only oral preparation, known in the UK as Levonelle®, commonly known as the 'morning after pill', although this terminology should be discouraged, as it is misleading.
- The ulipristal acetate oral preparation, known in the UK as ellaOne®, with increased effectiveness from 72h and up to 5 days post coitally over Levonelle®.
- A copper IUD.
  ❶ The 'Mirena' IUS should not be used for this purpose.

How do they work?
- These methods inhibit implantation, should unwanted conception have occurred.
- The primary action of ellaOne® is to delay or inhibit ovulation and alter the endometrium, which may also contribute to efficacy.
- This must be explained carefully, as personal beliefs about whether life begins at conception or at implantation may affect a woman's decision about whether to take the emergency contraception pill or to have an IUD inserted.

Oral pill
- The Levonelle® tablet is taken within 72h of unprotected sexual intercourse or contraceptive failure to give maximum protection, but it can be taken up to 5 days after intercourse. If taken within 24h, the efficacy rate is 99.6%, and 98.9% at 72h.
- The ellaOne® tablet is taken orally as soon as possible, but no later than 120h of unprotected sexual intercourse or contraceptive failure.
- In explaining the mode of action and efficacy of the emergency contraceptive pill, it is vital to ensure that the woman clearly understands that this relates only to the immediately preceding 72h, even if there are multiple episodes of intercourse within this period.[1]
- ❶ Any episodes in the current cycle occurring prior to this 72h period may have already resulted in pregnancy and render emergency contraception totally ineffective.
- Treatment with Levonelle®, may be repeated in any menstrual cycle, if necessary. However, ellaOne®, is not currently recommended to be used more than once per cycle, as the efficacy of repeated exposure has not been assessed.
- ellaOne® has been shown to be more effective compared to levonorgestrel in women who are categorized as overweight or obese.
- There is no evidence of any effect on the fetus, if taken in early pregnancy.
- If there is any doubt about whether pregnancy is possible, carry out a reliable pregnancy test prior to administration. The trophoblast embeds in the uterus in 5–7 days after conception and a reliable dipstick test, which takes a maximum of 5min, should give the answer.
- It is professionally responsible for the midwife to discuss ongoing reliable methods of contraception with the woman and to give her information or refer her to a contraception and sexual health clinic, or

a doctor trained and currently up to date with contraceptive methods, if hormonal methods are required, or to a midwife or nurse competent in the non-hormonal methods.

Side-effects
- Virtually none.
- The period may be heavier than normal but should occur at the expected time.

Contraindications
- Current or suspected pregnancy.
- No other absolute contraindications.

Follow-up
- Usually 1 week after the next expected period, i.e. approximately 3 weeks.
- If a normal period has not occurred, carry out a pregnancy test.

Intrauterine device
- It can be inserted up to 5 days following unprotected intercourse or up to 5 days after the earliest calculation of the day of ovulation. This latter point clearly relies on the woman knowing her own menstrual cycle pattern, in order for the doctor or nurse/midwife to calculate and fit the IUD, *in good faith*, e.g. up to day 20 in a 28-day cycle.
- Usually advise a copper IUD, normally one of the cheaper varieties, with the minimum 5-year lifespan on the copper component. This can then be removed at the end of the next period.
- Discussion with the woman may reveal that she would like to keep the IUD as a long-term method of contraception, longer than 5 years, in which case an IUD with an 8–10-year copper licence will be fitted.

Pre-insertion infection screen
- Not possible in this circumstance. Take swabs at the time of fitting, along with visual inspection for evidence of existing infection. Antibiotics are prescribed, if necessary.
- For further details about IUD insertion, see Intrauterine devices, p. 550.

Follow-up
- Normally 1 week after the next expected period.
- If a normal period has occurred, the IUD can be removed.
- If the period has not occurred, a pregnancy test should be carried out.
- It is good practice to offer an infection screen at this point, or to refer the woman to the appropriate clinic.

1 Faculty of Sexual and Reproductive Healthcare Clinical Effectiveness Unit (2009). *New Product Review (October 2009) Ulipristal Acetate (ellaOne®)*. London: Faculty of Sexual and Reproductive Healthcare Clinical Effectiveness Unit.

Part 6

Care of the newborn

Chapter 23

Care of the newborn

Examination of the newborn: monitoring progress

The purpose of the examination of the newborn is to monitor the normal progress of the baby and for early detection of deviations from normal.

During the examination advice can be given to the parents about minor disorders (📖 see Minor disorders of the newborn, p. 586) and safe baby care practice, such as the correct amount and type of clothing and bedding needed and correct sleeping position, to reduce the risk of sudden infant death syndrome (SIDS). Information can also be gained about the baby's overall feeding and sleeping pattern.

The midwife will monitor and record the following information.

- With the mother's permission the baby should be undressed and examined in a draught-free environment. Care is taken not to expose the baby longer than necessary and he/she should be re-dressed as quickly as possible to maintain body temperature.
- Colour: the baby should not be pale, cyanosed, or jaundiced. The skin is inspected for rashes and spots.
- Temperature: the chest and back should feel warm. If the hands and feet are cool mittens and bootees can be put on.
- Respirations: should be regular, up to 40 per min with no dyspnoea or expiratory grunt.
- Muscle tone should be neither floppy nor stiff.
- The eyes, nose, and mouth should be inspected for discharge or other signs of infection.
- The umbilicus is inspected for signs of cord separation and advice given about washing the umbilicus as part of the daily bath. The cord may need to be cleaned during the nappy change and warm tap water is sufficient for this purpose. The cord usually separates during the first 10 days of life.
- The nappy area is inspected for signs of rashes and the mother can be asked whether the baby is passing urine and stools regularly.
- The baby should pass urine during the first 24h after birth and then urine output is governed by the baby's intake of food and fluid. Wet nappies signify a good fluid intake.
- The first stools will be meconium, a soft black sticky substance which accumulates in the gut in fetal life. Passage of meconium confirms the patency of the lower gut.
- After a few days of feeding the stools change colour to green/brown as the milk starts to be digested. Passage of a changing stool confirms the patency of the upper digestive tract.
- Yellow stools confirm that milk is being fully digested. A breastfeeding baby may pass stools several times per day or only once every few days depending on its intake. Formula-fed babies should pass stools each day.
- Weight should be recorded on the 10th day to ensure the baby has regained its birthweight. Weight recording between birth and the 10th day would be performed if there were any other concerns about the baby's progress. Evidence-based local midwifery guidelines on weighing should be followed.

If the mother expresses any concerns that the baby is not progressing as expected, advice should be given and the baby re-examined later the same day. A baby showing signs of illness such as lethargy, poor tone, breathing or feeding difficulties, needs to be referred to a paediatrician as a matter of priority.

Reflexes in the newborn

Reflexes are incorporated into the neurological examination performed by the paediatrician or suitably trained midwife following birth. Reflexes are involuntary reactions to external stimuli such as touch, sound, and light. Certain stimuli evoke specific reactions that give reassurance regarding normal neuromuscular development. Inborn reflexes are movement patterns that develop during fetal life and are crucial for survival of the newborn. All reflexes have their own time span—an infant exhibiting reflexes after this time indicates neurological impairment.

Common reflexes observed in the newborn infant

- *Rooting reflex*: a very common reflex observed by midwives. When the cheek is brushed lightly with the finger, a soft object or the nipple, the baby's head will turn to the side being stimulated and he or she will open their mouth wide. A mother wishing to breastfeed will be advised to use this reflex to encourage the baby to open the mouth to receive the nipple and ensure successful attachment to the breast.
- *Grasping reflex*: stroking or applying pressure to the palm of the hand will result in the baby making a clenched fist. This reflex is very strong in the newborn baby. A weak reflex may indicate neurological disturbance.
- *Sucking reflex*: when the root of the baby's mouth is touched with a clean finger or a teat, the baby spontaneously starts to suck. This response begins at about 32 weeks' gestation, but is not fully developed until 36 weeks' gestation. Therefore premature babies may well have a weak sucking reflex.
- *Moro reflex*: also known as the 'startle' reflex. This reflex is initiated by startling the baby, usually by supporting the baby supine on the hand and forearm. When the baby is relaxed the head is suddenly dropped back a few centimetres. The baby then flings his or her arms open, with the hands open and fingers curled in slightly. This is followed by drawing the arms back towards the chest in an embrace like position. This may be accompanied by the baby grimacing or crying. This reflex may also be stimulated by sudden noise.
- *Walking or stepping reflex*: the significance of this reflex is not fully understood. When the baby is held under the arms in an upright position over a flat surface, the baby will make stepping movements forwards.
- *Tonic neck reflex*: with the baby lying on his or her back, when the head is turned to one side, one arm and leg are extended in the direction that the baby's head is facing. The opposite arm and leg are in a flexed position.
- *Babinski reflex*: stroking the sole of the foot from heel to toe will result in the baby's toes fanning out and the foot turns inwards. This reflex is present until the age of 2 years.

Screening tests

Screening tests aim to identify the likelihood of potential abnormality within a normal population. During the early neonatal period, various tests and examinations may be undertaken to detect specific abnormalities that could undermine the infant's health. Screening procedures are only appropriate when diagnostic tests are available that are inexpensive, simple, and specific to the condition. Effective treatment or intervention should also be readily available before the onset of symptoms or pathology is apparent. Early diagnosis of some conditions can result in curtailing disease processes that have devastating effects on the individual. An excellent example is the screening test for phenylketonuria (PKU)—early diagnosis of this inborn error of metabolism prevents severe mental impairment, by prescribing a specialized diet.

Hearing

Approximately 1–2 babies in 1000 are born with hearing loss in one or both ears. Recent technological advances have led to major improvements in screening methods for detecting hearing loss in the neonate.

Early detection of hearing loss in infancy ensures that full investigation into the cause and possible therapy or treatment can be commenced that will be important for the baby's speech development.

Oto-acoustic emissions (OAE) test

- This test is done as early as possible; many maternity units perform this test within the first 24h of birth.
- A trained hearing test screener or health visitor undertakes the test, which only takes a few moments to perform.
- The test is non-invasive, using a small soft tipped ear piece placed in the outer ear, which transmits clicking sounds to the inner ear. A computer detects how the ears respond to sound emissions.
- A strong response to the test indicates the unlikelihood of hearing impairment. The result of the test is given immediately to the parents by the screener.
- If there is no clear response to the test, then a second test is arranged. Various reasons may make it difficult to test a baby's hearing: baby was unsettled; an accumulation of fluid in the ear after birth; background noise at the time of the test.
- Parents may also be given checklists to monitor their baby's hearing at key stages of development.

Automated auditory brainstem response (AABR)

- This is a similar test to the OAE using computer technology; it takes slightly longer.
- Three small sensors are placed on the baby's head, headphones are placed over the ears, and a series of clicking sounds are transmitted. The computer measures how well baby's ears respond to sound.

If the second test shows a poor response, then referral to the audiology department is necessary for further tests and follow up.

Further reading

Department of Health (2004). *NHS Newborn Hearing Screening Programme. MRC Institute of Hearing Research in collaboration with The National Deaf Children's Society.* London: DH.

Growth

Due to physical and psychological limitations the baby is reliant on its mother to provide dedicated care to enable its ongoing survival, growth and development. Providing the baby has been born with no physical or neurological abnormalities it will require the following in order to grow and develop normally:
- Nutritional needs met
- Safe environment
- Adequate exercise, rest, and sleep
- Psychological/emotional stimulation.

To some extent the physical growth and development of the baby depends on the nutritional status of the mother before, during, and after pregnancy (especially if breastfeeding), as well as the adequacy of the infants diet if bottle feeding.
- Nutrition—establishing infant nutrition in the early days is an essential part of midwifery care of the newborn whether the baby is breast or bottle feeding. Observation of the baby's feeding technique is important to ensure correct attachment to the breast or the baby's sucking and swallowing behaviour if bottle feeding.
- Environment:
  - *Safety*: ensuring that the environment is free from potential hazards/dangers that may impair adequate growth, such as tight clothing. Over-swaddling the baby may restrict movement. Avoid a smoky environment. There is some debate about the practice of bed sharing; parents should be encouraged to carefully weigh up the risks and benefits.
  - *Thermoregulation*: in mature infants heat loss may pose a problem to the baby's survival and health status due to the immaturity of the heat regulatory system. Because of the baby's immobility and lack of ability to shiver, there is still a risk of hypothermia if the environment is not adequately warm. If the baby is cold the nape of the neck may still feel warm, therefore it is best to check the skin of the abdomen for a more reliable assessment of temperature. Observing the baby's behaviour is crucial; initially babies may generate more heat by crying and creating activity. However, in the later stages of hypothermia the baby may become lethargic, with a poor response to stimuli, even though their pallor may be deceivingly healthy.
  - *Prevention of infection*: during the first 6 months of life babies are at increased risk of infection due to immaturity of the immune system. Care should be taken to ensure sound hygiene standards when caring for or handling newborn babies. Infection can seriously undermine a baby's health and growth, leading to morbidity and sometimes mortality.
- Psychological development—although the baby sleeps for long periods during the first 6–8 weeks, it is important to communicate and provide sensory stimulation during the wakeful times and at feed time. It is well known that emotional deprivation results in poor growth and delayed development.

Indicators of sound nourishment and adequate growth are:
- Steady increase in weight and length
- Regular sleeping patterns
- Regular, daily elimination
- Active, alert, and responsive during wakeful times
- Firm muscles and moderate amount of subcutaneous fat.

Some pre-disposing/inhibiting factors may need to be considered when assessing growth.
- Cultural and hereditary factors-small/large stature, diet.
- Prematurity—it may take some time for the premature baby to catch up with the normal parameters. The baby may still be on a strict feeding regime on discharge from hospital: consequently parents may require extra support and reassurance from the midwife. The baby's stomach capacity is much smaller and the sucking reflex may still be weak. In some instances the baby may still be receiving partial nutrition via a nasogastric route, which may require the support of a neonatal nurse.
- Small for gestational age—depends on the reason for the lack of adequate growth *in utero*. If the baby is nutritionally deficient, this may have far reaching effects, which may not necessarily be rectified post delivery. Lack of essential minerals *in utero* and early neonatal life has been linked with suboptimal brain development and impaired physical growth. These babies are increasingly discharged home much earlier, therefore the parents may need extra support from the midwife/neonatal nurse until they are confident in their abilities to maintain the healthy growth and development for their baby.
- Babies of diabetic mothers—due to high glucose levels *in utero*, there may be a period of readjustment before normal feeding patterns are established.
- Congenital abnormalities—some abnormalities may deter the ability to feed properly, therefore potentially causing difficulty:
  - Cleft lip and cleft palate—special teats may need to be used
  - Oesophageal atresia
  - Pyloric stenosis—projectile vomiting occurs between the third and fifth week of life and affects males more than females.
- Twins—there may be inherited differences in feeding and growth patterns, it is therefore important to monitor both babies to ensure that they both progress along normal parameters. The mother will require extra support and input from the midwife to ensure she retains the healthy growth and development of both infants.

In order to monitor a baby's growth and development various checks may be carried out:
- Weight—in most units the routine weighing of healthy term infants is not carried out, as most babies may lose up 10% of their birthweight within the first week of life. Thereafter, most babies will have regained their birthweight by 10 days. It is usual for babies to gain approximately 200g per week although individual differences need to be taken into account as outlined above.
- Length—the measurement at birth gives a baseline for the baby's further growth. Debate about measuring length accurately is crucial

if using it to monitor adequate growth patterns. A correct supine stadiometer should be used and two people are required for the procedure.

- Head circumference—measurements for the head circumference at birth and up to 24h may be inaccurate due to moulding. Some units delay this measurement until 24–48h post delivery. The head circumference provides a good baseline for later comparisons. An unusually large or small head circumference indicates abnormality.
- Percentile charts are the most common means of assessing growth, usually these consist of graphs plotting the upper, lower, and midpoint levels of average growth patterns—the baby's weight, length, and head circumference readings can be plotted and compared with normal expectations. Babies below the 9th centile will have reduced glycogen stores and are therefore more prone to hypothermia and hypoglycaemia.
- Feed charts may be employed where strict feeding regimens are important to ensure that exact calorific requirement are provided.

Minor disorders of the newborn

Skin rashes

Babies commonly present with non-infective skin rashes within the first few weeks of life, which usually resolve spontaneously without treatment.

- *Erythema toxicum*: also known as urticaria neonatorum, is a blotchy red rash with pinhead papules, which usually occurs within the first week of life and normally disappears within a day or two.
- *Heat rashes*: appear as reddened areas, often in the skin folds and have hard pinpoint centres. The rash resolves quickly when the baby cools down.
- *Milia*: also know as a sweat rash, is seen in babies who become overheated and is due to blocked sweat glands. Less clothing and fewer cot blankets should be used and more fresh air may help.
  Other skin rashes that may occur but require remedial action include:
- *Chafing or intertrigo*: this is due to inadequate drying of the skin, particularly in the groin or axilla area, after washing or bathing. The skin should be dried using a dabbing movement with the towel and then a slight dusting of antiseptic power applied.
- *Sore buttocks*: presents as soreness and excoriation around the anus and buttocks and is usually a result of frequent loose stools. It is more common in formula-fed babies than breastfed babies. Other causes may include infrequent nappy changes, poor hygiene, incorrect laundering of nappies, diet, and infections such as candidiasis (thrush). It is usually very painful. Treatment includes identifying the cause, good hygiene, and exposure of the buttocks to the air. If candidiasis infection is thought to be present, the mouth should also be examined and treatment with local and oral nystatin is required. If sore buttocks persist for more than a day or two medical advice should be sought.

Any rash that presents as watery, filled pustules, or appears infected, should be seen by the paediatrician or family doctor without delay.

Nappy rash (ammoniacal dermatitis)

The skin beneath the nappy area becomes red and excoriated. This usually results from infrequent changing of the nappies (either cloth or disposable), hot weather, and the use of plastic pants. Increased contact of urine with the skin leads to production of ammonia and chemical burns. The condition is preventable by avoiding the precipitants and the use of commercial barrier creams. However, care should be taken with their application as they can cause the one-way process design of disposable nappies to become ineffective by blocking the perforations within the nappy linings. This will result in the urine not being able to soak through into the inner lining of the nappy, which may exacerbate the condition.

Treatment involves the protection of the damaged skin and exposure of the skin in a warm dry atmosphere to promote healing of the excoriated skin. Care needs to be taken to prevent secondary infection. If this occurs, refer for a medical opinion.

Breast engorgement

Breast engorgement may occur in both male and female babies on or about the third day of life. The drop in serum oestrogen levels following the separation of the mother and baby at birth stimulates the breasts to secrete milk. No treatment is required as the condition will resolve spontaneously. Mothers must be advised not to squeeze the breasts as this may result in infection.

Pseudo-menstruation

A blood-stained vaginal discharge may occur in baby girls. This is due to oestrogen withdrawal following separation of mother and baby. The mother should be reassured that it is a normal physiological process, which will resolve without treatment.

Constipation

Constipation is defined as the difficult passage of infrequent dry, i.e. hard, stools. A baby's constipated stool resembles rabbit droppings or gravel in its size and consistency. Not all hard stools are constipated. The stools of a formula-fed baby will be bulkier, firmer, and often drier than that of a breastfed baby. Babies will often appear to strain even when passing normal soft stools.

Constipation is unusual in breastfed babies although they may not pass a stool for 2–3 days once feeding is established, but this is quite normal, provided that the stool is of a normal soft consistency. Constipation most commonly occurs in formula-fed babies. If a formula-fed baby is constipated the following should be considered:
- Are the feeds being made-up correctly, i.e. is the formula is being added to the water and not vice versa?
- Is anything being added to the feed, e.g. baby rice, baby rusks?

All of these will result in a reduced fluid:solids ratio, which will result in the baby receiving inadequate fluids. If either is occurring, advise the mother appropriately. If neither of the above are occurring, advise the mother to offer the baby small amounts of extra boiled, cooled water between feeds and, if constipation still persists, to seek medical attention.

Regurgitation

Regurgitation is the effortless posseting of small amounts of milk following a feed. It usually occurs after a large feed and is usually of no importance. A newborn baby may have swallowed liquor amnii, blood, or mucus shortly before or during the process of being born. If following birth he or she vomits watery fluid or mucus, possibly streaked with blood, reassure the mother that it is usually of no significance.

Vomiting other than this may well be abnormal and should be referred to the paediatrician. Possible causes may be:
- Feeding errors
- Infection
- Intracranial injury
- Congenital malformation
- Haemorrhagic disease of the newborn
- Metabolic disorders.

The colour, quantity, frequency, and timing in relation to feeding should be observed and recorded, and whether or not it is projectile.

Neonatal temperature control

Temperature is controlled from the heat-losing centre and the heat-promoting centre of the hypothalamus, an area of the brain near to the pituitary gland. The mechanisms controlled by these centres are immature in the newborn, especially if premature.[1,2]

- The newborn temperature should be maintained between 36.5°C and 37°C.
- Hypothermia in the newborn is defined as a temperature below 35°C.[1,2]

Non-shivering thermogenesis

Newborns have a limited ability to sweat and shiver. Non-shivering thermogenesis (NST) is used by newborns to keep warm, and is initiated by:

- Oxygenation
- Separation from the placenta: cutting the cord maximizes NST
- Cutaneous cooling: cold receptors in the skin stimulate noradrenaline and thyroxine release, which stimulate brown fat.

Brown fat

- It is found around the neck and between the scapulae, across the clavicle line and the sternum.
- It also surrounds the major thoracic vessels and pads the kidneys.
- The cells contain a nucleus, glycogen, mitochondria (which release energy), and multiple fat vacuoles in the cytoplasm (a source of energy).
- The presence of the mitochondrial enzyme, thermogenin, means that, when the fat is oxidized, it releases heat rather than other forms of energy.
- It has a high concentration of stored triglycerides, a rich capillary network, and is densely innervated.
- It increases in amount during gestation.[2]

Heat loss

Heat is lost during birth, resuscitation, and transportation.
Mechanisms of heat loss are:

- *Conduction* from cold surfaces
- *Radiation* from surrounding objects
- *Convection* from the air
- *Evaporation*: insensible water loss from the skin, especially in the preterm infant.

Thermoneutrality is the environmental temperature at which minimal rates of oxygen consumption and energy expenditure occur.[2]

Effects of hypothermia (cold stress)

- Increases pulmonary vascular resistance, reducing oxygenation.
- Decreases surfactant production and efficiency, giving rise to atelectasis which worsens hypoxia.
- Poor perfusion causes an increase in anaerobic metabolism, worsening acidosis.

- Acidosis increases pulmonary artery pressure, decreasing the amount of flow of blood through the lungs, leading to hypoxia.
- Increased acidosis also leads to displacement of unconjugated bilirubin from binding sites, risking hyperbilirubinaemia.
- Increased use of glucose, due to the increase in metabolism, leads to hypoglycaemia and reduces the energy available for growth.
- Poor cardiac output and reduced blood flow to the gastrointestinal tract causes ischaemia, which can lead to necrotizing enterocolitis (NEC).
- Pulmonary haemorrhage can also occur due to left ventricular failure and damage to the pulmonary capillaries, leading to leakage of fluid and cells from the alveoli.[2]

Hyperthermia

Hyperthermia is unusual in the newborn and is normally the result of environmental factors or pyrexia due to sepsis.

Usually in sepsis there is a vast difference between core and peripheral temperatures. *Low core temperatures indicate thermal stress.* A difference between core and peripheral temperatures of >2–3°C indicates thermal stress can be due to:

- Sepsis
- Patent ductus arteriosus
- Hypervolaemia
- Catecholamine infusions.
  The factors that lead to hyperthermia are:
- Large surface area
- Limited insulation
- Limited ability to sweat.
  Sweating, seen on the forehead and temples, can occur in term babies in response to overheating. This can lead to:
- Hypotension, secondary to vasodilation
- Dehydration, following insensible water loss.[2]

Maintaining the neonatal temperature

Assessment

The different methods of assessing the baby's temperature are:

- Electronic axilla: most commonly used
- Rectal: occasionally used with caution as it can cause damage, but it can give a more accurate estimation of the core temperature in the newborn
- Skin probes: may also be used during resuscitation or incubation
- Infrared tympanic: can be used but is not very accurate in the newborn as the ears are still full of fluid from the delivery.[3]

Care at birth

- The temperature of the fetus is at least 1°C higher than that of the mother, due to heat exchange via the placenta.
- The drop in ambient temperature at delivery is more marked when the wet infant is delivered into a cool environment.
- A healthy term baby will respond by increasing heat production.

- Drying and wrapping the baby in warm towels will enable it to maintain its temperature.
- 'Kangaroo care' helps to keep the baby warm. Putting the baby in skin-to-skin contact on the mother's chest stimulates the mother to alter her temperature to the needs of the baby.[2,3]

Premature babies

- Delivery rooms can be cool and draughty, which increases convective heat loss.
- The body temperature of a 1kg infant can decrease by 1°C every 5min.
- Set the radiant warmer to maximum and have warm towels ready.
- Remember, the head is a large surface area for heat loss, so place a hat on the baby if he or she requires extensive resuscitation and transfer to the NICU.
- During resuscitation and transportation to the NICU use plastic bags to contain the infant's body. The plastic next to the skin helps to cut down the trans-epidermal fluid loss through the immature skin of premature babies.
- Once the baby is in the incubator environment, the 87% humidity will also help the baby to warm up.[2,3]

Equipment used to maintain temperature in the newborn

Radiant heaters

- Provide dry heat directly on to the skin.
- Are used mainly at delivery or during interventions.
- Increase insensible, evaporative, and convective heat loss.

The infant will increase its metabolic rate as it tries to produce neutral thermal conditions. Radiant heaters are not used for long with very premature or ill babies.

Incubators

- Provide an enclosed protected space.
- As a result of their double-glazed design, they reduce radiation heat loss, surrounding the infant with a 'curtain' of heat even when the doors are open.
- Enable the administration of humidity (87%) to help cut down evaporation (insensible) heat and fluid loss.
- Enable the administration of oxygen.
- Reduce noise, because the portholes and doors are cushioned.

Controlling temperature

Incubators control temperature in three ways:

- Servo control: if the infant's temperature decreases, the incubator will increase its heat automatically to compensate. This is not used for premature infants as the decrease in temperature needs to be observed as an early and subtle sign that the infant is becoming unwell, perhaps with an infection.
- Air temperature: this can be altered according to the changes in the infant's condition and is the method used for premature and ill babies as it allows for an observation to be recorded and recognized as a sign that the baby is unwell.
- Air temperature probe: this hangs near to the infant and maintains a consistent set temperature, leading to less fluctuation.

Radiant hood warmer

This can be used independently of the incubator's main source. It is preferred for very premature infants as it:

- Cuts down on handling.
- The hood warmer reduces oxygen consumption, which can be 8.8% higher under a standard radiant warmer.
- Provides a better thermal environment for controlling trans-epidermal water loss.[2,3]

If a baby in an incubator becomes cold

- Turn up the incubator temperature by 0.5°C.
- Put a hat on the baby.
- Check the baby's colour, heart rate, respiration rate, blood sugar, activity, feeding, and aspirate.
  If still cold after 1h:
- Turn up the incubator temperature by another 0.5°C.
- Inform the medical staff, especially if the baby remains unwell. This could be an early indication of infection and may lead to an examination and full infection screening.[2,3]

General points

- Most incubators will be double glazed to keep warm while the doors are open. Do not keep the doors open for longer than necessary.
- Check the baby's temperature before commencing cares or procedures. Let the baby warm up in between episodes of handling.
- Warm the air and oxygen.
- Overhead heaters provide dry heat only.
- Humidity may be required.[2,3]

Cot-nursed babies who become cold

- Use a hat.
- Add extra clothes and covers.
- Use an overhead radiant heater.
- Observe the baby closely for signs of infection.
- Inform the medical staff if the baby does not respond or if he or she appears unwell.[2,3]

1 Fleming PJ, Blair PS, Bacon C, *et al.* (1996). Environment of infants during sleep and risk for SIDS: Results of 1993–1995 case centred study for confidential enquiry into stillbirths and deaths in infancy. *British Medical Journal* **313**(7051), 191–5.

2 Fellows P (2001). Management of thermal stability. In: Boxwell G (ed.) *Neonatal Intensive Care Nursing*, 2nd edn. London: Routledge.

3 Bailey J (2000). Temperature measurement in the preterm infant: a literature review. *Journal of Neonatal Nursing* **6**(1), 28–32.

Hypoglycaemia

Healthy term newborns who are breastfeeding on demand *need not* be screened for hypoglycaemia and need no supplementary foods or fluids. They do not develop 'symptomatic' hypoglycaemia as a result of simple underfeeding.

Babies at high risk of hypoglycaemia can be identified as follows:

- Preterm baby <37 weeks
- Weight <2.5kg
- Apgar <5 at 1min and/or <7 at 5min
- Fetal blood sample pH <7.2
- Umbilical venous/arterial pH <7.1.

If a baby meets one or more of the above criteria the following protocol is instigated.

1. Breastfeed and give skin-to-skin contact as soon as possible after birth.

2. 2h post delivery, blood glucose analysis required.

3. Then 3h feeds and pre-feed blood glucose analysis for 12h.

4. Discontinue blood glucose analysis after 12h if pre-feed results are at/or >2.6mmol/L.

5. Continue 3h feeds and assessment of vital signs for 24h.

6. Document results and actions taken.

- If the baby fails to feed at 3h intervals assist the mother to express her milk.
- Offer expressed breast milk (EBM) obtained via cup/pipette.
- Leave baby to rest.
- After 24h if baby is well, extend feeds to 3–4h, then introduce demand feeding as tolerated.
- Assess baby's vital signs and feeding at each shift until transfer to community.
- Infants of diabetic mothers (insulin dependent or gestational diabetic) require active management.
- 30min post delivery, blood glucose analysis required, then offer baby a breastfeed irrespective of result.
- If baby fails to feed well, offer any EBM obtained with additional formula milk if required.
- The baby must receive as much milk as possible but at least 5mL/kg birthweight should be given. The total volume taken should be controlled by the baby's appetite.
- Then 3h feeds, pre-feed blood glucose analysis, and assessment of vital signs for 24h.
- Discontinue blood glucose analysis after 24h if pre-feed results are at/or >2.6mmol/L.
- Document results and actions taken.
- If pre-feed blood glucose analysis is <2.6mmol/L inform paediatrician.
- Offer baby a breastfeed. If baby fails to feed well, offer any EBM obtained with additional formula milk if required.

- The baby must receive as much milk as possible but at least 5mL/kg birthweight should be given. The total volume taken should be controlled by the baby's appetite.
- Repeat blood glucose analysis 1h post feed. If blood glucose is <2.6mmol/L, baby requires paediatric assessment.
- If blood glucose analysis is at/or >2.6mmol/L follow protocol as before.

Advice to parents: reducing the risk of sudden infant death syndrome

Cot death, or SIDS, is the sudden unexpected death of an apparently well baby aged from birth to 2 years. Over 300 babies still die of cot death a year in the UK. The UK rate was 0.55/1000 live births in 2007.[1]

Although there is no guaranteed method of preventing cot deaths the risk can be reduced by following Department of Health and Foundation for the Study of Infant Deaths (FSID) guidelines.[2] This leaflet should be given to and discussed with all new mothers prior to taking a baby home from hospital. Since parents and carers have been following the risk reduction advice, the number of babies dying has fallen by over 70%. Health professionals can explore the research behind the recommendations by downloading a fact file from the FSID website.[3]

▶ The recommendations that should be given to parents are as follows.
- Place your baby on their back to sleep, in a cot in a room with you.
- Do not smoke in pregnancy or let anyone smoke in the same room as the baby.
- Do not share a bed with your baby if you have been drinking alcohol, if you take drugs or if you are smoker.
- Never sleep with your baby on a sofa or armchair.
- Do not let your baby get too hot. Keep your baby's head uncovered. Their blanket should be tucked no higher than their shoulders.
- Place your baby in the feet to foot position (with their feet at the end of the cot or pram).

Other factors that can help reduce the risk[4] are:
- Breastfeeding.
- Keeping the baby in the same room as the parents for the first 6 months.
- Using sheets and lightweight blankets. Do not use duvets, quilts, pillows or similar thick bedding.
- Keeping the bedroom at a comfortable but not hot temperature (18°C).
- The baby should never sleep with a hot water bottle or next to a radiator, heater, or fire, or in direct sunlight.
- Using a dummy but if breastfeeding do not give the baby a dummy until they are 1 month old.

1 Foundation for the Study of Infant Deaths (2009). *Cot Death Facts and Figures.* London: FSID. Available at: ℘ http://fsid.org.uk/Document.Doc?id=42 (accessed 3 April 2010).

2 Department of Health (2009). *Reduce the risk of Cot Death.* London: DH and FSID.

3 Foundation for the Study of Infant Deaths (2009). *Factfile* [2]: *Research Background to the Reduce the Risk of Cot Death Advice from the Foundation for the Study of Infant Deaths.* London: FSID. Available at: ℘ http://fsid.org.uk/factfile_2 (accessed 3 Aril 2010).

4 National Health Service (2009). *Cot Death: How to Reduce the Risk.* London: NHS. Available at: ℘ www.nhs.uk/livewell/childhealth0-1/pages/cotdeath.aspx (accessed 3.4.10).

Bed sharing

Bed-sharing is a controversial issue and has been linked to cot deaths. Many mothers will take their babies into bed to feed and provide comfort without intending to fall sleep. Bed sharing has been shown to promote breastfeeding, therefore it is important that midwives give the mothers the correct information to enable mothers continue breastfeeding, while at the same time reducing the risk of cot death.[1]

Recommendations while in hospital

▶ Mothers should be constantly supervised if bed sharing and co-sleeping if they are:
- Under the effects of a general anaesthetic
- Immobile due to a spinal anaesthetic
- Taking drugs that may cause drowsiness
- Seriously ill, e.g. high temperature, large blood loss, severe hypertension
- Excessively tired
- Have a condition that affects mobility, sensory, or spatial awareness, e.g. multiple sclerosis, blindness
- Very obese
- Likely to have temporary loss of consciousness, e.g. if she is diabetic or epileptic.
  Bed sharing and co-sleeping is contraindicated if:
- A mother is a smoker
- The baby is preterm or ill.

Advise to mothers at home

Mothers should always be given the UNICEF leaflet 'Sharing a bed with your baby' prior to transfer home.[2] It is recommended that babies share their mother's room for at least the first 6 months, as this assists breast-feeding and protects against cot death.

When mothers should not sleep with their babies

If they or their partners:
- Are smokers
- Have drunk alcohol
- Have taken any drug (legal or illegal) which makes them drowsy
- Have a condition that affects their awareness of their baby
- Are overtired to the point that they could not readily respond to their baby.

Reducing the risk of accidents and overheating

- Parents should *never* sleep with their baby on a sofa or armchair.
- The bed must be firm and flat.
- Ensure the baby can not fall out of bed or get stuck between the mattress and wall.
- Make sure the room is not too hot (16–18°C is ideal).
- The baby should not be overdressed.
- Bedclothes must not overheat the baby or cover the baby's head.
- Never leave the baby alone in or on the bed.
- The partner should be informed if the baby is in bed.

- If an older child is also bed sharing, there should be an adult (you or your partner) between the child and the baby.
- Never share your bed with pets and your baby.

Mothers who are bottle feeding should be advised to put their babies back into their cot after feeding, as mothers who bottle feed can sometimes turn their backs on their babies when they have fallen asleep.

1 UNICEF UK Baby Friendly Initiative (2004). *Babies Sharing their Mothers Bed while in Hospital: A Sample Policy*. London: UNICEF UK Baby Friendly Initiative. Available at: ✍ www.babyfriendly.org. uk (accessed 5.1.11).

2 UNICEF/Foundation for the Study of Infant Deaths (2008). *Sharing a Bed with Your Baby: A Guide for Breastfeeding Mothers*. London: UNICEF UK Baby Friendly Initiative. Available at: ✍ www.babyfriendly.org.uk/pdfs/sharingbedleaflet.pdf

Neonatal infection

The incidence of infection in the newborn has declined over the past 10 years due to the increased use of antenatal antibiotics and more effective management of premature rupture of the membranes.[1]

Definitions

- Very early onset: <24h.
- Early onset: 1–7 days.
- Late onset: >7 days.
- Nosocomial infection: hospital acquired.
- Bacteraemia: the presence of viable bacteria in the blood.
- Septicaemia: systemic disease caused by the multiplication of organisms in the blood.
- Sepsis: the presence of pus-forming and other pathogenic organisms in the blood.[1]

Infections acquired in the antenatal period

Amniotic fluid has bactericidal properties and the membranes provide a physical barrier. If these defences are breached, the fetus will be infected by direct aspiration into the lungs, causing pneumonia and bacteraemia.

- GBS is the most common cause of early-onset septicaemia and meningitis.
- Mycoplasmas found in the maternal genital tract can cause premature labour.
- GBS and mycoplasmas have also been found where the membranes remain intact.

Other organisms that ascend the genital tract and contaminate the amniotic fluid are:

- *Bacteroides* spp.
- *Escherichia coli*
- *Clostridium* spp.
- *Peptococcus* spp.

Infections acquired via the placenta

- *Listeria monocytogenes* causes placentitis.
- Viruses, such as cytomegalovirus, herpes, and that causing rubella, and the parasitic protozoan *Toxoplasma* sp., also affect placental function, resulting in growth retardation and congenital abnormalities.
- Intrauterine infection with parvovirus B19 is associated with fetal anaemia.
- Vertical transmission of HIV from the mother to the fetus through the placenta is thought to be related to the maternal viral burden, disease stage, and immune response.

Intrapartum infection

Factors that increase the likelihood of intrapartum infection are:

- Premature labour
- Maternal pyrexia
- Prolonged rupture of the membranes.

Causative organisms include:
- GBS: the most common.
- Herpes simplex: acquired through contact with genital secretions.
- Hepatitis B: acquired through contact with vaginal secretions.
- HIV: attributed to contact with infected secretions.

Sexually transmitted diseases are on the increase in the UK and are transmitted during vaginal delivery. These include:
- Chlamydiosis
- Syphilis
- Gonorrhoea—in the newborn this can cause conjunctivitis, which can develop into pneumonia.[1,2]

▶▶ All healthcare workers are strongly advised to use universal precautions routinely when in contact with maternal and fetal blood and other body fluids.[3]

Late-onset and nosocomial infections

Occur due to:
- Maternal contact
- Contact with hospital personnel (cross infection)
- Contact with inanimate objects.

The most common causative organisms are:
- *Klebsiella* spp.
- *Escherichia* coli
- Coagulase-negative staphylococcus
- *Staphylococcus aureus*
- *Pseudomonas aeruginosa.*[3]

Risk factors for nosocomial infection are:
- Low birthweight with a depressed immunological function
- Underlying disease
- Raised gastric pH and poor nutritional status requiring total parenteral nutrition
- The excessive use of antibiotics
- Multiple IV site access, the presence of an endotracheal tube and central lines
- Long hospital stay
- Poor compliance of staff with infection control, and poor hand washing
- Shared equipment, overcrowding, and inadequate staffing
- The presence of opportunistic organisms.[1,2]

Defences

The physical defences
- The skin
- Mucous membranes
- Gastric secretions
- Tears
- Urine pH
- Ciliated epithelium.

Are all affected by immaturity, poor skin keratinization, and invasive procedures.

The non-specific defences
- Phagocytes (neutrophils and monocytes)
- Natural killer cells
- Inflammatory responses
- Antimicrobial proteins
- Complement activation
- Serum opsonins
- Polymorphonuclear neutrophils.

All of these are immature as there is little or no transmission via the placenta. Their ability to release complement is reduced until 6–18 months. This deficiency in phagocytosis and opsonization is pertinent in the case of GBS and is further compounded by prematurity.

T and B cells
- Generated from bone marrow.
- T cells are responsible for cell-mediated immunity.
- B cells confer humoral immunity from which antibodies are produced.

Humoral immunoglobulins
There is some evidence of transfer, which gives the newborn some protection:
- *Maternal IgG* is transferred from 22 weeks and increases by 30 weeks, giving the fetus passive immunity.
- *IgM* does not cross the placenta, so immunity to acute maternal infection at the time of delivery is not provided.
- *IgA* is secretory, present in saliva, sweat, tears, intestinal secretions, and colostrum.
- *IgD* is present on the surface of lymphocytes to control activation and suppression of B cells.
- *IgE* is present in low quantities in the serum but in higher quantities in the respiratory and gastrointestinal tracts.[1,2]

Signs of neonatal infection (Table 23.1)
▶ Early detection is crucial or the infection will overwhelm the baby leading to:
- Septicaemia
- Meningitis
- Death.

Indicators may be apparent in the maternal history, such as:
- Maternal pyrexia
- Prolonged rupture of membranes.
- Length of gestation of the fetus.

The midwife or nurse caring for the baby will often 'feel' that the baby is 'not as well as it was'. Neonatologists in practice will act on this observation, especially if it comes from an experienced neonatal nurse, and it often leads to examination and an infection screening.[1,2]

Table 23.1 Signs of neonatal infection

Common signs	Uncommon signs
Pallor	Purpura
Poor feeding	Omphalitis
Tachycardia/arrhythmia	Vasomotor instability
Decreased peripheral perfusion	Bleeding
Unstable blood pressure	Pustules
Abdominal distension	Bulging fontanelle
Apnoea	Splenomegaly
Lethargy	Rash
Hyperbilirubinaemia	Diarrhoea
Recession/grunting/cyanosis	Seizures
Tachypnoea	
Unstable temperature	

Investigations

- *Surface swabs* taken from multiple sites are useful when late infection is suspected or on admission to the NICU. The optimal site is a deep ear swab or a swab of obvious lesions in later-onset infection.
- *Blood cultures* are mandatory before starting antibiotics.
- *Total neutrophil count* is more reliable than a total white cell count. The immature to total ratio is a good indicator of infection.
- *CRP*: a level of >6 mg/L is a sign of infection. This is used to measure the course of infection and response to treatment. Levels should return to normal 96h after starting treatment.
- *Platelet count*: due to increased destruction, aggregation and adhesion occur, but this is usually a late finding in about 50% of cases.
- *CSF*: lumbar punctures are carried out to rule out bacterial meningitis.
  - The sample should be clear.
  - *CSF white cell level* <30mm,[3] with more than 66% neutrophils.
  - *CSF protein level* of >1g/L in a term baby or 2g/L in a premature baby are suspicious of meningitis.
  - *CSF glucose level* should be approximately 70–80% of the plasma glucose level.
- *Urine*: usually collected as a bag sample or suprapubic tap. The long-term effects of urinary infection can be renal scaring and atrophy.[1,2]

Management of the infected infant

- *Supportive therapy and broad-spectrum antibiotics:* begin as soon as the infection screening is complete.

- *Ventilation* may be needed and is mandatory in cases of GBS, due to associated pulmonary vasoconstriction and the development of pulmonary hypotension.
- *Cardiovascular support.* The infant will be shocked. Management of the blood pressure and perfusion are necessary. A decrease in circulating blood volume can cause prenal failure.
- *Peripheral perfusion and capillary refill time* must be kept within normal limits.
- *Volume replacement* with plasma or blood helps to provide immunoglobulins and clotting factors.
- *Dopamine and dobutamine and plasma*: are used to treat hypotension.
- *Acid–base balance*: maintained with ventilation, fluid replacement, and inotropes.
- *Sodium bicarbonate*: use with caution to help correct acidosis where all other treatments have failed. It can improve acidaemia, myocardial contractility, surfactant production, and lower pulmonary vascular resistance.
- *Fluid and electrolyte balance*: record carefully. This can be complicated by the inappropriate secretion of antidiuretic hormone due to severe hypoxia or meningitis.
- *Hyponatraemia* can result from inappropriate antidiuretic hormone secretion.
- *Sodium and potassium losses* increase when the baby has NEC or the diuretic phase of acute tubular necrosis following low renal perfusion rates.
- *Hypoglycaemia* can occur due to increased metabolic demands.
- *Haematological management*: keep a record of all blood taken and treatment with top-up transfusions, especially in small premature babies.
- *Bruising, oozing, and petechiae* due to consumptive coagulopathy: treat with platelet transfusions, plasma, and vitamin K.
- *Exchange transfusion*: in extreme cases this can wash out coagulation inhibitors and supply missing coagulation factors, opsonins, and increase the oxygen carrying capacity of the blood.[1,2]

Antibiotic therapies and sensitivities (Table 23.2)

Table 23.2 Antibiotics therapies and sensitivies

Penicillins	Aminoglycosides	Cephalosporins	Vancomycin
Streptococci	Gram-negative organisms	Gram-negative bacilli	Staphylococci
Pneumococci	Have a synergistic effect when used with penicillin to treat GBS	Meningococci	Enterococci
Meningococci		Gonococci	Gram-positive bacteria
Gonococci		*Haemophilus influenzae*	Used to treat meticillin-resistant *Staphylococcus aureus* (MRSA)
Treponema pallidum		*Pseudomonas* spp.	

- *Gentamicin levels*: check after five half-lives at steady state, or after three to five doses have been given, to avoid the occurrence of troughs in blood levels.
- *Metronidazole* is used to treat Gram-negative anaerobic bacilli such as *Bacteroides*, and is useful for the treatment of NEC.
- Despite the increase in MRSA, some penicillins are useful to treat *Staphylococcus aureus* and *Staphylococcus epidermidis*.
- *Vancomycin* is active against staphylococci, enterococci and other Gram-positive bacteria; it is also used for treating MRSA.
- Meticillin has been replaced by *nafcillin*.
- *Ticarcillin* is a semi-synthetic penicillin used for treating *Pseudomonas* spp.[2]

1 Boxwell G (2001). Neonatal infection. In: Boxwell G (ed.) *Neonatal Intensive Care Nursing*, 2nd edn. London: Routledge, pp. 260–80.

2 Stein CM, Dear P (1999). Infection in the newborn. In: Rennie JM, Roberton NRC (eds) *Textbook of Neonatology*, 3rd edn. London: Churchill Livingstone, p. 1093.

3 Department of Health (1990). *Guidance for Clinical Health-Care Workers: Protection Against Infection with HIV and Hepatitis Viruses: Recommendations of Expert Advisory Group on AIDS*. London: HMSO.

Neonatal jaundice

Jaundice is one of the most common problems in the newborn period as all infants undergo changes in bilirubin metabolism at birth.[1]

- *Physiological jaundice* is a normal process seen in about 40–50% of term and up to 80% of premature infants within the first week of life. It is a transitional change, leading to an excessive build-up of bilirubin in the blood, which gives the baby a jaundiced (yellow) colour.[1]
- *Pathological jaundice* refers to jaundice that arises from pathological factors that alter the usual processes involved in bilirubin metabolism, such as blood-group incompatibility, excessive bruising, and sepsis.[1]

Newborn physiological jaundice

- Newborns have high haemoglobin levels 18–20g/dL.[1]
- The short life of the baby's red blood cells produces a high rate of haemoglobin breakdown (haemolysis) compared to adults.
- Each gram of haemoglobin produces 34–35mg of indirect (unconjugated) bilirubin.
- β-glucuronidase from fetal life may still be active in the gut.
- This changes conjugated bilirubin into unconjugated bilirubin.
- *In utero*, this would have been excreted via the placenta and the maternal circulation. This is known as the enterohepatic circulation.
- After birth this unconjugated bilirubin can be reabsorbed into the enterohepatic circulation, causing a further build up in the baby's blood.

Indirect unconjugated bilirubin:

- Has not been unconjugated by the liver
- Is fat soluble and cannot be excreted in the bile or urine
- It builds up in the blood and can be deposited in the fatty tissue of the skin, leading to jaundice
- If levels rise very high, it is deposited in the fatty tissue in the brain, which can lead to kernicterus and brain damage
- The body metabolizes unconjugated (indirect) bilirubin in the liver, changing it into conjugated (direct) bilirubin.

Direct conjugated bilirubin:

- Is water-soluble
- Can be excreted by the biliary system into the intestines and stools
- A small amount can be reabsorbed in the colon and excreted in the urine.
  Newborns are also deficient in:
- Albumin for binding, which will carry the unconjugated bilirubin to the liver
- Ligandins (Y and Z carrier proteins) these are needed to transport the unconjugated bilirubin across the space of Diss, which surrounds the hepatocytes in the liver. The bilirubin is then able to cross the hepatocyte cell membrane.
- Glucuronyl transferase, an enzyme in the hepatocyte, which helps to conjugate the bilirubin.
- Glucose substrate is needed to provide energy for the enzyme reactions to take place.[1–3]

Patterns of jaundice

Jaundice developing within the first 24h may be due to:
- Rhesus disease
- ABO incompatibility
- Congenital infection
- Glucose 6-phosphate dehydrogenase (G6PD) deficiency.
  Those jaundiced at 48h may have:
- Physiological jaundice
- Acquired infection
- Undetected haemolytic disease.
  Jaundice lasting beyond 10 days may indicate:
- Breastfeeding jaundice
- Chronic or late infection
- Hepatitis
- Obstruction, e.g. biliary atresia
- Inborn errors of metabolism, e.g. PKU, cystic fibrosis
- Hypothyroidism.

ABO incompatibility

The incidence is 1:5 births. A mother who is group O and whose baby is group A or B has naturally occurring anti-A or anti-B lysins (antibodies), which destroy the fetal RBCs, leading to newborn jaundice.

G6PD deficiency

This is an X-linked recessive condition. G6PD maintains the integrity of the RBC membrane, so a lack of this enzyme leads to excessive haemolysis. This condition can be triggered by infection or sulphonomides.[3]

Breastfeeding jaundice

- Breast-feeding jaundice is early in onset, seen by 2–4 days.
- The majority of infants with raised serum bilirubin where no other cause can be found are usually breastfed.
- There is an increase in enterohepatic shunting. This process normally exists in the fetus where β-glucuronidase in the gut unconjugates the conjugated bilirubin in order to return unconjugated bilirubin via the placenta to the maternal circulation for excretion by the mother. The fetus is not able to excrete it through its bowel until after birth. Breastfed babies excrete less bilirubin in their stools, keeping conjugated bilirubin in the intestines for longer, thus increasing the chance that the β-glucuronidase will unconjugate it before if is excreted.
- Decreased fluid intake leads to altered liver conjugation and clearance.
- Inadequate calorific intake causes an increase in fat metabolism, to meet energy needs, which interferes with bilirubin uptake by the liver.
- Human milk also contains β-glucuronidase, which increases enterohepatic shunting and indirect bilirubin levels in the blood.
- Supplementation of breastfeeding infants with water is counterproductive as it decreases milk intake, and therefore lowers production due to a lack of stimulation of the breast.[3]

Assessment of infants with jaundice

All infants are at risk of jaundice. Factors that increase this risk must be identified.

Factors that increase the risk
- Feto-maternal blood-group incompatibility (haemolysis).
- Birth trauma (RBC destruction and increased bilirubin production)
- Delayed cord clamping increases the RBCs in the baby's circulation.
- Congenital abnormalities of the gastrointestinal tract.
- Delayed passage of meconium /delayed feeding (increases enterohepatic shunting).
- Sepsis (leads to RBC destruction and altered hepatic clearance).

Other risk factors
- Low birthweight
- Prematurity
- PROM
- Increased weight loss, delayed feeding, and dehydration
- Swallowed/sequestered blood from trauma, cephalic haematoma, and surgery.[1,3]

Problems that interfere with bilirubin metabolism
- Hypoxia
- Asphyxia
- Hypoglycaemia
- Hypothermia.

Preventative strategies
- Give Rh D immunoglobulin to Rh D-negative mothers within 72h of delivery of each baby.
- Avoid trauma in labour.
- Prevention of hypothermia.
- Prevent hypoxia and hypoglycaemia.
- Early feeding/increased frequency of breastfeeding.[1,3]

Examination

Assess:
- Skin and sclera
- Activity.
  Note:
- Birth trauma
- Length of gestation.

NICE[4] now recommends that all babies who are more likely to develop jaundice in the first 72h should be assessed at every opportunity, in order to identify those needing intervention.
- Measure and record bilirubin level within 2h of all babies with suspected jaundice especially in the first 24h of life.[4]
- Continue to measure the bilirubin level every 6h for all babies with suspected or obvious jaundice.[4]

- Use a transcutaneous bilirubinometer (TBM), which is a small hand-held device placed against the baby's chest as this is more accurate than visual inspection alone. If a TBM is not available or it indicates a level >250mmol/L check the result by measuring the serum bilirubin.[4]
- Serum bilirubin is used to determine bilirubin levels in the first 24h and for babies <35 weeks' gestation. It is also a guide to treatment.[4]

Investigations

Laboratory estimation of serum bilirubin levels is required for all ill term and premature infants. The levels are reported as total bilirubin and the direct (conjugated) component.
- Haemoglobin/haematocrit
- Reticulocyte count
- Maternal and infant blood groups.

Investigate cases of prolonged jaundice for liver function and thyroid problems. To detect spherocytes and a diagnosis of congenital spherocytosis, carry out an RBC smear.

Total bilirubin
- This is an accurate reflection if the indirect (unconjugated) bilirubin because the direct (conjugated) component is usually very low.
- Exceptions can occur where there is significant Rh incompatibility or infants with elevated bilirubin levels after 2 weeks. The bilirubin in these cases will be mainly direct (conjugated).

Blood-group testing
Direct Coombs' test
This is a measure of antibody-coated blood cells. It is a direct measure of the amount of maternal antibody coating the infant's RBCs.
- If antibody is present it will be a *positive direct result*.
- Infants with Rh incompatibility will have a positive direct response.
- Infants with ABO incompatibility will have a negative or weakly positive result.

Indirect Coombs' test
This measures the effects of a sample of the infant's serum, thought to contain antibodies, on the RBCs of an unrelated adult. If antibody is present, the components will interact and coat these adult RBCs, giving a *positive indirect result*.

Kleihauer's test
This detects the presence of fetal blood cells in the maternal circulation. This normally occurs during separation of the placenta from the uterus following delivery of the baby. The presence of fetal cells in the maternal circulation indicates a risk of antibodies being formed if the mother is Rh negative and the fetal blood cells are rhesus positive.[1,3]

Management
- Phototherapy.
- Exchange transfusion will be used in cases where the rise in bilirubin levels cannot be controlled by the use of phototherapy.

Phototherapy

The light used in phototherapy reduces bilirubin levels by:

- *Photoisomerization*, which converts indirect bilirubin to water-soluble photoisomers. The light energy rearranges the molecules in the chemical group to produce photobilirubin and rearranges the atoms to produce lumirubin. These can be excreted in the bile without conjugation. This isomerization is thought to be the most important in terms of bilirubin elimination.
- *Photosensitized oxidation* is a minor pathway, by which the bilirubin molecule absorbs light energy which is then transferred to oxygen, forming a reactive oxygen molecule. Bilirubin is then oxidized, forming a water-soluble product which is excreted in the urine with no need for conjugation.[2,5,6]

Strength of light

A blue light, of wavelength in the of range 425–475 nanometers is used. White light can be used, but it is less effective. Recommended irradiance is between 5 and 10mcW/cm^2.[2]

Light sources

- *Overhead strip lights* incorporated into a unit which is designed to fit closely over the incubator hood to give maximum efficiency, maintaining the effectiveness of the treatment.
- *Fibreoptic paddles* used underneath the baby, often used in conjunction with overhead lights.
- *Fibreoptic blankets* ('Biliblankets®') can be used if the baby is well enough to be held. The light source, a tungsten halogen lamp, is linked to a woven fibreoptic pad via a fibreoptic cable.
- *Bilibed*, a bed with lights incorporated into the base. The baby lies on the bed and is covered with a sleeping bag attached to the base.[7]

Recording the levels

- The bilirubin levels are plotted on a chart to indicate when treatment is needed.
- The charts differ for gestational age and for the degree of illness.
- The more premature, ill baby will be treated at lower levels than a term, well infant, who may not need any treatment.
- Incorporated into the charts are also levels at which an exchange transfusion may be required if phototherapy is not enough to control the rising levels of bilirubin.[6]

In practice

- Commence phototherapy as soon as bilirubin levels start to rise, using the charts as a guide.
- Give the parents a full explanation of the cause and treatment.
- Turn the incubator temperature down to accommodate extra heat from the lights and record the infant's temperature frequently.
- The baby should be naked, but cover the gonads.
- Turn the baby regularly to get maximum exposure.
- Protect the baby's eyes with goggles.
- Change nappies frequently, because of diarrhoea.

- Calculate extra fluid into the daily requirements of premature babies, to allow for insensible water losses.
- Do not use creams on the skin, because of burning.
- Observe for skin rashes and irritation.
- Treatment is continuous until levels start to fall, usually by 3–4 days from starting treatment.
- Physiological jaundice should have resolved by 10 days. If the jaundice persists beyond this time, investigate other causes.[7]

Advantages
- Cheap.
- Effective.
- Non-invasive.

Disadvantages
- Makes observation difficult.
- Can upset the baby's water and electrolyte balance.[5,6]

1 Blackburn S (1995). Hyperbilirubinaemia and neonatal jaundice. *Neonatal Network* **14**, 7.

2 Edwards S (1995). Phototherapy and the neonate; providing a safe and effective nursing care for jaundiced infants. *Journal of Neonatal Nursing* **1**(5), 9–12.

3 Rennie JM, Roberton NRC (eds) (1999). *Textbook of Neonatology*, 3rd edn. London: Churchill Livingstone, pp. 715–30.

4 National Institute for Health and Clinical Excellence (2010). *Neonatal Jaundice*. Clinical guideline 98. London: NICE. Available at: ℞ www.nice.org.uk/cg98 (accessed 29 June 2010).

5 Hey E (1995). Neonatal jaundice; how much do we really know? *MIDIRS Midwifery Digest* **5**, 1.

6 Hey E (1995). Phototherapy: Fresh light on a murky subject. *MIDIRS Midwifery Digest* **5**, 3.

7 Day C (1995). Phototherapy for neonates: A step by step guide. *Journal of Neonatal Nursing* **3**, 4.

Vomiting in the newborn

- Vomiting small amounts of milk after feeding is a common event in healthy babies during the first 2 weeks of life. It is physiological and universal.
- The normal baby swallows a variable amount of air during a feed which can be expelled easily by sitting the baby upright and gently rubbing his or her back.
- A teaspoon or two of milk is often regurgitated within the first 10min after feeding. This is known as poseting and is considered to be a normal response.[1,2]
- Vomiting has many possible causes, most of which are simple and benign. Should the vomiting become persistent then more serious causes will be considered.[1]

Causes

The causes of vomiting can be non-organic or organic.

- Non-organic:
  - Overfeeding
  - Incorrect preparation of feeds
  - Overstimulation and excessive handling
  - Crying
  - Air swallowing.
- Organic:
  - Infection
  - Gastroenteritis
  - Meningitis
  - Otitis media
  - Gastro-oesophageal reflux
  - Gastritis from swallowed meconium or blood
  - Bowel obstruction
  - Pyloric stenosis
  - Hiatus hernia
  - Feeding intolerance/allergy
  - Metabolic disorders.

Bile-stained vomiting may indicate malrotation of the bowel.[2,3] Bile stained or projectile vomiting may indicate intussusception of the bowel.

The cause can be determined by a taking a history of:

- Feeding technique
- Description of the vomiting
- Preparation of the feed
- Other symptoms.

Investigations

If the history and physical examination of the baby prove inconclusive, the following investigations are carried out:

- U/E
- Abdominal X-ray for bowel obstruction
- Oesophageal pH monitoring

- Barium swallow and follow through for:
  - Oesophageal anomalies
  - Hiatus hernia
  - Gut malrotation
- Abdominal ultrasound examination for:
  - Malrotation
  - Gastric outlet obstruction
- Infection screen, including:
  - Blood cultures
  - Urine microscopy
  - CSF culture
- Arterial blood gases for:
  - Alkalosis with pyloric stenosis
  - Persistent acidosis with inborn errors of metabolism serum electrolytes
  - Hypokalaemia in paralytic ileus
  - Hypochloraemic alkalosis in pyloric stenosis[2]
- Metabolic screen for:
  - Urine amino and organic acids
  - Plasma amino acids
  - Lactate.[2,3]

Management

Management involves identifying and treating the cause and maintaining the baby's fluid balance.

▶ Throughout the period of investigation and management the midwife must remember the need for accurate and detailed documentation, and the need for advice, support, and clear explanations to the parents.

The above list of investigations is not necessary for every vomiting baby. Vomiting can often be transient and attention to the frequency and volume of feeds is enough to improve the situation.[2,3]

Abdominal distension

Feeding should be stopped where there is vomiting accompanied by mild to moderate abdominal distension. Carry out an abdominal X-ray. If this is satisfactory but the baby continues to vomit when feeds are reintroduced, stop feeding for 3 days to rest the gut and provide fluids and electrolytes via an IV line, then gradually reintroduce enteral feeding again.

Feeding intolerance

This is not common in the newborn but should be considered where simple remedies have failed to improve the baby's condition, or if there is a family history of feeding intolerance. It may then be necessary to introduce the baby to a soya-based formula.

Irritation due to swallowed fluids

During birth amniotic fluid, meconium, and mucus can be swallowed, which can irritate the stomach, causing gastritis and the rejection of early feeds. A small stomach wash-out via a nasogastric tube can usually cure the problem.[1]

Vomited blood

Vomited blood in the first few days is usually swallowed maternal blood. This can be distinguished easily from the baby's own blood as it will not contain any fetal haemoglobin.

Vomited bile

▶ Vomited bile is more serious and can indicate intestinal obstruction, which can occur at different levels in the gut. Abdominal X-rays will confirm or exclude this as the problem. Bile-stained vomiting may also occur with a cerebral disorder such as intracranial bleeding or meningitis.[1]

Gastro-oesophageal reflux

This is characterized by repeated small vomits occurring shortly after feeds. It is caused by an incompetent lower gastro-oesophageal sphincter and is common in:

- Premature babies
- Babies who have neurological abnormalities causing hypo- or hypertonia
- Following surgery for repair of diaphragmatic hernia or oesophageal atresia.

The baby may fail to thrive due to loss of calories in the vomit and there is a risk of aspiration into the lungs. The problem can be treated in several ways:

- Thickening feeds with:
  - Nestargel®
  - Carobel®
  - Thixo-D®
- Nursing the baby in a prone position with the cot tilted up 30–40°
- Drugs, such as:
  - Gaviscon® 1–2g with each feed, but this can cause constipation
  - Cisapride (discontinued), a prokinetic drug, to improve gastric emptying, but this can cause arrhythmias
  - Antacids, such as cimetidine, can help to relieve gastritis.

Where medical treatment fails, fundoplication will be tried.

The natural history is for a gradual improvement as the baby grows and the condition is usually better by the end of the first year of life.[1,3]

Projectile vomiting

Projectile vomiting usually indicates pyloric stenosis. This is more common after the first month of life and rarely occurs in the first week. There is usually a family history and it is more common in boys.

Diagnosis can be made by observing visible peristalsis and a palpable 'tumour' in the area of the pyloric sphincter (the muscle that regulates the flow of milk from the oesophagus into the stomach).

Because this muscle is too tight, the milk stays in the oesophagus for longer. The amount of milk in the oesophagus increases as the baby feeds and it is forcibly ejected. Treatment usually involves surgery to split the muscle (Ramstedt's operation).[3]

1 Johnston PGB (1998). *The Newborn Child*, 8th edn. London: Churchill Livingstone, pp. 88–9.

2 Mupanemunda RH, Watkinson M (2000). *Key Topics in Neonatology*, 2nd edn. Oxford: Bios Scientific, pp. 275–7.

3 Levene MI, Tudehope DI, Thearle MJ (2000). *Essentials of Neonatal Medicine*, 3rd edn. London: Blackwell, pp. 93–115.

Metabolic disorders and the neonatal blood spot test

Although these conditions can present in the neonatal period, diagnosis is difficult or delayed because the clinical signs may not be specific to an individual disorder or to an inborn error of metabolism. Routine screening is designed to detect the affected infants before symptoms develop, allowing treatment to be initiated as soon as possible.[1]

Genetic inheritance

These conditions are usually inherited as autosomal recessive conditions, which have the following pattern:[1]
- Both parents are normal and do not have the condition
- Both parents are carriers of a faulty gene
- Both carrier genes from both parents must be inherited to produce a child with the condition
- This gives a 1:4 risk of having an affected child with the condition with each pregnancy
- 2:4 will be normal, but carriers of the faulty gene
- 1:4 will be normal, non-carrier.

Clinical presentation
- There may be a family history of neonatal death or siblings with a known inborn error of metabolism.
- A period of 'well-being' followed by illness and collapse.
- Infection may be suspected and a full infection screening done, but the baby will not respond to treatment.
- Parental consanguinity.[1]

General signs and symptoms
- Unexplained metabolic acidosis
- Reducing substances in the urine
- Feeding difficulties/vomiting/diarrhoea
- Hepatomegaly
- Convulsions/cerebral oedema
- Ketosis/hypoglycaemia/hyperglycaemia
- Respiratory distress
- Bradycardia/apnoea
- Hypothermia
- Abnormal tone (hypertonia or opisthotonus)
- Axial hypotonia
- Smelly urine
  Don't forget that antibiotics also make the urine smell of yeast.[1]

Initial investigations
- *Non-specific* blood and urine tests, with the test results available within a few hours, can place the error within a diagnostic category, allowing appropriate emergency treatment to be instigated. These are available in all units providing neonatal care:
  - FBC
  - U/E

- Blood gas
- Blood ammonia
- Urine-reducing substances
- Urine ketones.
- A *presumptive diagnosis* from the urine and blood can be available within a few days. Second-line investigations available in each region:
  - Urine amino acids
  - Urine organic acids
  - Plasma amino acids
  - Blood and CSF lactate
  - Beutler test for galactosaemia
  - Plasma carnitine.
- A *definitive diagnosis* requires specific enzyme or genetic analysis and can take weeks or months. Specialized investigations available at a supra-regional level are:
  - Specific enzyme assays on blood or skin fibroblasts, e.g. lysosomal enzyme studies
  - DNA mutation analysis
  - Special metabolite studies, e.g. long-chain fatty acids, bile acid analysis.[1]

Screening

Routine neonatal screening is offered for five disorders:
- PKU
- Congenital hypothyroidism
- Cystic fibrosis
- Medium-chain acyl CoA dehydrogenase (MCAD) deficiency
- Sickle-cell disorders and thalassaemia major.[1]

Collecting the sample

Parents will receive an information leaflet, and have the reasons for the test explained to them, in the third trimester of the pregnancy. The reasons should also be discussed with them again just before the procedure is carried out.

The health professional responsible for the baby will usually take the sample on day 6 of milk feeding, and will also record the event in the maternity notes.

Gather equipment
- Parent information leaflet
- Blood spot card and envelope
- Gloves
- Automated lancet device
- Cotton wool
- Spot plaster
- Maternity record.[2]

The procedure
- With the consent of the parents, offer the baby a pacifier with sucrose on it, to lessen pain responses.
- Wash the heel with sterile water and an alcohol swab, then leave to dry for 30s.

- Lance the heel on the planter surface beyond the lateral and medial limits of the calcaneus. Avoid the posterior curvature of the heel.
- Allow the blood to fill the circle by natural flow.
- Apply the drop to one side of the card.
- Fill all the circles completely. Avoid layering the blood and ensure that the blood permeates through to the back of the card.
- Wipe the foot and apply gentle pressure and the plaster if required.
- Comfort the baby.
- Complete the records and inform the parents how and when they will receive the results.
- Send the card within 12h of the sample being taken.[2]

Phenylketonuria

- The incidence in Britain is 1:10 000 births.
- ❶ If it is not treated it leads to permanent brain damage.
- It is treated with a diet restricting phenylalanine.
- The baby is born with a normal blood phenylalanine level.
- There is a block in the normal metabolic pathway, preventing conversion of unused phenylalanine into tyrosine.
- The baby quickly shows a marked rise in blood phenylalanine when given feeds containing protein.

Screening

▶ It takes a few days for levels of blood phenylalanine to accumulate, therefore the screening test is usually done after 6 days of milk feeding or at least 48h of intravenous feed containing protein.

Guthrie's test

Introduced by Dr Robert Guthrie, this test was originally based on inhibition of bacterial growth. It is now carried out using a fluorometric assay to test for PKU. A 6.25mm diameter disc is punched out of a dried blood spot on a blood-screening card. Water is added and the sample is then left to dry. Reagents are added to cause the phenylalanine to fluoresce and the fluorescence is measured. Any rise in serum phenylalanine above a given standard stands out on the chart. This will be followed up with further tests on the original sample before confirmation of the diagnosis with the parents.[3,4]

Congenital hypothyroidism

- The incidence in Britain is 1:3500 births.
- It is due to an absent or small thyroid gland and reduced/absent thyroxine production.
- TSH levels will be increased.
- ❶ If it is not treated, the individual will have a decreased IQ.
- Treatment is a regular daily dose of thyroxine to replace the missing hormone.[4,5]
- The baby may
  - Have prolonged jaundice, beyond 10 days
  - Be lethargic
  - Be feeding poorly
  - Be constipated

- Have an odd appearance with a large tongue
- Have a hoarse cry.

Screening

The test involves punching a small hole out of the blood-screening card. A radioactive marker is added to the blood spot, the sample is left overnight and the TSH is measured the next day.

Cystic fibrosis

- Affects about 1 baby in 2500.
- It affects the digestion and causes chronic lung disease.
- There is no cure for cystic fibrosis, but early detection improves the quality of life.

Screening

- The initial screening test measures immunoreactive trypsinogen (IRT) in the blood, which will be increased if the baby has cystic fibrosis.
- The IRT can be raised in normal babies due to other factors.
- If levels are raised, a DNA test is carried out.
- It is estimated that 1 in 25 people in the UK carry the cystic fibrosis delta F508 gene mutation.
- If the delta F508 gene is found on both alleles in the child, then he or she definitely has cystic fibrosis.
- If the delta F508 gene is found on one allele, the child will be a carrier.
- If the IRT is still raised at this time, it confirms the diagnosis of cystic fibrosis.[4,6]

Sickle cell disorders and thalassaemia major

- In *sickle cell disorders* the RBCs become sickle shaped, causing anaemia and making the baby more prone to serious infections.
- These cells can also block the small blood vessels, causing pain.
- A baby with sickle cells needs treatment with antibiotics to prevent serious infections.
- In *thalassaemia major* the baby does not make enough haemoglobin and becomes severely anaemic, needing regular blood transfusions to remain well.

All parents in these situations will be carriers and are usually offered genetic counselling. CLIMB—Children Living With Inherited Metabolic Diseases—is a support group for parents and health professionals.[4,7]

Medium-chain acyl CoA dehydrogenase deficiency (MCADD)

- Incidence: 1:10 000–20 000 births.
- About 1:80 people are carriers and do not have any symptoms.
- It is due to a lack of an enzyme needed to metabolize fat into energy.
- It becomes apparent if the child has long periods between meals:
  - Children with MCADD cannot break down the fat quickly enough to provide energy.
  - This leads to a hold-up in the breakdown of medium-chain fats, due to the lack of the correct enzyme.

- The banked-up medium-chain fats form toxic substances, which lead to life-threatening symptoms or death.
- MCADD has no apparent symptoms at birth.
- The most acute presentations occur within the first 2 years of life.
- It is not possible to predict which children will develop symptoms.
- Symptoms occur if the child is not feeding well or is ill with an infection.
- The child becomes:
  - Drowsy, and may vomit
  - Hypoglycaemic
  - Comatose, due to low blood sugar and also the build up of the toxins.
- Most children with this condition will be well as long as they eat regularly. The main problem occurs when the child has additional viral illnesses with a sore throat, vomiting, and diarrhoea, which makes them reluctant to eat or drink.
- The body also requires increased energy to cope with the infection, so children with MCADD need to eat more often during such infections.

Management of MCADD

- The main focus for treatment is to prevent a 'metabolic crisis'.
- Closely monitor the child to determine 'safe' time periods between meals.
- Follow a strict feeding schedule.
- If the child becomes unwell, drowsy or vomits, give glucose supplements and refer to a doctor.
- There is no cure for MCADD, but with early detection and monitoring the child can lead a normal life, and the 'safe' time between meals increases with age.[4,8]

1 Wraith JE (1999). Inborn errors of metabolism in the neonate. In: Rennie JM, Roberton NRC (eds) *Textbook of Neonatology*, 3rd edn. London: Churchill Livingstone, pp. 986–1002.

2 UK Newborn Screening Programme Centre (2004). *Proposed standards and Policies for newborn blood spot screening—an integrated consultation.* London: DH.

3 National Society for Phenylketonuria. *Phenylketonuria.* London: NSPKU. Available at: ℜ www.nspku.org.uk (accessed 14.4.10).

4 General information. Available at: ℜ www.newbornscreening.bloodspot.nhs.uk (accessed 14.4.10).

5 UCL Institute of Child Health. *Congenital Hypothyroidism.* London: UCL. Available at: ℜ www.ich.ucl.ac.uk/factsheets (accessed 14.4.10).

6 Cystic Fibrosis Trust. *Cystic Fibrosis.* Kent: Cystic Fibrosis Trust. Available at: ℜ www.cftrust.org.uk (accessed 14.4.10).

7 Sickle Cell Society. *Sickle Cell Disease.* London: Sickle Cell Society. Available at: ℜ www.sickle-cellsociety.org (accessed 14.4.10).

8 National Information Centre for Metabolic Diseases. *MCADD.* Crewe: National Information Centre for Metabolic Diseases. Available at: ℜ www.climb.org.uk (accessed 14.4.10).

Developmental dysplasia of the hip (DDH)

In its severest form, developmental dysplasia of the hip is one of the most common congenital malformations.[1] Neonatal screening programmes, based on clinical screening examinations, have been established for more than 40 years but their effectiveness remains controversial. The longer-term outcomes of developmental hip dysplasia with its contribution to premature degenerative hip disorders in adult life, and the benefits and harms of newborn screening are not clearly understood. High quality studies of the adult outcomes of developmental hip dysplasia and the childhood origins of early degenerative hip disease are needed, as are randomized trials to assess the effectiveness and safety of neonatal screening and early treatment.[2]

It is becoming more common for midwives with appropriate training to be responsible for screening the hips as part of the holistic assessment of the newborn. Approximately 1.5 per 1000 babies is born with a dislocatable or subluxable hip. This used to be called congenital dislocation of the hips but the terminology has changed to reflect its potentially progressive nature.

If the condition remains untreated the hip will function well initially but ultimately lead to problems with walking and premature degenerative disease of the hip.

Risk factors
- Breech presentation
- Family history of hip dysplasia
- Increased birthweight
- Females more at risk than males
- First baby more at risk than subsequent babies.

Diagnosis
The diagnosis is made in the first instance by physical examination and then confirmed by ultrasound scan. Two methods are used.
- Ortolani's manoeuvre detects a dislocatable but reducible hip.
- Barlow's manoeuvre is a provocation test for an unstable hip.

Carrying out the examination
- Consent is obtained from the parents before the test is carried out and then performed in their presence.
- Ortolani's—the baby must be relaxed and on a firm surface.
- The hip is flexed to 90° and then gently abducted (an outward movement away from the body).
- The examiner's finger on the outer part of the hip can detect the 'clunk' as the head of the femur slides into the hip socket.
- This differs from the benign click of soft tissues snapping over bony prominences during the manoeuvre.
- Barlow's—the hip is flexed to 90° and then the leg adducted (an inward movement towards the body) and the leg gently pushed backwards.

- The hip will 'clunk' as the head of the femur dislocates.
- ▶ These tests are not forceful and should not cause any discomfort.

Should either test be positive the result should be sensitively explained to the parents and arrangements made to confirm the diagnosis by ultrasound scan. Following diagnosis the most common treatment is for the baby to wear a Pavlik's harness or hip spica cast which gently keeps the hips in abduction until the hip capsule tightens and the hips are kept in place by the normal action of the ligaments.

Recommended reading

Stricker SJ, Barone SR (2001). Tips about hips in children. *International Pediatrics* **16**, 196–206.

1 Dezateux C, Rosendhal K (2007). Developmental dysplasia of the hip. *Lancet* **369**, 1541–52.

2 Sewell MD, Rosendhal K, Eastwood DM (2009). Developmental dysplasia of the hip. *British Medical Journal* **339**, b4454.

Birth injuries

Birth injuries are most commonly caused by trauma or mechanical difficulty at delivery. Head injuries are most common, followed by injury to limbs, internal organs, and the skin.

Head injury

- **Cephalhaematoma and caput succedaneum** are common birth injuries (📖 see Examination of the newborn: monitoring progress, p. 578).
- **Hypoxia** is the most common cause of cerebral injury following birth. This may result in intracranial haemorrhage or oedema. Occasionally cerebral trauma may result in cerebral palsy; this is often linked to pregnancy complications such as pre-eclampsia.
- **Tentorial tears**: these are due to the fetal skull being exposed to excessive, rapid, or abnormal moulding, which exerts pressure and stress on the cranium. If this pressure is stretched to its limit, the underlying soft tissues of the brain are vulnerable to tearing (the tentorium cerebelli and the falx cerebri). The source of the bleeding is usually from rupture of the great cerebral vein.
- **Fractured skull**: serious fracture to the skull is extremely rare. Where a woman may have a severely immobilized sacrococcygeal joint and coccyx, this can cause abnormal compression to the fetal head, which may result in a small depressed fracture of one of the frontal bones. Unusual or excessive moulding may produce a fine linear fracture of the cranial bone. Neither of these injuries requires treatment.
- **Facial paralysis**: this injury is usually caused by trauma at delivery. Damage to a branch of the seventh cranial nerve occurs when pressure is applied on the facial nerve as the head emerges at delivery. The affected side shows no movement when the baby cries, the eye is permanently open, and the mouth droops. This may affect the baby's feeding ability if severe. Invariably full recovery occurs within hours or up to several days. Care of the affected eye is important to prevent corneal damage.

Other injuries

- **Dislocations and fractures**: the humerus or clavicle may be fractured in a difficult shoulder dystocia. Occasionally, the femur may be fractured, and in a mismanaged breech delivery the fetal hip may be dislocated.
- **Sternomastoid haematoma**: this may occur following traction to expedite delivery of the head or shoulders. Swelling occurs to the sternomastoid muscle due to blood oozing from a torn blood vessel. Shortening of the muscle results in the head twisting to one side, this is commonly known as torticollis or wry neck. This condition takes several weeks to subside and rarely causes permanent damage.
- **Klumpke's palsy**: this is caused by traction on the arm when delivering the shoulders, resulting in damage to the lower brachial plexus. Paralysis to the hand and wrist drop occurs and sometimes a fracture is also apparent. Physiotherapy is the main treatment and recovery is usually slow.
- **Erb's palsy**: this is caused by excessive traction on the neck during a breech or cephalic presentation, resulting in damage to the upper

brachial plexus. The arm hangs loosely from the shoulder with the palm of the hand turned backwards in the 'waiter's tip' position. Physiotherapy is the main treatment, again this may be slow but the condition does usually resolve completely.

- **Injury to abdominal organs:** this usually occurs after inappropriate handling of the baby during a breech delivery, causing rupture of the liver or spleen.
- **Skin injuries:** bruising and/or abrasions are sometimes a result of application of forceps. More extensive bruising accompanied by soft-tissue swelling may result from a ventouse delivery, this usually resolves within a few days. Abrasions may also be noted due to application of a scalp electrode in labour. Small superficial haemorrhages of the head, face, and neck may resemble cyanosis, but are due to congestion of blood vessels in the head. This may occur due to trauma or a precipitate delivery—no treatment is required.

Practice points

- ► Birth injuries still cause a significant number of unnecessary perinatal deaths.
- ► Good antenatal surveillance and skilful labour care may go some way to prevent such injuries.
- ► Careful observation of the newborn in the postnatal period, particularly after a traumatic or difficult birth, is essential, to enable abnormal signs and symptoms to be detected promptly.

Congenital abnormalities

The incidence of congenital abnormalities varies between 2% and 7% of livebirths. They are classified into two groups, malformations and deformations. Malformations result from disturbed early embryonic growth, e.g. congenital heart disease. Deformations result from late changes to normal structures by pathological processes or intrauterine forces.[1]

Causes

- Teratogens: substances like chemicals, drugs, viruses or radiation
- Excessive alcohol intake: fetal alcohol syndrome
- Infections: e.g. rubella
- Chemicals: e.g. mercury
- Maternal disease: e.g. diabetes, maternal PKU.

Examination

The most obvious defects will be detected shortly after birth during the neonatal examination.[2]

The face

- There is a wide range of recognizable features called dysmorphic features which may suggest congenital abnormality.
- The position of the eyes in relation to the nasal bridge should be noted. If they are too far apart this is called hypertelorism and if they are too close together this is called hypotelorism.
- Low-set ears are seen in a variety of conditions including Potter's syndrome.
- Cleft lip and/or palate occurs in 14.6 per 10 000 births.
- A large or protruding tongue may suggest hypothyroidism or Down's syndrome.
- An underdeveloped jaw, called micrognathia, is seen in Pierre Robin syndrome.

The chest

- It should be symmetrical and move equally on respiration.
- A small chest may occur with hypoplastic lungs and in a variety of rare syndromes.

The abdomen

- Distension suggests intestinal obstruction.
- A scaphoid abdomen suggests diaphragmatic hernia.
- An umbilical hernia may be present.
- The anus should be patent.

The genitalia

- Testes should be present in the scrotum in 98% of full term boys.
- Hypospadias occurs if the opening of the urethra is on the underside of the penis.
- Epispadias occurs if the urethral opening is on the upper side of the penis.
- A hydrocele (fluid filled cyst) may be present in the scrotum. No treatment is required as they usually spontaneously resolve.

- The size of the outer labia in girls is governed by gestational age. By term they should completely cove the inner labia.
- The clitoris is variable in size. If large consider adrenogenital syndrome, especially if the labia are also fused.

The extremities

- Mild postural deformities may be present in the feet. The ankle joint should be able to be passively moved through its range of normal movements. Abnormalities include talipes.
- The hips are examined to detect a dislocatable or dislocated hip.
- There should be a range of normal movements in the arms.
- Examination of the hands may reveal a single palmar crease in Down's syndrome.

Recommended reading

Davies L, McDonald S (2008). *Examination of the Newborn and Neonatal Health: A Multidimensional Approach.* Edinburgh: Churchill Livingstone.

1 Levene MI, Tudehope DI, Thearle MJ (2000). *Essentials of Neonatal Medicine*, 3rd edn, Oxford: Blackwell, 25–31.

2 Baston H, Durward H (2001). *Examination of the Newborn. A Practical Guide.* London. Routledge, 65–91.

Heart murmurs in the newborn

Murmurs are caused by the sound of turbulent blood flow into the chambers and vessels of the heart. This will usually be detected during the neonatal examination undertaken prior to the baby being discharged home from hospital after the birth.

Increasingly this holistic examination is being performed by suitably trained midwives as part of the continuing care given to all mothers and babies. Community midwives undertaking the assessment in the mother's home have clear referral guidelines to follow if a problem is detected. It is common for babies to have a heart murmur in the first 24h following birth. This is the time during which two structures of the fetal circulation complete their closure in response to onset of respirations and the establishment of a normal pulmonary circulation.

The two structures are:
• The foramen ovale—an opening in the atrial septum
• The ductus arteriosus—a vessel connecting the pulmonary artery to the aorta. This normally closes within 24h.

Another examination is carried out at the age of 6 weeks on all babies, during which the heart is examined again.

Significance of heart murmurs

In one study murmurs were detected in 0.6% of babies, of whom around half had a cardiac malformation.[1] Some babies who were later diagnosed with cardiac malformations had a normal neonatal examination.[2] The study concluded that the neonatal examination only detects 44% of cardiac malformations, but if a murmur is heard there is a 54% chance of it being due to a cardiac malformation. Occasionally heart murmurs are not diagnosed for several months.

Management

▶ Babies presenting with a murmur during examination should be referred to a consultant paediatrician. This needs to be sensitively explained to parents who are waiting to go home with their baby after this examination takes place.

If the consultant suspects an abnormal murmur an echocardiogram is arranged. If a problem is suspected, the baby will be referred to a cardiologist for more detailed investigations.

Other signs that may become apparent in the baby in the first few days of life if there is a cardiac malformation are:
• Tachypnoea
• Feeding difficulties
• Cyanosis around the lips
• Failure to gain weight.

Provided the baby is otherwise well and there are no feeding problems parents may take the baby home in the interim period while awaiting appointments and tests.

The two most common cardiac defects in children are:
- Ventricular septal defect
- Atrial septal defect.

1 Ainsworth SB, Wylie JP, Wren C (1999). Prevalence and clinical significance of cardiac murmurs in neonates. *Archives of Diseases in Childhood* **80,** 43–5.

2 Azhar AS, Habib HS (2007). Accuracy of the initial evaluation of heart murmurs in neonates: Do we need an echocardiogram? *Pediatric Cardiology* **27**, 234–7.

Management of the small for gestational age baby

Definition

A small for gestational age baby is any baby whose weight falls below the 10th percentile for its gestational age.[1]

A baby can be premature and small for dates, or term and small for dates, for example:

- A baby born at 28 weeks who weighs 500g
- A term baby who weighs 2500g.

Determination

- Gestational age is calculated using ultrasound scanning, where measurement and comparison of the fetal skull and femur enable determination of the age in days, size and weight.
- Whether the baby is the correct size for its gestational age or if it is growth restricted can also be determined.[2]

Causes

The small for gestational age baby will have been starved *in utero* due to poor placental supply of nutrients. Some of the causes relate to poor maternal health, others relate to socio-economic factors, and some are fetal, for example:

- Pregnancy-induced hypertension
- Antepartum haemorrhage
- Congenital infection
- Multiple pregnancy
- Some congenital abnormalities
- Poor diet
- Smoking
- Alcohol
- Drug abuse
- Poor housing
- Unemployment.[3]

There may be genetic and racial inheritance reasons why babies appear small when weighed and measured using standard percentile charts designed for the average European Caucasian population. This is often the case for babies of Asian origin. Also, occasionally, it may also be linked to poor diet and health, where the mother, living in a different culture, finds it difficult to obtain food she would normally enjoy.[2]

Due to poor nourishment from the placenta, the fetus is unable to lay down any spare stores of fat or glycogen and, once born, the baby will have difficulty in maintaining temperature and blood glucose levels.

- Although the baby will be small, his or her organs will be mature, especially if it is near to term.
- If the baby is also preterm, then the problems will be compounded by immaturity of the main organs and, depending on its gestation, this baby will also be at risk of the complications of prematurity and will

need to be managed as a preterm baby (📖 see Management of the preterm baby, p. 634).

Poor fetal growth may indicate placental failure and, without intervention, the fetus may die. Caesarean section may be carried out when the fetus reaches a viable age.[3]

Growth restriction

Growth of a fetus is referred to as symmetrical or asymmetrical, and is diagnosed using ultrasound scanning, when various measurements are taken:

- Bi-parietal diameter
- Head circumference
- Limb lengths
- Abdominal circumference.[2]

Asymmetrical babies

- Are diagnosed later in pregnancy.
- They have a normal sized head and brain for gestation. The brain has received sufficient nutrients to grow normally. Referred to as 'brain sparing syndrome'.
- The abdominal circumference is small because of depleted fat and glycogen stores in the liver.
- These babies normally make up their growth in the first 2 years and do not appear to have any adverse effects in the long term.

Symmetrical babies

- Are diagnosed early in the pregnancy from the first scan.
- The head and abdominal circumference are decreased but in proportion.
- This situation is more serious as it indicates a longer period of time without nutrition to the brain and major organs, and the baby will be slow to make up the deficiency after birth.
- As the baby will have missed out on the biologically timed periods of brain growth and development, the long-term prognosis is guarded as to their intellectual development.[2]

Congenital abnormalities

Small for gestational age may also be associated with some congenital abnormalities, such as trisomies (where there is an extra chromosome), leading to conditions such as Down's and Edward's syndromes.[3]

Congenital infections

Babies with congenital infections tend to be small for dates.

- These infections are usually transferred to the baby from the mother.
- They are viral and are the only infections capable of crossing the placenta.
- They can affect placental function, leading to diminished growth.
- Exposure to these infections can also lead to early miscarriage and fetal abnormalities.
- Handling babies born with these infections also presents a risk to the midwives, nurses, medical staff, and family.

- The use of universal precautions are recommended for all personnel handling newborn babies.[4]

Taking the first letter from each name of an infection in this group spells out the word **TORCH**:

- **T**oxoplasmosis
- **O**thers (chicken pox, measles)
- **R**ubella
- **C**ytomegalovirus
- **H**erpes.

TORCH screening is the test carried out on the placenta and blood to detect these infections.[1]

Characteristics of a small for gestational age baby

At birth the baby:

- Will probably be active and wide awake
- Tends to look anxious and wizened
- Has a loud cry, possibly fuelled by hunger
- Has lax, dry, and cracked skin
- Has a flat or scaphoid abdomen, due to poor liver storage of glycogen and a lack of subcutaneous fat
- Has a dull, yellow, thin and stretchy cord
- May be jittery, due to a low blood sugar
- Has an apparently large head, disproportional to body size
- Is at increased risk of meconium aspiration:
  - Due to poor oxygenation through the placenta, the fetus may have become distressed and passed meconium before birth
  - The baby's skin may also be stained with old meconium.[2,3]

Management at birth

Taking the above factors into consideration, management will depend on the gestation and condition of the baby at birth.

- If the baby is also premature (<37 weeks' gestation) it may need to be admitted to the NICU or SCBU, where he or she will receive full support.
- Babies near to term may require intensive care if they have major problems e.g. meconium aspiration. If this has occurred, the baby must be taken to the NICU to clear the meconium from the lungs and to administer a course of antibiotics.
- If no major problems are apparent, then the baby can be managed in a transitional care setting, where he or she can be observed by the midwife but can be kept with or near to the parents.

If on examination major problems are ruled out, care will entail management of:

- Temperature
- Glucose homeostasis
- Nutrition
- Prevention of infection
- Care of the family.

Glucose homeostasis

Small for gestational age babies have long been identified at risk of hypoglycaemia, due to:

- High brain-body mass ratio, with a corresponding increase in glucose consumption
- Reduced fat stores
- Failure of counter-regulation (the process that ensures the availability of glucose and other fuels, regulated by glucagon and adrenaline)
- Delayed gluconeogenesis
- Hyperinsulinism.

Some evidence suggests that babies with abnormal metabolic adaption have had abnormal end diastolic flow velocities (EDVs) in the umbilical artery.[3]

Not all small for gestational age babies are at risk of hypoglycaemia. Those at risk:

- Are below the 3rd percentile in weight, which is a weight 2 standard deviations from the mean for gestation
- Have an increased head circumference-body weight ratio (disproportionate)
- Have abnormal artery Doppler flow velocity profiles.[5]

Frequent blood sampling is not necessary to identify those at risk. Laboratory measurements of cord blood glucose and blood glucose at 4–6h of age (before the second feed) are recommended.[6]

Each maternity unit will have its own protocol for identifying and treating babies at risk of hypoglycaemia, based on the recommendations from WHO.[6]

Prevention of hypoglycaemia

- Avoid excessive infusions of glucose to the mother during labour.
- Dry and warm the baby immediately to avoid heat loss due to evaporation, which increases energy demands.[6]
- Provide skin-to-skin contact for maintenance of the baby's core temperature.

Early enteral feeding

- Start at a rate of 90mL/kg as 3h feeds, increasing by 30mL/kg daily.[5]
- Breast milk is preferred as it promotes ketogenesis.
- Blood glucose levels are lower in formula-fed babied due to the insulinogenic effects of the protein in formula milks.[6,7]

Temperature control

- The baby may need to be nursed in an incubator if temperature maintenance is difficult, or if the baby is premature or ill with other problems.
- If the baby is otherwise well, he or she can be cared for in a cot near the mother once feeding is established and the blood sugar level is maintained.
- The parents can be encouraged to give skin-to-skin care to help the baby to maintain their temperature. This also helps to stimulate the

mother's lactation, and promotes bonding between the baby and the parents as the father can also provide skin-to-skin care.

Prevention of infection
- The baby may have been exposed to congenital infection. Depending on the baby's condition, a TORCH screening at birth will confirm or eliminate such infection.
- The baby's skin may be in a poor condition. If it is dry and cracked and stained with meconium, the baby will be at increased risk of infection.
- Close observation of the baby's condition will detect any changes that indicate a developing infection. If suspected, this will be treated following a full infection screening.
- Breast milk from the baby's mother will help to give the baby some protection *against* infection. Breast milk confers some immunity due to its high IgA content (🕮 see Neonatal infection, p. 598).

Follow-up
- If the baby is well and able to maintain its temperature and blood glucose level then he or she will be discharged home as soon as possible.
- Those who are premature or who have other problems will stay in the NICU/SCBU until they have recovered.
- There may be a need for follow-up to assess the baby's future development.

Parental support
- If the baby is ill at birth and needs care within the NICU/SCBU, then the parents will need the same level of support as discussed in 🕮 Management of the preterm baby, p. 634. Where congenital abnormality is confirmed, the parents will be referred for genetic counselling.

1 World Health Organization (1992). *International Statistical Classification of Diseases and Related Health Problems*. 10th revision. Geneva: WHO.

2 Yeo H (ed.) (2000). *Nursing the Neonate*, 2nd edn. Oxford: Blackwell, pp. 1–17.

3 Rennie JM, Roberton NRC (eds) (1999). *Textbook of Neonatology*, 3rd edn. London: Churchill Livingstone, pp. 133–40.

4 Department of Health (1990). *Guidance for Clinical Health-care Workers: Protection Against Infection with HIV and Hepatitis Viruses: Recommendations of Expert Advisory Group on AIDS*. London: HMSO.

5 Hawdon JM, Ward-Platt MP (1993). Metabolic adaptation in small for gestational age infants. *Archives of Diseases in Childhood* **68**, 262–8.

6 World Health Organization (1997). *Hypoglycaemia of the Newborn: Review of the Literature*. Geneva: WHO.

7 Beresford D (2001). Fluid and electrolyte balance. In: Boxwell G (ed.) *Neonatal Intensive Care Nursing*, 2nd edn. London: Routledge, p. 220.

Management of the preterm baby

Definitions
- A preterm baby is any baby born before 37 completed weeks of gestation.[1]
- The legal age of viability is 24 weeks.[2]

These definitions indicate a wide range of babies between 24 and 37 weeks of gestation who will potentially need specialist management in a NICU or a SCBU.

Main aims of management
- To provide an appropriate environment where normal homeostasis can be maintained and where emergencies can be responded to in an appropriate way.
- To support the physical, developmental, psychological, and emotional welfare of the babies.
- To provide support for the families of babies nursed within these contexts.

As there is a vast difference in maturity between a baby of 24 weeks gestation and a baby of 37 weeks gestation, the care provided will be tailored to each individual baby's needs.

- As the baby approaches 34–37 weeks there is less need for intensive or invasive care, and these babies will be treated as normal term infants, provided they do not have any other problems.
- Babies of 24–34 weeks will need specialist care, with the smaller, sickest babies needing intensive care from birth.

Management and care
Initially most preterm babies will be nursed in an incubator for:
- Temperature control
- Humidity control
- Easier observation
- Oxygenation
- Barrier to infection
- To cut down on handling.

Ventilation and surfactant replacement
A baby of 30 weeks or less will require ventilation and surfactant replacement from birth, due to surfactant deficiency and immaturity of the lungs (☐ see Respiratory distress syndrome in the newborn, p. 640). The need for ventilation will be assessed according to the baby's gestation and condition at birth. The main aim is to prevent the baby's condition becoming worse because of tiredness.

Several different methods of ventilation are available, which have been developed especially for use with premature babies.

Different techniques of ventilation
- *High-frequency oscillation ventilation (HFOV)* has been developed to cut down on the use of high-pressure ventilation, which can lead to long-term damage to the immature lungs. HFOV provides breaths or cycles of 240–3000 per min. It facilitates the diffusion of gases and

improves ventilation and perfusion matching. It is used where there is poor gas exchange, as in RDS that has not responded to conventional ventilation.
- *Continuous positive airway pressure (CPAP)* delivers a predetermined continuous pressure and supplemental oxygen into the airways of a spontaneously breathing infant. It splints the chest, preventing collapse of the alveoli on expiration and maintaining a residual capacity that will improve ventilation and perfusion.
- *Patient-triggered ventilation (PTV) and synchronous intermittent ventilation (SIMV)* have been developed to provide ventilator breaths that will coincide with the infant's own breathing pattern.
  - In PTV the ventilator rate is controlled by the baby. Every time the baby's breath exceeds a critical level the machine will deliver a breath. If the infant does not breathe within a predetermined period, the machine will deliver a breath. Every breath initiated by the baby will be ventilator assisted.
  - SIMV can help to prevent the problems caused by asynchronous breathing. The ventilator breaths can be delivered to coincide with the baby's breathing. A total number of breaths are decided and any further breaths that the baby takes will be unsupported by the ventilator.
- *Nitric oxide.* Inhaled nitric oxide is used as treatment for persistent pulmonary hypertension following meconium aspiration, and in babies with severe RDS. It produces localized vasodilation in the pulmonary circulation and is used when the baby is not responding to conventional or HFOV.[3]

Temperature and blood sugar

As well as management of babies' ventilation needs, management of their temperature and blood sugar levels are fundamental to their survival.

Nutrition

Provision of nutrition can be difficult due to:
- Poorly developed sucking and swallowing reflexes
- A lack of coordination.

Tube and intravenous feeding. Total parenteral nutrition may be required.

Minimal enteral nutrition is small amount of milk given continuously via a nasogastric tube which will help to mature the gut and prepare it for receiving full milk feeds when the baby has matured enough to tolerate feeding.

Once the baby improves, breast or bottle feeding can be introduced. Breastfeeding, or the provision of expressed breast milk, is preferred as it has many benefits for the premature baby, especially for protection against infection and the prevention of NEC. It has also been shown to improve the longer-term development of the brain.[4]

Physiological jaundice

This occurs because of an immature liver and will probably need treatment with phototherapy and or exchange transfusions (see Neonatal jaundice, p. 604).

Preventing infection

The baby's immune system will be immature, resulting in an increased susceptibility to infection.

- Early recognition and treatment with antibiotics is important.
- If infection is suspected, carry out a full infection screen and commence the baby on a 10-day course of antibiotics (📖 see Antibiotic therapies and sensitivities, p. 603).
- Scrupulous handwashing and drying by staff and visitors has been proved to be the most effective way of reducing the risk of infection.[5]
- All equipment is sterilized and used only for one baby.
- Each baby has its own personal equipment for day-to-day care.

Visiting policies

- These are in place to protect the baby from too many visitors.
- Parents are encouraged to be with the baby at all times.
- Other visitors are allowed at the discretion of the parents.
- Special arrangements are made for siblings to visit with parental support.

Observations

Make constant observations of:

- Colour/activity
- Temperature/respirations/blood pressure and oxygen saturation
- Incubator and inspired oxygen humidity and temperature
- Fluid intake
- Ventilator settings and oxygen concentrations.

Record all of these hourly over a 24h period. It is important to keep an accurate record of events, as even the slightest change can be very significant in detecting the problem as early as possible.

Physiotherapy and suction

While the baby is on ventilation this is carried out by specialist physiotherapists who prescribe a daily treatment for each baby following individual assessment of its requirements.

The physiotherapist will advise the nursing staff and parents about how to correctly position the baby according to his or her gestation and medical needs. This is often referred to as 'supported positioning'.

The importance of supported positioning

- The muscle tone of premature babies is poor and their movement is limited because of underdeveloped muscles.
- They tend to lie in a 'frog-like' posture with the limbs extended.
- Being left to lie for long periods of time without a position change can lead to long-term muscular skeletal and developmental problems.
- Several supported positions are used, including prone, supine, and lateral.[6]
- The prone position is considered to be the best for preterm babies who are being monitored, as it promotes oxygenation and energy conservation.[7,8]
- Once the baby is ready to go home, advise the parents to use the supine position as advocated by the DH campaign for the prevention of cot death.[9]

Environment

Babies can be affected by constant exposure to:
- Noise
- Light
- Pain from invasive procedure
- Excessive handling
- Separation from their parents.

Much research has been done into the possible short- and longer-term effects that these factors have on the baby and how to soften the nursery environment by reducing levels of noise and light, and ways of assessing and reducing the discomfort and distress caused by painful procedures.

The use of therapeutic touch

Premature babies have a poor tolerance to the excessive handling they are often subjected to, but have been shown to have a positive response to parental handling.

Baby massage techniques have been modified for use for premature ill babies. These have become an important way of helping the parents to become involved with their baby by providing a positive loving touch.[10]

Parental needs

The application of family-centred care for parents with a baby in the NICU or SCBU presents a challenge for the nursing and medical staff. These parents:
- Have yet to get to know their baby, and they may be parents for the first time
- Have to develop their relationship with their new baby in a very public way, in an alien environment which is also influenced by input from a variety of nursing and medical personnel
- Are faced with separation, which is not normal for most parents with a new baby
- Require a constant stream of up-to-date information and reassurance about their baby's progress
- Need an honest and realistic prognosis, which is difficult at first and can alter drastically if the baby develops any problems
- Need facilities for rest, sleeping, food, and drinks
- Need open visiting and a gradual involvement with the decision making as their understanding of their baby increases
- Need access to other medical personnel, such as health visitors and social workers
- Need help to give the baby its care and to take on more as their confidence increases
- Need to involve the baby's siblings and the support of their wider family.

1 World Health Organization (1992). *International Statistical Classification of Diseases and Related Health Problems*, 10th revision. Geneva: WHO.

2 Roberton NRC (1993). Should we look after babies less than 800 grams? *Archives of Diseases of Childhood* **68**, 326–9.

3 Cameron J (2001). Management of respiratory disorders. In: Boxwell G (ed.) *Neonatal Intensive Care Nursing*, 2nd edn. London: Routledge, pp 101–3.

4 Wheeler J, Chapman C (2000). Feeding outcomes and influences within the neonatal unit. *International Journal of Nursing Practice* **6**(4), 196–206.

5 Yeo H (ed.) (2000). *Nursing the Neonate*, 2nd edn. Oxford: Blackwell.

6 Downs J (1991). The effect of intervention on development of hip posture in very preterm babies. *Archives of Diseases of Childhood* **66**, 797–801.

7 Heimler R. Langlois J, Hodel DJ, Nelin LD, Sasidharan P (1992). Effects on the breathing pattern of preterm infants. *Archives of Diseases of Childhood* **67**, 312–14.

8 Turrill S (1992). Supported positioning in intensive care. *Pediatric Nursing* **4**(4), 24–7.

9 Department of Health (1991). *Sleeping Position and the Incidence of Cot Death*. London: HMSO.

10 Appleton S (1997). 'Handle with care': An investigation of handling received by preterm infants in intensive care. *Journal of Neonatal Nursing* **3**(3), 23–7.

Respiratory distress syndrome in the newborn

- RDS is one of the main causes of morbidity and mortality in preterm infants.
- The lungs of babies born at 28 weeks or less will be immature, having few alveoli and reduced surfactant production.[1]

Surfactant

- A substance produced in the type 2 alveolar cells in the lungs.
- It is composed of 95% lipid and 5% protein. The lipid adsorbs rapidly to the air–water interface and is responsible for the majority of the surface-active properties of pulmonary surfactant.
- Surfactant coats the entire surface of the lung.
- It equalizes the surface tension.
- It prevents collapse of the alveoli when breathing out.
- It stabilizes the size of the alveoli.
- It is produced in the fetal lungs from 20 weeks' gestation.
- It is present in small amounts from 24 weeks' gestation.
- It increases steadily up to 34 weeks, when there is a surge in production to prepare for birth.

RDS occurs because of a deficiency of surfactant, which in turn causes atelectasis, and high pressures are needed to reinflate the lungs.

In preterm babies the diaphragm and intercostal muscles are still developing, so that the baby's efforts to breathe will often be inadequate and the baby will soon become tired, needing mechanical support to help with breathing.[1]

The lack of surfactant leads to:

- Alveolar collapse on expiration.
- The alveolar walls are thickened due to them not being fully expanded on inspiration, which leads to a decreased amount of oxygen diffusing into the blood, which further leads to hypoxia.
  ▶ The associated hypoxia can cause:
- Right-to-left shunting through the foramen ovale.
- Left-to-right shunting through the ductus arteriosus.
- Failure to make the transition from intrauterine to extrauterine life.
- Pulmonary ischaemia.
- Further damage to the developing lungs.[1]

The onset of RDS

Usually within 4h of birth as the baby becomes increasingly tired.

The signs of RDS

- Grunting on expiration caused by the baby trying to force air past a partially closed glottis. This effort can keep air in the alveoli at the end of each breath and prevent atelectasis.
- Increased rate of breathing.
- Intercostal, sternal and subclavicular recession; where the soft tissues around the clavicles, ribs and sternum are sucked in on inspiration (chin tug).

- Nasal flair.
- Chin tug: where the baby's chin is pulled downwards on inspiration. This is related to the effort of breathing and the need to suck in the soft tissues around the neck and the ribs (known as recession) because the baby is unable to fully expand its lungs on inspiration due to the lack of surfactant. The soft tissues fill the vacuum left by the unexpanded lungs and as everything is connected from the trachea to the diaphragm the chin is tugged downwards.
- Cyanosis.
- Apnoea.
- Diminished breath sounds because of poor air entry.[1]

Diagnosis

- A chest X-ray 4h after birth shows a 'ground glass' effect of contrasting white and black areas.
- The black areas are alveoli which have air in them, due to the presence of surfactant, in contrast to the white areas, which are collapsed due to the lack of surfactant.
- A chest X-ray before this time would probably be normal, but may be carried out to rule out other respiratory problems e.g. infection, which will be apparent at an earlier time.
- Babies who develop RDS are usually premature, <34 weeks.
- RDS is also associated with:
  - Perinatal asphyxia due to hypoxia
  - Acidosis
  - Hypothermia (a temperature <35°C decreases surfactant production and efficiency even further).
- Maternal diabetes suppresses surfactant production and there is a higher risk of intrapartum asphyxia due to the size of the baby. Babies of diabetic mothers tend to be larger than normal due to the maternal fluctuating blood sugar levels, which allows higher than normal levels of sugar to be transferred to the fetus via the placenta.[1]

Treatments

Include:
- The administration of maternal steroids prior to the baby being born, in an attempt to initiate a stress response in the fetus, which will mature the fetal lungs, stimulating an increase in normal surfactant production
- Surfactant replacement therapy at birth
- Ventilation at birth if the baby is <30 weeks' gestation.[1]

Surfactant replacement

Most preterm babies of 28 weeks' gestation or less will be given surfactant at birth in measured doses directly down the endotracheal tube into the lower trachea.
- Exogenous surfactant therapy has been shown to reduce the severity of RDS.
- Early administration is more effective than rescue treatment.
- Animal surfactants are more effective than synthetic ones in reducing the need for ventilation.[2,3]

Curosurf®

This is an animal-based surfactant made from pigs' lungs and is one of only two licensed for use in the UK for the treatment of surfactant-deficient RDS, the other being Survanta® from calf's lungs.

Curosurf® is expensive, a single-dose vial 1.5mL costs £281. The 3mL vial costs £547.

- The dose is 100–200mg/kg (1.25–2.5mL/kg).
- The baby must be lying supine and flat.
- The vials need to be warmed immediately prior to use, as they will have been stored in the fridge.
- Apply the surfactant directly down the endotracheal tube.
- Give the baby 1min of ventilation using a Neopuff® ventilation system (📖 see Neonatal resuscitation, p. 454) to disperse the surfactant as far as possible into the lungs, then reconnect to the ventilator.
- Give further doses in the same manner.
- If the baby has a closed suction device attached, give the surfactant through a catheter passed via the suction port. The baby can remain connected to the ventilator during this procedure.
- Following administration, pulmonary compliance can improve rapidly, requiring prompt adjustment of the ventilator settings and inspired oxygen concentrations to avoid hyperoxia.
- Avoid suction for at least 4h after administration.[2,3]

Prophylaxis

If the baby is deemed suitable for prophylaxis, the surfactant is given immediately and a chest X-ray is obtained as soon as possible.

The aim is to give the surfactant within the first 30min after birth if the baby is <26 weeks' gestation.

The criteria for prophylaxis are:
- Gestational age 28 weeks or less
- Ventilated
- Receiving supplementary oxygen >30%
- Clinical judgement that the baby is unlikely to wean rapidly from the ventilator
- Chest X-ray compatible with RDS.

The criteria for rescue treatment are:
- Ventilated
- X-ray diagnosis of RDS
- Inspired oxygen >40%
- PaO_2 <7 kPa.[2,3]

Nursing care

- *Incubator care* provides warmth, humidification, observation, oxygen therapy, protection from infection, and easy access.
- *Vital signs*: monitor hourly.
- *Temperatures* of incubator and inhaled gases: monitor hourly, along with the baby's temperature.
- *Blood pressure and blood gases:* monitor via an arterial line 4–6h, backed up by continuous saturation monitoring.
- *Blood sugar*: check whenever blood samples are taken.
- *Fluid intake/output*: record hourly and evaluate every 24h.

- *Nutritional requirements*: work these out daily. This usually involves IV infusion of 10% glucose, followed by total parenteral nutrition if the baby's condition is unstable. When the baby's condition improves, commence continuous gastric feeding with breast milk or formula milk as soon as possible.
- *Early initiation of feeding* is important to stimulate the premature gut and digestive hormones.
- *Minimal enteral nutrition* is used where feeding is delayed. It stimulates the gut with small amounts of milk given continuously via a nasogastric tube.
- *Chest physiotherapy and suctioning* are not necessary for the first 24h. Assess after this time and give according to individual needs.
- *Minimal handling* and the reduction of light and noise help to promote periods of rest.
- *Supported positioning* helps to achieve flexion and support in a variety of positions. The premature baby has immature and weak muscles and skeleton, and will therefore need help with support, to prevent the development of longer-term problems.
- *Care for the family*: encourage them to visit and care for the baby with help and support from the nursing and medical staff. Provide constant explanation and reassurance, as well as practical support, such as 'rooming in' and facilities for food and drinks. Involve all family members in support of the parents.[1]

Recovery from RDS[1]

- Usually occurs between 48h and 72h after birth, as surfactant production increases and the need for ventilation decreases.
- A very preterm baby will require specialized care and mechanical ventilation for some weeks, due to other complications of prematurity.

1 Cameron J (2001). Management of respiratory disorders. In: Boxwell G (ed.) *Neonatal Intensive Care Nursing*, 2nd edn. London: Routledge, pp. 101–3.

2 Ainsworth SB (2004). Exogenous surfactant and neonatal lung disease: An update on the current situation. *Journal of Neonatal Nursing* **10**(1), 6–11.

3 OSARIS Collaborative Group (1992). Early versus delayed administration of synthetic surfactant— the judgment of OSARIS. *Lancet* **340**, 1363–9.

Respiratory problems in the newborn

Respiratory problems manifest as respiratory distress are the commonest cause of admission of newborns to the neonatal unit in the perinatal period.[1]

Respiratory distress is a general term used to describe respiratory symptoms and is not synonymous with respiratory distress syndrome[2] (📖 see Respiratory distress syndrome in the newborn, p. 640). Respiratory distress arises from:

- Inadequate *in utero* maturation of the lungs and the mechanisms controlling respiration.
- Disease processes present before or after birth which compromise respiratory function.[1]
  The clinical signs of respiratory distress are:
- Tachypnoea: respiration rate greater than 60 breaths/min.
- Expiratory grunt: the baby expires against a closed glottis, which helps to maintain a higher lung residual lung volume preventing alveolar collapse at the end of expiration thus improving oxygenation.
- Central cyanosis.
- Chest recession which can be intercostals, lower costal, sternal or sub-clavicular.
- Nasal flaring and chin tug: these along with chest recession represent the baby's use of accessory respiratory muscles.
- These may be superseded by apnoea or acute collapse.[2]
  Additional signs may include:
- Cardiac murmurs
- Abnormal peripheral pulses
- Signs of cardiac failure may also be present if there is an underlying congenital heart defect.[1]

Diagnosis

If two or more of the symptoms persist for 4h or more then respiratory distress is the likely cause and a diagnosis will be made following:

- A full clinical history
- Physical examination including:
  - Observation
  - Vital signs
  - Auscultation of the lungs for air entry, symmetry and breath sounds
- Palpation of dextrocardia and hepatomegaly
- Appropriate investigations (📖 see p. 645) including a chest X-ray
- Perinatal history including:
  - Gestational age
  - The presence of poly/oligohydramnios
  - Anomalies on ultrasound
  - Risk factors for sepsis
  - The passage of meconium
  - Respiratory depression at birth
  - Duration of membrane rupture.[2]

Investigations

- Pulse oximetry to measure the arterial saturations. This gives an indication of the severity of hypoxia and the urgency of intervention.
- Temperature to exclude hypothermia or hyperthermia.
- Blood glucose to exclude hypoglycaemia.
- Arterial blood gases to determine the degree of respiratory failure and to decide on appropriate interventions such as the need for assisted ventilation and supplementary oxygen. A persistent metabolic acidosis may lead to a diagnosis of a metabolic disorder (📖 see Metabolic disorders and the neonatal blood spot test, p. 614).
- Chest X-ray to rule out:
  - Pneumothorax
  - Effusions
  - Pulmonary oedema
  - Abnormal cardiac silhouette
  - Congenital diaphragmatic hernia
  - Bell-shaped chest as seen in neuromuscular disorders
  - A 'ground glass' appearance seen with idiopathic RDS, congenital pneumonia, or aspiration.
- An FBC to detect infection suggested by a high or low white cell count and thrombocytopenia.
- Full infection screen where infection is suspected.
- ECG and echocardiogram where congenital heart disease is suspected.[1]

The causes and management of respiratory distress vary depending on the gestation and chronological age of the baby. The management is determined by the underlying diagnosis.[1,2]

Causes

These include:
- RDS:
  - Surfactant deficiency seen in premature babies with RDS (📖 see p. 634)
- Pneumothorax:
  - Pneumomediastinum
  - Pulmonary interstitial emphysema
  - Pleural effusions
- Pulmonary haemorrhage following:
  - Asphyxia
  - Hypothermia
  - Rhesus disease
  - Left-sided heart failure
- Transient tachypnoea of the newborn:
  - Retained or slow absorption of fetal lung fluid at birth
- Infection:
  - Pneumonia
  - Septicaemia
  - Meningitis
- Aspiration syndromes:
  - MAS
  - Milk
  - Blood

- Pulmonary hypoplasia: Potter's syndrome (renal agenesis and diminished amniotic fluid (oligohydramnios) leads to a lack of lung fluid which prevents the development of the lungs)
- Surgical conditions:
  - Choanal atresia
  - Pierre Robin syndrome
  - Diaphragmatic hernia
  - Lobar emphysema
  - Oesophageal atresia with tracheo-oesophageal fistula
- Following birth asphyxia
- Persistent fetal circulation (persistent pulmonary hypertension of the newborn (PPHN))
- Congenital heart abnormalities leading to heart failure:
  - Hypoplastic left heart syndrome
  - Obstructed total anomalous pulmonary venous drainage
  - Severe coarctation of the aorta
- Congenital lung malformation: cystic adenomatoid formation
- Congenital malformations:
  - Pulmonary lymphangiectasia
  - Pulmonary hypoplasia
  - Congenital nasolacrimal duct obstruction (congenital dacryocystocele)
- Congenital surfactant protein B deficiency
- Cold stress
- Hypoglycaemia
- Anaemia
- Polycythemia
- Cerebral damage
- Neuromuscular disorders:
  - Spinal muscular atrophy type1
  - Myotonic dystrophy
- Inherited metabolic disease (📖 see Metabolic disorders and the neonatal blood spot test, p. 614)
- Maternal drugs (e.g. opiates)
- Chronic causes of respiratory distress:
  - Bronchopulmonary dysplasia
  - Wilson–Mikity syndrome
  - Chronic pulmonary insufficiency of prematurity.[1,2]

Management

The aims of management are to identify the underlying cause and to provide supportive care with appropriate interventions. The care needed is similar regardless of the aetiology.[1,2]

- Correct acid–base balance.
- Alleviate hypoxaemia and respiratory failure.
- Warm cold babies (📖 see Neonatal temperature control, p. 588).
- Correct hypoglycaemia.
- Give supplemental oxygen if needed.
- Intubate and give surfactant to premature babies with RDS (📖 see Respiratory distress syndrome in the newborn, p. 640).

- Provide mechanical ventilation or CPAP where necessary based on the blood gas results (□ see Management of the preterm baby, p. 634).
- Site an arterial line for blood gas monitoring.
- Observe for the signs of infection and treat with broad-spectrum antibiotics (□ see Neonatal infection, p. 598).
- Observe for the signs of pneumothoraces and effusions and provide drainage procedures.
- Chest and abdominal X-rays to monitor effectiveness of treatments and progress.
- Babies with congenital heart abnormalities requiring surgery need to be transferred to a specialist cardiac surgical unit as soon as they are stabilized.
- Babies with other abnormalities which require surgery need to be stabilized and transferred into a unit specializing in surgery.
- Provide appropriate fluids and nutrition.
  - IV infusion of 10% glucose for the first 24h during initial stabilization and assessment of the condition.
  - IV infusion of total parenteral nutrition may be used from 48h if the baby is very unstable or if there is an underlying abnormality which requires surgery.
  - If the condition stabilizes and the condition does not require surgery then early enteral nutrition via a naso-gastric tube is recommended preferably with expressed breast milk especially if the baby is premature.
- Continuous monitoring and recording at regular intervals of:
  - Temperature
  - Blood pressure
  - Heart and breathing rates
  - Blood gases:
    — Umbilical or radial arterial samples
    — Pulse oximetry
    — Transcutaneous pO_2 and pCO_2
  - Oxygen needs
  - Ventilation requirements
  - Fluid intake and output.
- Incubator care provides:
  - Thermal stability
  - Warmth and humidity
  - Administration of oxygen
  - Observation
  - Isolation
  - Protection from excessive handling.[1,2]

The parents will need to be given support and an explanation of the condition and treatment required. They will also need to be with or near to their baby during transfer and admission to the neonatal or surgical unit (□ see Management of the preterm baby, p. 634).

1 Mupanemunda RH, Watkinson M (2000). *Key Topics in Neonatology*, 2nd edn. Oxford: Bios Scientific, pp. 275–7.

2 Levene MI, Tudehope DI, Thearle MJ (2000). *Essentials of Neonatal Medicine*, 3rd edn, London: Blackwell, pp. 93–115.

Neonatal abstinence syndrome

- Neonatal abstinence syndrome results from prenatal exposure to opioids, such as the morphine derivative, heroin.
- Specific receptors in the CNS are associated with neurotransmitters called endorphins and encephalins, which are sometimes referred to as endogenous opioids, as they are produced naturally in the brain and activate analgesia. Long-term exposure to opioid drugs results in adaptation of these receptors, leading to tolerance.
- Physical dependence occurs as the CNS adapts and larger amounts of the drug are required to achieve the same physiological effects.
- Following birth, the baby is no longer exposed to maternal levels of the drug and therefore shows acute withdrawal. Physical symptoms are experienced, as the naturally occurring opioids have been suppressed.[1]
- The onset, duration, and severity of symptoms vary according to type of drug, length of the mother's dependency, timing and amount of the mother's last dose before birth, clearance of the drug by the baby and his gestational age.[1]
- The symptoms are less severe if the mother has been on a methadone substitution programme during the pregnancy.[1]

Common symptoms

Typically the symptoms involve the CNS and the respiratory, gastrointes-tinal, and vasomotor systems:
- Hyperactivity and hyper-irritability
- High-pitched cry
- Increased muscle tone
- Exaggerated reflexes
- Tremors
- Hiccups and yawning
- Disorganized vigorous sucking, hyperphagia (wanting to feed very frequently)
- Vomiting/posseting
- Diarrhoea
- Drooling
- Excess secretions and stuffy nose
- Flushing of the skin and sweating.[1]

Principles of care

- Withdrawal symptoms may appear between 24h and 3 weeks after the birth.
- A social model of care following birth, where mothers and babies can be cared for together on the postnatal wards, even if babies require medical support for neonatal abstinence syndrome, has been advocated. By following this model:
  - Mothers are encouraged to develop appropriate parenting skills
  - They receive support from midwives
  - They are not separated from their babies.
- ▶ Breastfeeding is not contraindicated as it aids the withdrawal process.

- Soothing interactions can help with some of the more distressing symptoms:
  - Cuddle the baby
  - Keep the baby wrapped up
  - Avoid overstimulation
  - Keep the baby in a quiet environment.
- Feed the baby slowly, with small, frequent amounts, allowing rest periods between feeds. This helps to overcome gastrointestinal symptoms.
- Medication may be required to relieve and control symptoms.
- Assess the baby's status regularly (2–3 times daily) and monitor the mother-baby interaction and bonding. Record keeping is vital as this information is used to plan follow-up care.
  - Use score charts to monitor symptoms and their control. Some units have adapted or designed their own.
- The length of hospital stay will depend on the severity of withdrawal and the baby's response to interventions.
- The multidisciplinary team will decide whether the mother and baby go home together, and whether the mother is adequately prepared and supported.
- Mother and baby will continue to receive extra support once transferred home. Care is coordinated between social services, the health visitor, and the community midwife.
- Child protection may be an issue and must be considered by the midwife. (📖 See Safeguarding children, p. 650 for further details.)

Further reading

Winklbaur AB, Jaqsch R, Peternell A, et al. (2007). Management of neonatal abstinence syndrome in neonates born to opioid maintained women. *Drug and Alcohol Dependence* **87**, 131–8.

1 Women and Children's Health Service (2004). *Neonatal Abstinence Syndrome*. Available at: ℜ http://wchs.health.wa.gov.au (accessed 20.1.2011).

Safeguarding children

Definitions

- A number of terms are commonly used, i.e. child abuse (now outdated), child protection, safeguarding children, and children in need. 'Safeguarding children' is now the term used to cover all aspects.
- Legislation and guidance referred to here is that currently operating in the UK.
- The Children Act (2004) is an amendment of the Children Act (1989), largely as a result of the Victoria Climbié inquiry, to give boundaries and help for local authorities to better regulate official intervention in the interests of children. The Act also made changes to the laws pertaining to children, notably on adoption agencies, foster homes, baby sitting services, and the handling of child related crimes and crimes against children.
- A child is defined as a person <18 years (Children Act 1989). However, it is important to remember that a married woman >16 but <18 is not regarded as a child.
- In current British law an individual has no legal entity until the moment of birth, i.e. the fetus has no legal rights. This is not the case in all parts of the world.
  Safeguarding children is a complex topic and general principles are given here for guidance.
- ▶The guiding principle in any consideration of the child's needs is that their welfare and interests are paramount. In other words, the current and future quality and safety of the child's physical, emotional, psychological, and cultural upbringing must be central to any decisions that may be made in this respect by a court.
- ▶ As a midwife, you must ensure personal familiarity with your national legislation and resulting local policies, procedures and guidance in the child protection process, and update your understanding regularly.
- In the UK, each NHS trust has a specialist named nurse and midwife, who can be consulted and must be involved in all stages of child protection procedures, for specialist support, guidance, and leadership. A named midwife, usually the head of midwifery, is the named Midwife for Safeguarding Children within the local maternity service, and must also be consulted and involved at all stages of the procedure in individual cases. Any midwife dealing with an established safeguarding children situation or who has concerns about any child's safety must make that concern known to these people in the first instance.
- A key, valuable role in safeguarding children situations is that of the supervisor of midwives and the local supervising authority midwifery officer, in supporting the midwife and facilitating a system of tracing mothers of 'at risk' newborn babies.
- The Local Safeguarding Children Board (LSCB) has overall responsibility for managing the interagency functioning, developing policies and procedures at senior management level, identifying training needs, and conducting reviews of difficult cases or where a child dies as a result of abuse or neglect in their area. The LSCB maintains the local child protection register.

The key features of the Children Act

- A universal duty to promote and safeguard the welfare of the child. The child's welfare is paramount in all decisions made.
- Children are brought up with their own family, and local authorities have a duty to support and facilitate this, wherever possible.
- Wherever possible, professionals should work in partnership with parents, involving them in the care and decisions made about their children.
- The race, religion, culture, and language of the child are to be taken into account in the provision of services.
- Intervention by the statutory services should occur when it is in the child's best interest, and legal measures are only used as a last resort.
- The wishes and feelings of the child should be sought (depending on his age and level of understanding) and taken into account when decisions are made about his/her future.

The midwife's role

- Current guidance on implementation of the legislation that midwives should be familiar with are *Working Together to Safeguard Children*,[1] the *Framework for the Assessment of Children in Need and Their Families*,[2] and the *National Service Framework for Children and Young People*.[3] This guidance requires all relevant agencies to work together with children and families. Midwives have a central role in this process, ensuring that the parents and families are involved in discussions and in the preparations for the care of the newborn baby.[4]
- The midwife has an accepted role within society with pregnant mothers, their families and their newborn babies, and will frequently undertake an advocacy role to support the parent(s) and baby, giving additional parenting education support, as necessary. In the case of teenage mothers, both the mother and her baby, and possibly the baby's father, may be regarded as children in need and require services in their own rights.
- Within the multi-professional context, the midwife contributes significantly to the assessment, planning, and intervention required, particularly in pre-birth assessments and post-birth care, in terms of the child's development needs, parenting capacity and family and environmental factors. The close contact with the mother, including home visiting, places the midwife in the ideal situation to be aware of the care of the newborn and other children in the family, conditions in the home, parenting, lifestyle, and injuries to the mother or children.
- A midwife working in an independent capacity should know how to seek advice, support, and training and should consult her supervisor of midwives for guidance.

Pre-birth assessment

Examples of issues that may trigger a pre-birth assessment or a referral to social services are:

- Young and vulnerable mothers, who have no support mechanism—a girl herself 'in need', looked after by the local authority, recently left local authority care, or subject to a Care Order

- Extreme poverty or inadequate housing
- Social exclusion
- A mother with physical or learning disability, making it difficult for her to care for her baby
- Concern about the mental health of the mother or adult likely to have care of the child
- Substance abuse: persistent use of illegal drugs or alcohol by the mother or within her environment
- The mother lives with, or has frequent social contact with, someone who has been convicted of an offence against children
- Families where a child has previously been placed on the child protection register
- Pregnancy as a result of rape.

Making a referral

You should identify vulnerable children and decide whether to refer them to social services for assessment, consulting the supervisor of midwives and named midwife (safeguarding children) before taking any action.

Assessment of risk and significant harm

- Significant harm is defined in the Children Act (1989) as 'ill treatment or impairment of health or development'. Abuse and neglect are considered under the following categories:
  - Physical abuse
  - Emotional abuse
  - Sexual abuse
  - Neglect.
- The local authority has a duty to make enquiries, to decide whether or not any action to promote or safeguard the child's welfare is required. Each case is assessed individually. The decision as to whether or not the harm is significant is judged against what is reasonably expected for a child. A range of factors is considered and legal advice will normally be sought when the assessment determines that there is significant risk.
- Assessment under the *Framework for the Assessment of Children in Need and Their Families*[2] is child centred, so that the impact of parenting capacity, family, and environment on the child can be clearly identified. A quarter of the reasons identified refer to the child, whereas more than half relate to factors in respect of the parents.

Emergency Protection Order (EPO)

Section 44 of the Children Act (1989) allows emergency action if there is reasonable cause to believe that a child is likely to suffer harm unless the child is removed to other accommodation.

In respect of young babies, an EPO may be applied for at birth if there are concerns that the parent will remove the child. This usually applies when the baby is subject to *Safeguarding Children* proceedings and the parent(s) are threatening to remove the child.

Other powers allow the perpetrator to be removed from the home/baby's environment through an Exclusion Order attached to an EPO, or Interim Care Order.

Female genital mutilation

FGM has been illegal in the UK since 1985. The possibility of FGM is a legitimate reason for safeguarding children investigation and proceedings, as it constitutes physical injury and abuse and can take place any time from 1 week after birth to 12 years of age.

It can provide evidence for an EPO or a Care Order.

Practice points

- The safety and welfare of the child is paramount.
- The Children Act protects the rights of children within society and provides the protection of children at risk.
- ▶ You must be aware of the context of working with vulnerable families and the impact on practice.
- You have a crucial and integral role in the interprofessional team, notably in pre-birth and post-birth assessments.
- ▶ Always seek guidance and support from the named professional nurse and midwife for child protection whenever dealing with actual or possible cases.

Further reading

Department of Health (2003). *Every Child Matters*. London: DH.

1 Department of Health (2006). *Working Together to Safeguard Children*. London: DH

2 Department of Health (2000). *Framework for the Assessment of Children in Need and Their Families*. London: DH.

3 Department of Health (2004). *National Service Framework for Children, Young People and Maternity Services*. London: DH.

4 Nursing and Midwifery Council (2008). *Child Protection and the Role of the Midwife*. Advice Sheet. London: NMC. Available at: www.nmc-uk.org (accessed 12.4.10).

Part 7

Feeding

Breastfeeding

Constituents of breast milk

Colostrum

- Provides complete nutrition for the healthy term baby until lactation is established, provided frequent feeds are offered and supplements are not considered medically necessary.
- Produced in the first 3 days after delivery.
- Volume: 2–10mL daily.
- Transparent and yellow, due to high β-carotene content.
- Easily digested and absorbed.
- Energy content: 58kcal/100mL.
- Rich in immunoglobulins responsible for passive immunity.
- Contains higher levels of protein and vitamins A and K than mature milk.
- Contains lower levels of sugar and fat than mature milk.
- The presence of lacto bifidus factor provides favourable (acidic) conditions, which encourage colonization of the infant's gut with the beneficial microbe, *Lactobacillus bifidus*.
- Stimulates the passage of meconium.

Breast milk

Breast milk is a complex fluid that contains above 200 known constituents,[1] and changes to meet the needs of the infant, from:

- Colostrums to transitional then mature milk
- The beginning to the end of the feed
- Morning to evening.[2]

Nutritional composition

- *Carbohydrate*: the main type being lactose, a disaccharide.
- *Fat*: the most variable constituent. Provides 50% of the energy supplied by breast milk. Linoleic and linolenic acids are converted into long-chain polyunsaturated fatty acids, which are essential for development of the nervous system.
- *Protein*: in the form of whey protein, required for growth and energy. Consists of anti-infective factors, including lactalbumin, immunoglobulins, lactoferrin, lysozyme and other enzymes, hormones and growth factors.[3]
- *Non-protein nitrogens*: the three most important are taurine, nucleotides and carnitine. Taurine is important for bile acid conjugation, brain, and retinal development.[2] Nucleotides are important for the function of cell membranes and for normal development of the brain.[2] Carnitine plays an important part in lipid metabolism and is thought to be important in thermogenesis and nitrogen metabolism.[4]
- *Minerals and trace elements*: the major ones are sodium, calcium, phosphorus, magnesium, zinc, copper, and iron. The quantities and ratios of these elements are species specific; human and cow's milk differ significantly.
- *Vitamins*: human milk contains all the vitamins required for a term neonate, with the possible exception of vitamins D and K.

- *Enzymes*: breast milk contains at least 70 enzymes.[3] They contribute to digestion and development. Possibly the two most important are amylase and lipase. Their presence in breast milk compensates for the limited pancreatic amylase and lipase activity in the newborn and therefore aids digestion.

For a comprehensive breakdown of the composition of breast milk, see Henschel and Inch[2] and Coad.[4]

Immunological properties of breast milk

Human milk also has a non-nutritive protective role for the infant and also for protecting the breasts from infection. Important constituents are as follows.

- *Immunoglobulins*: IgA, IgG, IgM, IgD, and IgE, which are active against specific organisms, e.g. *Salmonella* species and poliovirus.
- *Cells*: B lymphocytes, T lymphocytes, macrophages, and neutrophils. The actions of these cells include:
  - Production of antibodies against specific microbes
  - Killing of infected cells
  - Production of lysozyme and activation of the immune system
  - Phagocytosis of bacteria.
- *Lacto bifidus factor*: promotes an acidic environment suitable for the growth of *Lactobacillus bifidus* and inhibits the growth of pathogenic organisms.
- *Lactoferrin*: reduces iron availability for bacterial growth, by binding to iron. It also acts as a bacteriostatic agent.
- *Binding proteins*: increase the absorption of nutrients, therefore reducing those available to be utilized by bacteria.
- Complement, lipids, fibronectin, γ-interferon, mucins, oligosaccharides, bile salt-stimulated lipase, epidermal growth factor, and many more.[4]

The immunological properties of breast milk are increased with better maternal nutrition.[5]

1 Jessen RG (ed.) (1995). *Handbook of Milk Composition*. London: Academic Press Inc.

2 Henschel D, Inch S (1996). *Breastfeeding Guide for Midwives*. Hale: Books for Midwives Press.

3 Lawson M (1992). Non-nutritional factors of human breastmilk. *Modern Midwife* **2**(6), 18–21.

4 Coad J (2001). *Anatomy and Physiology for Midwives*. Edinburgh: Mosby.

5 Chang SJ (1990). Antimicrobial proteins of maternal and cord sera and human milk in relation to maternal nutritional status. *American Journal of Clinical Nutrition* **51**, 183–7.

Advantages of breastfeeding

An ever-increasing amount of quality research has demonstrated the advantages of breastfeeding for both infant and mother.[1]

Advantages for the infant:
- Optimal nutrition
- Reduced risk of mortality from necrotizing enterocolitis and sudden infant death
- Reduced infection: gastrointestinal, respiratory, urinary tract, ear, meningitis, intractable diarrhoea
- Reduced atopic disease: eczema, asthma
- Optimal brain development
- Reduced risk of autoimmune disease
- Enhanced immunity
- Reduction in childhood obesity.

Advantages for the mother:
- Convenience, cost, and lack of contamination
- Reduced risk of maternal breast and ovarian cancer
- Reduced risk of hip fractures in women over 65
- Losing pregnancy weight gain if feeding for 6 months or longer,
  📖 see also Health risks associated with formula feeding, p. 728.

For the infant breastfeeding also may have positive effects on:
- Interpersonal relationships and sleep patterns[2]
- Reduced crying if they stay close to the mothers and breastfeed from birth.[3]

1 Coad J (2009). *Anatomy and Physiology for Midwives*, 2nd edn. Edinburgh: Mosby.

2 Renfrew M, Fisher C, Arms S (2000). *The New Bestfeeding: Getting Breastfeeding Right for you, The Illustrated Guide*. California: Celestial Arts.

3 Christensson K, Winberg J (1995). Separation distress call in the human neonate in the absence of maternal body contact. *Acta Pediatrica* **84**, 468–73.

Contraindications to breastfeeding

- *Drugs.* Most drugs will pass into breast milk in a greater or lesser degree. The majority of drugs can be taken safely, but there some are drugs where breastfeeding is contraindicated.
- *Cancer.* Anticancer treatments are normally highly toxic and will make it impossible to breastfeed without harming the baby. The mother could, if she wishes, express and discard her milk for the duration of treatment and resume breastfeeding later. If the mother has had a mastectomy, she may successfully breastfeed from the other breast. If the mother has had a lumpectomy, she should seek advice from her surgeon as she may be able to feed from the treated breast.
- *Breast surgery.* Breast reduction and augmentation are not contraindications to breastfeeding, but this depends upon the surgical techniques used. Advice should be sought from the surgeon. Following unilateral mastectomy it is perfectly possible to breastfeed using the other breast.
- *Breast injury.* Serious damage caused by burns and accidents may have caused scarring that makes breastfeeding impossible.
- *HIV infection.* HIV may be transmitted in breast milk.
  - Current WHO recommendations are that when breast milk substitutes are acceptable, feasible, affordable, sustainable, and safe, then mothers should be advised not to breastfeed. Therefore in the UK mothers would be advised against breastfeeding.[1]
  - In developing countries, or in countries, where artificial feeding is a significant cause of infant mortality, exclusive breastfeeding may be less of a risk.

1 Department of Health (2004). *HIV and Infant Feeding. Guidance from the UK Chief Medical Officers' Expert Advisory Group on AIDS.* London: DH. Available at: ℞ www.dh.gov.uk/en/ Publicationsandstatistics/Publications/PublicationsPolicyAndGuidance/DH_4089892 (accessed November 2009).

Management of breastfeeding

Initiation of breastfeeding

'All mothers should be given their baby to hold with skin-to-skin contact in an unhurried environment for an unlimited period as soon as possible after delivery. All mothers should be offered help to initiate a first breastfeed when their baby shows signs of readiness to feed'.[1]

The need to suckle is common to all mammalian young and the human baby is no different. If the mother and baby are given a peaceful, unhurried environment and the baby is placed on the mother's abdomen following delivery, it will crawl to the breast and initiate suckling.[2] A number of studies have shown that satisfying the infant's early urge to suckle positively influences the success and duration of breastfeeding.[3,4]

Skin-to-skin contact

- Initiate as soon as possible after birth.
- Place the naked, dried baby against their mother's skin.
- Place a blanket around them both to ensure neither becomes cold.
- Very small babies may also need a hat.
- If the mother so wishes, place the baby inside her nightgown.
- Provide a calm, unhurried atmosphere.
- Ensure that the mother and baby are uninterrupted during this time.
- Skin-to-skin contact should last until after the first breastfeed or until the mother chooses to end it.[1]

The midwife is responsible for ensuring that the mother and infant have a successful first feed. It is also their responsibility to provide information about breastfeeding, although the timing of this should be decided on an individual basis.

Positioning and attachment

Before commencing a feed, the comfort of the mother should be ensured. Talk the mother through the process as far as possible, to help develop her confidence and ability in breastfeeding. For the infant to suckle successfully at the breast, two processes need to be correct. These are positioning and attachment.

Positioning of the baby at the breast

Correct positioning is the secret of successful breastfeeding. Good positioning will enable the baby to achieve and maintain attachment at the breast. This, in turn, will enable the baby to feed effectively for as long as he or she needs. Good positioning is fundamental to successful breastfeeding and the prevention of problems. The mother should position the baby at the breast although some mothers may need guidance.

Principles of effective positioning

- The baby's head and body should be in a straight line.
- The mother should hold the baby's body close to hers. 'Tummy to mummy' may not be the appropriate position for all babies, as this will depend upon the shape and size of the mother's breasts.
- The baby should face the breast with the nose opposite the nipple.

- The position should be sustainable for both the mother and the baby.
  Support may sometimes be required to assist good positioning. This may be in the form of cushions to support a comfortable position for the mother or to raise the baby to the level of the breast.
  The following should be avoided:
- Holding the back of the baby's head—this will cause the baby to push their head backwards away from the breast
- Holding the breast away from the baby's nose—this can disturb the attachment and also prevent drainage from some lobes of the breast
- Holding the baby in a bottle-feeding position—this necessitates the baby to turn their head, which can cause friction to the nipple
- Taking the breast down to the baby rather than bringing the baby to the breast—this alters the shape of the breast and can cause problems, including ineffective suckling by the baby and backache for the mother.

Biological nurturing

This is a new, non-prescriptive, mother-centred breastfeeding approach that refers to a range of semi-reclined maternal breastfeeding postures and innate feeding behaviours.[5] The positions used are similar to those used in skin-to-skin contact. The baby is held instinctively and cuddled in a natural way. This can be done with the baby held long ways, sideways or slanting. The baby always has close contact with the breast and can have unrestricted access to the breast for feeding. This is a useful approach for many mothers and especially those encountering problems with latching on. The Baby Friendly Initiative (BFI) recommends that those working towards BFI accreditation should inform themselves about biological nurturing and to look for ways to incorporate this information within a framework of care that provides women with a range of skills to enable them to adapt their breastfeeding to a variety of situations.[6]

Attachment of the baby at the breast

Attachment is the term used to describe how the baby's mouth fits around the mother's nipple and areola to suckle at the breast.[7]

The three main reflexes required for a baby to attach effectively are:

- Rooting reflex
- Sucking reflex
- Swallowing reflex.

If any of these reflexes is absent, the baby will not be able to attach and feed effectively. Premature babies frequently are unable to coordinate the reflexes.

Process of attachment

In order to attach correctly, the baby needs to:

- Open their mouth in a wide gape with their tongue down and forward (Fig. 24.1)
- The lower lip, then the tongue, should be the first point of contact
- The first contact should be well away from the base of the nipple
- They should then reach up and bring their mouth over the nipple, taking in a large portion of breast tissue to form the teat (Fig. 24.2).

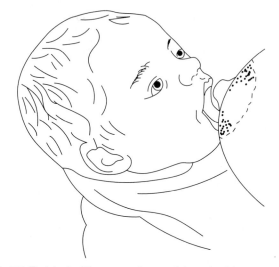

Fig. 24.1 The baby should be encouraged to open their mouth widely.

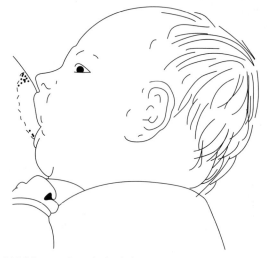

Fig. 24.2 Baby correctly attached at the breast.

Recognizing correct attachment
- The baby's mouth is wide open (wider than 100°) and they have a large mouthful of breast.
- The chin should indent the breast.
- There should be more areola visible above his top lip than below the baby's bottom lip.
- The nose should be close to the breast but not squashed.
- The cheeks are round and full.
- The whole of the lower jaw moves.
- The lower lip is curled outwards but this is not always easily visible if the baby is close to the breast.
- The mother feels a strong, and sometimes uncomfortable, 'drawing' sensation as the baby scoops up the nipple and breast tissue, draws it into his or her mouth and commences suckling.
- Swallowing may be heard but this only indicates that milk is flowing, not that the positioning and attachment are correct.

Exaggerated attachment at the breast
This is useful if:
- The baby is unable to attach and feed effectively
- The baby has a 'tongue tie' and has difficulty staying attached
- The baby has a cleft palate
- The baby is premature
- The nipples are sore or cracked and feeding is almost unbearable.

How to attain an exaggerated attachment
If the mother is going to feed from her left breast, she needs to cup the breast underneath with her left hand, keeping her fingers well away from the areola. There is always a tendency to want to move the fingers up, but this will affect the success of the attachment. The thumb should tilt the nipple back so it looks like it is pointing away from the baby. This will have the effect of making the breast under the nipple bulge forwards. The baby's bottom lip should make contact with the breast well away from the base of the nipple.

Pattern of sucking
Normally once the baby is attached he or she will take a few quick sucks at the breast which will initiate the oxytocin reflex. As the milk begins to flow and fills the mouth, the baby's sucks will become slower and deeper. The baby will pause occasionally. If a baby continues to take frequent short sucks or there are audible 'smacking' noises as the baby sucks, this is a good indication that the attachment is incorrect.

Recognizing incorrect attachment
- The mouth is not wide open.
- The bottom lip is not curled outwards, or it is less curled than the upper lip.
- There is the same amount of areola below the bottom lip as above the top lip.
- There is a gap between the breast and the chin.
- The nose is either squashed into the breast or a wide distance from the breast.

- The cheeks are drawn in as the baby sucks.
- The breast tissue is puckered.
- The breast tissue moves in and out of the baby's mouth as he feeds.
- The baby makes little sucks as if he is sucking a dummy.
- There is no change in the rhythm of feeding.
- The baby will show frustration at not having his hunger satisfied, by either becoming sleepy and ceasing to suck or by coming off the breast and crying.
- The colour of the stools may change back to green/brown from yellow.

Results of ineffective attachment

The mother may:
- Feel pain when feeding
- Experience sore nipples, especially cracks across the tip of the nipple or at the base of the nipple
- Experience engorgement of the breast.

The baby may:
- Appear unsatisfied
- Cry a lot and want frequent feeds, or may feed for protracted lengths of time
- Receive insufficient milk and fail to gain or even lose weight
- Become frustrated and refuse to feed
- Receive adequate nourishment for the first few weeks by feeding frequently if the oxytocin reflex works well but then will fail to thrive.

Measures shown to enhance breastfeeding success

A comprehensive systematic review conducted by NICE[8] has identified what practices enable a mother to breastfeed for longer, and these should be used in conjunction with the following information.

Baby-led feeding

Baby-led feeding, or demand feeding, simply consists of feeding the baby whenever he or she wishes and for as long as he or she wishes.

There is substantial evidence that the timing and duration of breastfeeds should be responsive to the needs of the baby.[9] Babies will feed at the breast for very different lengths of time if left undisturbed, and it is thought that the length of a feed is determined by the rate of milk transfer between mother and baby.[10]

Limiting the duration of the feed or removing a baby from the breast before they finish spontaneously, may prevent the baby from receiving adequate calorific intake causing failure to gain weight despite frequent feeds and an apparently good milk supply.

Unrestricted frequency of feeds is also advocated. Observation studies have demonstrated that the frequency of feeds in the first few weeks appears to be unpredictable and random, varying between 1h and 8h. Babies who regulate the length and frequency of feeds gain weight more quickly.

Advice to the mother to restrict or limit suckling time or frequency at the breast will not only do no good, but could do harm. However, a baby that has protracted feeds without coming off spontaneously, or a baby that feeds very frequently, may be attached to the breast incorrectly.

A baby that is poorly attached can also cause nipple trauma, which may give rise to engorgement and/or mastitis.[11]

Night feeds
The advantages of night feeds include:
- Prolactin levels are higher at night, and a breastfeed at night will result in a greater prolactin surge than would occur with a feed given during the day. Night feeds therefore ensure good milk production.[12]
- Exclusive breastfeeding that incorporates night feeds raises prolactin levels which, in turn, inhibits luteinizing hormone release, this prevents ovulation.[12]
- Frequent feeds, including night feeds, help to prevent/reduce engorgement when the milk first comes in.
- There is a soporific effect on the mother, which improves the quality of sleep. This results from the release of dopamine, which is believed to be involved in the mechanism of oxytocin release.[13]

Rooming-in
Rooming-in, which allows mother and babies to remain together for 24h a day, has been shown to:
- Improve breastfeeding outcomes, especially duration; this is partly because rooming-in facilitates demand feeding[14]
- Improve mother–baby relationship, regardless of feeding method
- Be preferable to nursery care for both mother and baby.[14]
  Common reasons to not room in, e.g. it interferes with the mother's sleep, do not appear to be valid.[14]

Staff training
Healthcare professionals who have not been trained in breastfeeding management cannot be expected to give mothers effective guidance and to provide skilled counselling. It is necessary to increase their skills to enable their knowledge to be used appropriately. Education and training sessions need to incorporate elements that enable health professionals to address bias that will hinder breastfeeding.

In-service training needs to be mandatory to be successful and requires a strong policy supported by senior staff.[14]

Inconsistent or conflicting information and advice disempowers women, reducing their self-confidence and ability to breastfeed successfully.[15]

Breastfeeding and growth monitoring
NICE[16] recommends that GPs, paediatricians, midwives health visitors, and community nursery nurses should:
- As a minimum, ensure babies are weighed (naked) at birth and at 5 and 10 days, as part of an overall assessment of feeding. After this healthy babies should be weighed (naked) no more than fortnightly and at 2, 3, 4, and 8–10 months in their first year. Ongoing weekly weighing is unnecessary for healthy babies who give no cause for concern. Unnecessary weighing may lead to an inappropriate intervention and undermine parents' confidence.
- Ensure infants are weighed using digital scales which are maintained and calibrated annually, in line with medical devices standards (spring scales are inaccurate and should not be used.

- It is important that support staff are trained to weigh infants and young children and to record the data accurately in the child health record held by the parents.

Breastfeeding patterns of growth
- Breastfed babies show a different pattern of growth from formula fed babies.
- Growth rate is not constant and slowed growth is not always indicative of growth failure.
- Breastfed infants grow more quickly in the first few weeks and more slowly from about 4–5 months than formula fed infants. The difference is on average ½ to 1 centile channel.[17]

New UK growth charts, based on breastfed babies, were introduced in May 2009 to plot the weight, height, and head circumference of children from birth to 4 years of age.[18] These charts should be used for all new births and new referrals to health professionals. The UK90 Growth charts will continue to be used for children born before this date and for children over 4 years. Fact sheets about the new charts are available at the Royal College of Paediatrics and Child Health website (⌘ www.growthcharts. rcpch.ac.uk).

Weight loss of more than 10% from birthweight should be a cause for concern. Check that the baby is having plenty of wet and dirty nappies. Poor urine and stool output indicates the need for the baby to be weighed naked on digital scales even if outside the recommended weighing guidelines. A breastfeeding history should be taken and a breastfeeding assessment form recorded prior to advice being given for strategies to improve feeding. Weight loss of 15% or more requires urgent investigation, paediatric referral, and experienced breastfeeding support.

1 UNICEF UK Baby Friendly Initiative. *Step 4—Help Mothers Initiate Breastfeeding Soon After Birth.* Available at: www.babyfriendly.org.uk/page.asp?page=64 (accessed November 2009).

2 Righard L, Frantz K (1992). *Delivery Self Attachment.* California: Video Giddes Productions.

3 Perez-Escamilla R, Pollitt E, Lonnerdal B, Dewey KG (1994). Infant feeding policies in maternity wards and their effect on breastfeeding success: An analytical overview. *American Journal of Public Health* **84**(1), 89–97.

4 Righard L, Alade MO (1990). Effects of delivery room routines on the success of first breast-feed. *Lancet* **336**, 1105–7.

5 Colson S (2007). A non-prescriptive recipe for breastfeeding. *Practising Midwife* **10**(8), 42, 44, 46–47.

6 Baby Friendly Initiative (2009). *The Baby Friendly Initiative's Position on Biological Nurturing: Statement 18 February 2009.* Available at: ℘ www.babyfriendly.org.uk/items/item_detail. asp?item=558 (accessed November 2009).

7 UNICEF (2004). *Breastfeeding Management Course Workbook.* London: UNICEF.

8 Renfrew M, Dyson L, Wallace L, D'Souza L, McCormick F, Spiby H (2005). *Breastfeeding for Longer—What Works?* Systematic review summary. London: NHS National Institute for Health and Clinical Excellence. Available at: http://www.nice.org.uk/nicemedia/pdf/breastfeeding_ summary.pdf (accessed 19.1.11).

9 Renfrew MJ, Woolridge MW, McGill HR (2000). *Enabling Women to Breastfeed: A Review of Practices Which Promote or Inhibit Breastfeeding—With Evidence-Based Guidance For Practice.* London: The Stationary Office.

10 Woolridge MW, Baum JD, Drewett RF (1982). Individual patterns of human milk intake during breastfeeding. *Early Human Development* **7**, 265–72.

11 Henschel D, Inch S (1996). *Breastfeeding: a Guide for Midwives.* Hale: Books for Midwives Press.

12 Howie PW, McNeilly AS, Houston MJ, Cook A, Boyle H (1982). Fertility after childbirth: Infant feeding patterns, basal prolactin levels and postpartum ovulation. *Clinical Endocrinology* **17**, 315–22.

13 Bourne MA (1982). Sleep in the puerperium. *Midwives Chronicle and Nursing Notes*, March, 91.

14 World Health Organization (1998). *Evidence for the Ten Steps to Successful Breastfeeding.* Geneva: WHO.

15 Simmons V (2002). Exploring inconsistent breastfeeding advice. *British Journal of Midwifery* **10**(10), 616–19.

16 National Institute for Health and Clinical Excellence (2008). *PH11 Maternal and Child Nutrition: Guidance.* London: NICE.

17 Cole TJ, Paul AA, Whitehead RG (2002). Weight reference charts for British long-term breastfed infants. *Acta Paediatrica* **91**(12)1296–1300.

18 Royal College of Paediatric and Child Health. Available at: ℘ www.rcpch.ac.uk/Research/ Growth-Charts (accessed November 2009).

The 10 steps to successful breastfeeding[1]

The 'Ten Steps to Successful Breastfeeding' are the foundation of the WHO/UNICEF Baby Friendly Hospital Initiative (BFHI). They are a summary of the maternity practices necessary to support breastfeeding. The BFHI was developed to promote the implementation of the second operational target of the Innocenti Declaration.[2]

Every facility providing maternity services and care for newborn infants should:

- Have a written breastfeeding policy that is communicated routinely to all health care staff
- Train all health care staff in skills necessary to implement the policy
- Inform all pregnant women about the benefits and management of breastfeeding
- Help mothers initiate breastfeeding within half an hour of birth
- Show mothers how to breastfeed, and how to maintain lactation even if they are separated from their infants
- Give newborn infants no food or drink other than breast milk, unless *medically* indicated
- Practice rooming-in: allow mothers and infants to remain together 24h a day
- Encourage breastfeeding on demand
- Give no artificial teats or pacifiers (also called dummies or soothers) to breastfed infants
- Foster the establishment of breastfeeding support groups and refer mothers to them on discharge from the hospital or clinic.

Evidence in support of the above steps can be found in the WHO publication *Evidence for the Ten Steps to Successful Breastfeeding.*[2]

The seven-point plan for the protection, promotion, and support of breastfeeding in community healthcare settings

All providers of community healthcare should:

- Have a written breastfeeding policy that is communicated routinely to all healthcare staff
- Train all staff involved in the care of mothers and babies in the skills necessary to implement the policy
- Inform all pregnant women about the benefits and management of breastfeeding
- Support mothers to initiate and maintain breastfeeding
- Encourage exclusive and continued breastfeeding, with appropriately timed introduction of complementary foods
- Provide a welcoming atmosphere for breastfeeding families
- Promote cooperation between healthcare staff, breastfeeding support groups, and the local community.

The UNICEF UK Baby Friendly Initiative University Standards programme

This is an accreditation programme aimed at university departments responsible for midwifery and health visitor/public health nurse education.

The purpose of the programme is to ensure that newly qualified midwives and health visitors are equipped with the knowledge and skills needed to support breastfeeding effectively. Accreditation is awarded to an individual course, not to the institution itself. Higher education institutions (HEIs) can apply for accreditation for each of the courses they provide for the training of midwives or health visitors/public health nurses.

1 World Health Organization (1989). *Protecting, Promoting and Supporting Breastfeeding: The Special Role of the Maternity Services*. Geneva: WHO.

2 World Health Organization (1998). *Evidence for the Ten Steps to Successful Breastfeeding, Division of Child Health and Development*. Geneva: WHO.

Support for breastfeeding

The support the woman receives from her partner, family members, friends, health professionals, and support networks can affect the uptake and continuance of breastfeeding. Emotional support as well as practical support is needed to empower mothers to breastfeed successfully. Various levels of support may be required by breastfeeding mothers, depending upon their social circumstances. Caregivers may find it easier to support breastfeeding mothers effectively if they have had the opportunity to come to terms with their own breastfeeding experiences.[1]

Partners

- The male partner has a strong influence upon the choice of infant feeding method.[2]
- The partner's positive attitude to breastfeeding is important for the mother initiating and continuing to breastfeed.[3]
- Women need to talk to their partners antenatally about breastfeeding, as a woman's guesses about her partner's ideas of breastfeeding have often been found to be inaccurate.[4]
- Partners need to be informed of the benefits of breastfeeding for both baby and mother.
- Partners should be involved in antenatal preparation for breastfeeding whenever possible.
- Partners are invaluable in providing emotional and practical support for breastfeeding mothers.
- Partners wishing to undertake shared care of the baby should be encouraged to look at alternatives to feeding, e.g. bathing the infant, skin-to-skin contact.

Family and friends

- Family and friends exert a strong influence on a mother's decision about breastfeeding.
- About one in four mothers are helped by a relative or friend when they have problems breastfeeding.
- First-time mothers are more likely to turn to relatives and friends for assistance.
- Breastfeeding mothers who were breastfed themselves are more likely to be breastfeeding at 4 weeks than those who had been bottle fed.
- Breastfeeding mothers whose friends mostly bottle fed are more likely to discontinue in the first 2 weeks postnatally.[5]

Peer support

NICE[6] recommends that there should be easily accessible breastfeeding peer support programmes and that appropriately trained breastfeeding peer supporters should be part of a multidisciplinary team. It is also recommends that breastfeeding peer supporters should contact mothers directly within 48h of their transfer to the community and offer them ongoing support according to their individual needs. This could be via telephone, texting, face-to-face, local support groups or the internet.

Breastfeeding peer support projects have been shown to:
- Demonstrate a positive trend towards increasing continuation of breastfeeding
- Help mothers at a time when they were strongly considering stopping breastfeeding
- Empower those living in socially excluded communities.[5]

Specialist infant feeding advisors

Many maternity units now employ specialist infant feeding advisers. Their role varies depending upon the needs of the local population and the requirements of the maternity units. There is very little research related to the role of the specialist feeding advisors but they can improve the care and support breastfeeding women receive by:
- Developing and monitoring infant feeding policies and guidelines
- Providing in service training for health professionals and support workers
- Auditing infant feeding practices
- Ensuring up-to-date evidence-based practice related to infant feeding
- Ensuring that leaflets and information for women are accurate, in line with breastfeeding policies and do not advertise formula milk companies
- Organizing and running breastfeeding workshops for women in the antenatal period
- Organizing and running breastfeeding drop-in services
- Supporting health professionals in their clinical area
- Supervising health professionals who are undertaking breastfeeding courses e.g. BFI Breastfeeding Management Course
- Taking the lead role when maternity units and communities are working towards the BFI Award
- Liaising with local and national organizations to promote, protect, and support breastfeeding
- Providing a contact person for liaising with formula milk companies.

Their role is not to deskill the health professional, by taking over the carer role for breastfeeding women, but to develop their skills and increase their knowledge base to ensure that all breastfeeding women are provided with evidence-based, sensitive, and consistent information and support.

Voluntary groups

There are a number of breastfeeding voluntary organizations, or organizations that have expertise in supporting breastfeeding mothers in special circumstances in the UK, including:
- National Childbirth Trust
- Breastfeeding Network
- Twins and Multiple Births Association
- La Leche League (Great Britain)
- Baby Milk Action
- Association of Breastfeeding Mothers.

These organizations supply information and support, by telephone and in leaflets and books. Mothers should be offered leaflets or cards giving details about support organizations prior to leaving the postnatal ward.

1 Smales M (1998). Working with breastfeeding mothers: the psychosocial context. In: Clement S (ed.) *Psychological Perspective on Pregnancy and Childbirth.* Edinburgh: Churchill Livingstone.

2 Losch M, Dungy CI, Russell D, Dusdicker LB (1995). Impact of attitudes on maternal decisions regarding infant feeding. *Journal of Pediatrics* **126**(4), 507–14.

3 Fraley K, Freed GL, Schanler RJ (1992). Attitudes of expectant fathers regarding breast-feeding. *Pediatrics* **90**, 224–7.

4 Freed GL, Fraley K, Schanler RJ (1993). Accuracy of expectant mothers predictions of fathers' attitudes regarding breastfeeding. *Journal of Family Practice* **37**(2), 148–52.

5 Bolling K, Grant C, Hamlyn B, Thornton A (2007). *Infant Feeding Survey 2005.* London: The Information Centre.

6 National Institute of Health and Clinical Excellence (2008). *PH11 Maternal and Child Nutrition: Guidance.* London: NICE.

Practices shown to be detrimental to successful breastfeeding

Inconsistent information

Despite efforts to ensure that appropriate advice and information are given to breastfeeding mothers, there is still evidence that, for many mothers, difficulty in establishing breastfeeding is compounded by inconsistent advice.[1] Conflicting advice does exist and persist, mostly as inaccurate information and practice.

Conflicting advice and information:
- Reinforce a mother's lack of self-confidence in her ability to breastfeed
- Disempower women.[2]

In order to prevent inconsistent advice, midwives need to:
- Have in-depth knowledge and understanding of the physiology of lactation
- Be able to communicate effectively
- Acknowledge their own subjective bias
- Provide consistent information and support in line with the best available evidence.[2]

An authoritarian approach to communication is unhelpful and even detrimental.

Use of pacifiers

The use of pacifiers (dummies) has become a widespread cultural practice in the UK. They are used to settle, soothe, or otherwise occupy a fretful or distressed baby.

Reasons given for using pacifiers have included:[3]
- Mothers who used them were more sensitive to their baby's crying than mothers who did not use them
- Mothers used them to space feeds, which they perceived to be too frequent
- They were used in the past to reduce the number of breastfeeds as part of the weaning process.

The use of pacifiers has been implicated in:
- Reducing the duration of breastfeeding[4]
- Increasing the risk of otitis media[5]
- Oral candida infection[6]
- Reduced jaw muscle activity[7]
- Reduced intellectual attainment[8]
- Greater incidence of abnormal jaw development.[9]

No research to date explores the effect of bottle teats and/or pacifiers on the initiation of breastfeeding. However, there is concern by health professionals that their use may adversely affect initiation and establishment of breastfeeding. Conversely some evidence suggests that the use of pacifiers can reduce the incidence of cot death.[10]

The use of nipple shields

The use of nipple shields is sometimes advocated as treatment for sore nipples; however, little evidence is currently available to support this practice.

The use of nipple shields:[11]
• Has been found to be unacceptable to mothers
• May lead to a conditioned rejection of the breast by the baby
• May adversely affect the mother's milk supply.

Clinical experience suggests that judicious use of a thin silicone shield may benefit mothers with severely traumatized nipples, but they should never be used as a substitute for teaching the mother how to correct the problem of sore nipples by improving positioning and attachment. They should never be used in the early postnatal days before the milk has 'come in'.

Supplementary feeding

Supplementary feeding is the practice of giving extra feeds of formula, glucose, or water. A recent study found that 33% of breastfed babies were given supplementary feeds while in hospital.[12] This study also found that breastfeeding mothers whose babies were given bottles were more likely to discontinue breastfeeding in the first 2 weeks postnatally than were other mothers.

Supplementary feeds have been associated with:[4,12,13]
• Interference with the supply and demand mechanism, therefore reducing milk supply
• Interference with the development of normal immunological mechanisms
• Allergic conditions in some babies
• Reactive hypoglycaemia
• 'Nipple confusion'
• Reduced maternal confidence.

Extra fluids

Giving extra fluids, either in the form of water or dextrose, to babies with jaundice has not been shown to reduce peak serum bilirubin levels, and may, in fact, cause levels to rise by reducing the milk intake and therefore delaying the evacuation of meconium.[14]

In a breastfed baby, filling the stomach with water will reduce the number of feeds and interfere with the establishment of breastfeeding. Women whose babies are given extra fluids are more likely to discontinue breastfeeding.

1 Health Visitor Association and the Royal College of Midwives (1995). *Invest in Breast Together*. Milton Keynes: Health Visitor Association and the Royal College of Midwives.

2 Simmons V (2002). Exploring inconsistent breastfeeding advice. *British Journal of Midwifery* **10**(10), 616–19.

3 Victora CG, Tomasi E, Olinto MTA, Barros FC (1997). Pacifier use and short breastfeeding duration: cause, consequence or coincidence? *Pediatrics* **99**(3), 445–53.

4 World Health Organization (1998). *Evidence for the Ten Steps to Successful Breastfeeding*. Geneva: WHO.

5 Watase S, Mourino A, Tipton G (1998). An analysis of malocclusion in children with otitis media. *Pediatric Dentistry* **20**(5), 327–30.

6 Darwazeh AM, al-Bashir A (1995). Oral candidal flora in health infants. *Journal of Oral Pathology and Medicine* **24**(8), 361–4.

7 Sakashita R. Kamegai T, Inoue N (1996). Masseter muscle activity in bottle feeding with the chewing type bottle teat: evidence from electromyographs. *Early Human Development* **45**, 83–92.

8 Gale CR, Martyn CN (1996). Breastfeeding, dummy use, and adult intelligence. *Lancet* **347**(9008), 1072–5.

9 Ogaard B, Larsson E, Lindsten R (1994). The effect of sucking habits, cohort, sex, intercanine arch widths, and breast or bottle feeding on posterior crossbite in Norwegian and Swedish 3-year-old children. *American Journal of Orthodontics and Dentofacial Orthopedics* **106**(2), 161–6.

10 FSID (2009) Factfile 2. Research background to Reduce the risk of cot death advice by the Foundation for the Study of Infact Deaths. ℘ http://fsid.org.uk/Document.Doc?id=42 (accessed 20.1.2011).

11 Royal College of Midwives (2002). *Successful Breastfeeding*. Edinburgh: Churchill Livingstone.

12 Bolling K, Grant C, Hamlyn B, Thornton A (2007). *Infant Feeding Survey 2005*. London: The Information Centre.

13 Henschel D, Inch S (1996). *Breastfeeding: A guide for Midwives*. Hale, Cheshire: Books for Midwives Press.

14 Nicoll A, Ginsburg R, Tripp JH (1982). Supplementary feeding and jaundice in newborns. *Acta Paediatrica Scandinavica* **71**, 759–761.

Expression of breast milk

Why express?

Expression of breast milk should be taught to all mothers as it helps them to understand how the breasts work. It can aid the mother's understanding of effective attachment and may help her to recognize and overcome many breastfeeding complications.[1] Health professionals should be able to teach the skills of both hand expression and mechanical expression to breastfeeding mothers.

Expression of breast milk can be helpful in a variety of situations.[1]

- General breast comfort:
  - To relieve discomfort from overfull breasts if a feed has been missed
  - To prevent leakage if mother and child are apart
  - To maintain healthy skin or to assist healing: if damage has occurred to the nipple, a small amount of breast milk may be applied to the nipple and areola.
- To assist a baby to breastfeed:
  - Expressing a small amount of breast milk will encourage a reluctant baby to breastfeed by enabling him to smell and taste the milk
  - By softening an overfull or engorged breast, enabling attachment
  - Milk may be expressed gently into the baby's mouth if he or she has a weak suck.
- To prevent or relieve breast conditions:
  - Overfull breasts due to a feed being missed
  - Engorgement
  - Blocked duct
  - Mastitis.
- To stimulate milk supply:
  - When mother and baby are separated or baby unable to suckle
  - If additional stimulus is required to increase or induce lactation.
- To maintain milk supply:
  - When mother and baby are separated, e.g. hospitalization, return to work
  - When the mother has to suspend breastfeeding temporarily, e.g. due to medication that may be harmful to the baby.

Methods of expression

Hand or manual expression

- Hand expression is usually gentler than using a pump, it can be undertaken anywhere and no/minimal equipment is needed.
- Hand expression requires skill, and some mothers find it difficult and prefer to use a pump.
- The risk of cross-infection is reduced with hand expression as less equipment is required.
- Hand expression is useful as a self-help method if blocked ducts, engorgement, or mastitis occurs.
- Inform the mother that when she first starts to express her breasts only small amounts will be expressed, but with practice it will become easier and she will be able to express more.

How to hand express

The mother should:
- Wash her hands
- Use a wide-mouthed sterile container to collect the milk
- Sit comfortably in a warm, peaceful and relaxing environment if possible
- Lean very slightly forward.
- Encourage the let-down reflex by:
  - Relaxing with a warm drink, music, or TV
  - Being near the baby or a photo of the baby
  - Warming the breasts
  - Gently pulling or rolling the nipples
  - Gently massaging the breasts by stroking with the finger tips, rolling with the knuckles, or using circular movements.

The mother should then:
- Make a 'C' shape with her thumb above and her fingers below the breast near the edge of the areola but away from the nipple (Fig. 24.3)
- Gently press her thumb and fingers together, release the fingers and repeat in a rhythmic pattern (Fig. 24.4)
- Sometimes it is helpful to press inwards and back towards the chest wall while squeezing
- The fingers should be repositioned at intervals to allow drainage from all the lactiferous ducts.

The length of time for expressing depends on the reason why the mother is expressing. If she wants to express all the milk she can from the breast, she should continue until the flow subsides.

The mother may express from the second breast by repeating the above process. A mother who wishes to express as much milk as possible should continue to switch between breasts for as long as milk is being obtained.[1,2]

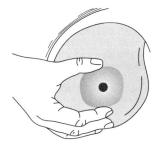

Fig. 24.3 Make a c-shape with finger and thumb.

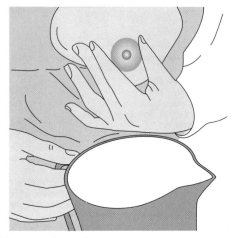

Fig. 24.4 Expressing breast milk.

Breast pumps

Mothers who use a mechanical pump may find they are able to express larger volumes, especially if using an electrical pump.[1]

Numerous pumps are available to hire or buy, but they fall into three types:

- *A hand pump* that is mainly for relieving the breasts. These are usually of simple design and work on a simple vacuum principle. They are not suitable for expressing milk which is to be stored and given to a baby because they can not be sterilized effectively.[1]
- *Battery-operated pumps* vary widely in design, all produce a rhythmic vacuum, although some are also designed to give a degree of compression. Some mothers find these pumps useful if they are expressing on a regular basis, as they are less tiring than a hand pump.
- *Electric pumps* are usually heavy and bulky and therefore less portable. As they are efficient, they are commonly used within hospitals, but they are usually shared by several mothers and therefore maintenance and cleanliness are essential. Ideally all mothers should be given their own equipment for the machine, which should include a collection beaker, tubing, and sterilizing equipment.[1]

Using breast pumps

Women may find that their let-down reflex is more difficult to induce with a pump than with hand expressing. Massaging the breast and hand expressing for a short time prior to using the pump may help. A photograph, item of the baby's clothing or toy may also help.

Dual pumping

Dual pumping is when both breasts are expressed at the same time. This can be done either by hand expression or using a pump. It has been shown to shorten the time required for expressing and increases the mother's prolactin levels.[1] If using a pump, a Y coupling is required. It is particularly helpful if a large amount of milk is required, e.g. with twins and multiple births, or if there is a need to increase the milk supply rapidly.

Principles of expression

Establishment of lactation:
- Expression should commence as soon as possible after the birth.
- Express frequently, 6–8 times in 24h, more if possible.
- Express at least once during the night.
- Avoid set patterns of expressing, instead aim to imitate the irregular feeding pattern adopted by most babies.

If lactation is already established, and there is a need to express to maintain lactation because of separation of the mother and baby, the last three of the above principles should be applied. It is important to remember that expressing does not provide the same stimulus to the breast as the baby suckling, and the milk supply may begin to diminish. If this is the case, the mother should be encouraged to increase the number of expressions.

To increase the milk supply, for example if the baby is not feeding sufficiently or if the mother wishes to build up a milk supply before returning to work, the mother should be encouraged to:
- Express after and/or between feeds or, if the baby is not feeding, to increase the number of expressions
- Express at least once in the night
- Avoid set patterns of expressing; rather, expressing whenever she can. It takes appropriately 24h for the supply to increase.

Recommendations for storage of breast milk

For use in the home[3]
- Fresh breast milk can be:
  - Kept for up to 5h at room temperature
  - Stored in a refrigerator at a temperature 2–4°C for up to 5 days.
- If milk is not to be used within 24h, freezing is recommended:
  - Milk can be kept frozen in an ice-making compartment for 2 weeks
  - Milk can be kept safely up to 6 months in a domestic freezer.
- Any plastic container that can be sterilized and made airtight, is suitable for storing breast milk. Many commercial products are available.[3]

Storing breast milk for use in hospital
- Some types of plastic are not suitable for storing breast milk for preterm or sick babies.
- Use up-to-date guidelines, e.g. UK Association for Milk Banking Guidelines,[4] for advising mothers which containers to use and how to store the milk.
- Hospitals often pasteurize milk for use in a milk bank but this is not usually necessary if the milk is for the mother's own baby.

Reheating expressed breast milk at home

- Frozen milk can be:
  - Thawed slowly in a refrigerator but must be used within 24h or discarded
  - Thawed at room temperature and used immediately
- Frozen milk should never be thawed or heated in a microwave.[5]
- Some prefer to warm the milk to body temperature.
- Never re-freeze breast milk.

1 UNICEF UK (2004). *Breastfeeding Management Course*. London: UNICEF UK Baby Friendly Initiative.

2 Breastfeeding Network (2004). *Expressing and Storing Breast Milk Leaflet*. Paisley: Breastfeeding Network.

3 UNICEF/Department of Health (2007). *Off to the Best Start*. London: DH. Available at: ℘ www. dh.gov.uk/publications (accessed 12.4.10).

4 United Kingdom Association for Milk Banking (2001). *Guidelines for the Collection, Storage and Handling of Breastmilk for a Mother's Own Baby in Hospital*. London: United Kingdom Association for Milk Banking (UKAMB), Queen Charlotte's and Chelsea Hospital.

5 Sigman, M. Burke KI, Swarner OW, Shavlik GW (1989). Effects of microwaving human milk. *Journal of the American Dietetic Association* **89**(5), 690–2.

Breastfeeding and returning to work

Mothers who are returning to work may find this a stressful time, especially if they are breastfeeding. The longer a mother breastfeeds, the more benefits there are for both mother and baby. Mothers may wish to consider different working options, e.g. part-time work, job sharing, working different hours, working partly at home. Health professionals should give mothers information and assistance to try to make the return to work as easy as possible.

Three practical ways to combine breastfeeding and work are:
• Expression of breast milk while at work
• Childcare near the mother's place of work
• Partial breastfeeding.

There are advantages and disadvantage to all three options and it will depend upon the mother's circumstances which option is most appropriate for her.

If the mother decides to express breast milk at work, she will need to:
• Practise expressing milk prior to returning to work (if possible she should wait until breastfeeding is fully established, when the baby is about 2 months old). The expressed breast milk (EBM) can be stored in the freezer to give the mother a back-up supply
• Ensure she has equipment for expressing at work, which will include a pump, storage containers, sterilizing equipment, spare breast-pads, and a cool bag for transportation (many commercial products are being produced now to make this easier for mothers)
• Consider dual pumping, as this reduces the time required to express
• Have spare batteries and vacuum seals at work if using a pump
• Ask at work for the following facilities:
  • Use of a room that is warm, clean, and has a lockable door
  • Facilities for hand washing
  • Somewhere clean to leave equipment for sterilizing
  • Use of a fridge to store EBM
  • A low comfortable chair
• Store milk safely.

The law relating to breastfeeding at work

In the UK, mothers do not have statutory rights to paid breastfeeding breaks, but do have certain legal protection under the health and safety laws. While breastfeeding, she and her baby have special health and safety protection, the same as that for a pregnant woman. However, to use this protection she must inform her employers in writing. Employers are also obliged to provide 'suitable facilities' where breastfeeding employees can 'rest'. If the woman is working with hazardous substances, the employer should take appropriate actions to make the job safe. If this is not possible, an alternative job should be offered or she should be suspended on full pay.[1]

When to express

This will depend upon the individual and the type of work, but also depends upon the employer's attitude. It is not essential to have regular breaks, as it is better to aim to imitate the irregular feeding pattern that most babies adopt.

Childcare near the mother's workplace

If the baby is in childcare near the mother's place of work, the mother could visit the baby during breaks and breastfeed normally. Although this is the best option, it may prove difficult to demand feed around working hours, and the baby may be upset by the mother coming and going.

Partial breastfeeding

This is when the mother breastfeeds normally when at home but the baby receives formula milk while the mother is at work. This can work very well when the mother is unable to express or visit the baby. However, her milk supply may diminish and she may still have to continue with formula feeds for those feeds that are normally missed when working. Partial breastfeeding is not possible before the milk supply is fully established at around 2 months.

1 Maternity Action (2009). *Information Sheet: continuing to breastfeed when you return to work*. London: Maternity Action. Available at: ℘ www.maternityaction.org.uk/workingparents.html (accessed 12.4.10).

Discontinuation of breastfeeding

The DH recommends exclusive breastfeeding for the first 6 months (26 weeks) of an infant's life, and 6 months is the recommended age for the introduction of solid foods for infants.[1] However, the time when mothers discontinue breastfeeding is very variable and depends upon many factors. Sudden cessation should be avoided if possible to maximize the mother's comfort and to avoid mastitis. The mother should be advised to slowly drop one feed at a time, allow several days before dropping a further feed, and to feed on alternate days when down to one feed. This helps the milk supply to adjust and allows the milk to diminish naturally. There are circumstances that need special consideration.

Mother going into hospital
- If possible, arrange for the baby to accompany the mother and continue feeding.
- A family carer may need to assist the mother with baby care if the hospital can not provide assistance.
- If this is known in advance, the mother can express and freeze EBM, especially if she is to undergo a general anaesthetic.
- The mother needs to ask about equipment and facilities for expressing, sterilizing, and storing breast milk. She may need to take in her own pump.
- If a mother has to stop feeding temporarily due to medication, the supply can be maintained by expressing.
- The mother should ask if safe alternative drugs are available.

Baby going into hospital
- If possible, the mother should accompany the baby.
- If not possible, e.g. because of other children at home, the mother should express and send the milk to the hospital.
- If the baby is unable to suckle and/or receive breast milk, the mother should express to maintain the supply and reduce the risk of mastitis.
- If stopping breastfeeding, this should be done gradually.

Sudden cessation, due to cot death or illness
- A small amount should be expressed, just to relieve pressure.
- Support the breasts well with a firm bra, binding has not been shown to help and may increase the risk of mastitis.
- Use cold compresses.
- Mild analgesics, e.g. paracetamol, may help relieve the discomfort.
- Slightly reduce fluids, but do not drastically reduce fluids as this may temporarily increase the supply.

---

1 Department of Health (2004). *Infant Feeding Recommendations*. London: HMSO.

Breastfeeding problems

A problem-solving approach should be taken when managing common breastfeeding problems. This should include;

- Listening to the mother
- Taking a breastfeeding history. Use of the UNICEF BFI Breastfeeding Assessment Form is advised[1]
- Observing a breastfeed
- Offering information on appropriate solutions and alternatives to enable a mother to make her own decision
- Offering the ongoing support of a breastfeeding peer supporter.

Sleepy/non-feeding baby

There are a number of reasons why a baby will not feed in the first few days following delivery and these include:

- Drugs given to the mother in labour, e.g. pethidine and epidural
- Unpleasant experience at the breast, e.g. force applied to the head when fixing
- Frustration as a result of not obtaining nourishment due to poor fixing at the breast
- Jaundice
- If lethargic when awake the baby may not be receiving adequate nutrition
- Baby is ill.

Actions

The first two actions should be addressed with all babies and the following actions acted upon as relevant to the history.

- A breastfeeding history should be taken to see if the reason can be identified.
- A breastfeed should be observed and positioning and attachment improved.
- If necessary wake the baby and give additional feeds (EBM or colostrum if possible) until the situation has improved.
- If the baby is jaundiced encourage the baby to feed as frequently as possible.
- Feed the baby when he or she is half asleep.
- Encourage the baby to stay awake whilst feeding by keeping the baby cooler during feeds.
- Switch feed—that is change the baby from one breast to the second as the baby becomes sleepy.
- Change the baby's position while feeding to stimulate the baby to suckle more vigorously.
- Encourage mother to adopt skin-to-skin as much as possible—do not offer the breast let the baby find it.
- Change nappy to wake the baby.
- Bath the baby.
- Sit in a warm bath to feed the baby.

Sore/cracked nipples

Breastfeeding should be comfortable and pain-free although some mothers may experience some discomfort at the beginning of the feed for the first few days. This usually resolves spontaneously. However, 24% of mothers who discontinue breastfeeding in the first week postnatally do so because of sore or cracked nipples.[2] It is very likely that the majority of sore nipples could be prevented and treated by correct positioning and attachment of the baby at the breast.

The causes of sore and cracked nipples include:

- Poor positioning and attachment of the baby at the breast.
- Engorgement, which may prevent good attachment.
- Physiological causes that include a baby with a short tongue or tongue tie, a high palate or a mismatch between the size of the mothers nipple and the baby's mouth.
- Pulling the baby off the breast without first breaking the seal between the baby's mouth and the mother's breast.
- The use of substances that may trigger a skin reaction or increase its susceptibility to damage, e.g. soap and scented bath products, antiseptic sprays.
- Thrush infections (📖 see Candida (thrush) infection, p. 696).
- Expressing too vigorously with a breast pump.

Action

- Observe a feed and assist the mother to attain better positioning and attachment.
- Provide emotional support to the mother.
- If engorgement is present, express a small amount of milk to soften the area immediately behind the nipple area.
- If the baby has a short tongue, or tongue-tie an exaggerated fix may help (📖 see Exaggerated attachment at the breast, p. 665). This is where the mother slightly compresses the breast in the same direction as the baby's mouth thus narrowing the width of the breast to enable the baby to attach easier. It may be appropriate to refer the baby for separation of the frenulum.
- Avoid the use of soap and similar products, which remove the natural oils.
- Teach the mother how to break the suction by inserting a finger gently in to the baby's mouth before removing the baby from the breast.
- Alter the position of the baby at different feeds.
- If the nipple is cracked, correct positioning usually enables the mother to feed without severe pain. In severe cases, short-term topical treatment may assist healing and be soothing for the mother. Moist wound healing promotes granulation and the use of an oil-based preparation may be advocated, e.g. highly purified lanolin.

Inverted nipples

Nipples usually protrude but appropriately 10% of pregnant women who wish to breastfeed have inverted or non-protractile nipples. Currently there is no evidence that any antenatal nipple treatment or preparation contributes to successful breastfeeding. No prediction of success of breastfeeding should be made on antenatal inspection.

Action
- The mother should be reassured that the baby breast feeds not nipple feeds.
- Skilled help with attachment is important for these women in the first few days postpartum.
- If difficulty is encountered attaching the baby, expressing a small amount of milk to soften the area around the areola can sometimes be helpful.
- Lactation can be initiated and sustained with a breast pump and further attempts made at attaching made when the milk has 'come in' and the breasts are softer.
- Dummies and nipple shields should be avoided as they require a different action and may confuse the baby.
- Mothers with inverted nipples can be as successful breastfeeding as mothers with protractile nipples.

Engorgement

There are two types of engorgement:
- Milk arrival engorgement
- Secondary engorgement.

Milk arrival engorgement

This occurs usually around the 2–4th days postnatal as the milk 'comes in.' It can result from poor attachment, restricting feeds in the early days, or not waking the baby enough. It is caused by increased blood supply to the breasts and extra lymph fluid. The mother will have red, painful, and swollen breasts. She may also have a mild pyrexia and flu-like symptoms. If action is not taken it may result in mastitis.

Secondary engorgement

The mother presents with the same symptoms of painful, swollen breasts but this can occur at any time and is due to the ineffective drainage of the breasts. It may result from a variety of causes including:
- The mother missing a feed
- Reduced appetite in the baby
- Over-stimulation of the supply
- Too rapid weaning
- Baby sleeping through the night.

Action

The actions taken are the same in both types of engorgement:
- Warm flannels can be used to aid the milk flow
- Expressing a small amount of milk will also help to get the milk flowing and make it easier for the baby to attach
- Improve positioning and attachment
- Encourage the baby to feed frequently
- Analgesia may be required (paracetamol is usually the drug of choice). Reassure the mother that it is a temporary situation.

Blocked duct/s

The woman will generally feel well but she will present with a localized tender lump or a feeling of bruising. It usually occurs in one breast and can occur at any time during the breastfeeding period. The woman's temperature is not usually raised.

Actions
- Ensure effective positioning and attachment.
- Feed from the affected side first for the next two feeds, then alternate.
- Ensure the baby feeds frequently.
- Use warm flannels, the shower or bath to bathe in warm water.
- Massage the lump gently towards the nipple during a feed, after a feed or while in the bath.
- Remove any white spot from the nipple.
- Use alternate positions.
- Feed the baby with its chin on the same side as the affected duct.
- Avoid bras that dig into the breast.

Mastitis

Mastitis means inflammation of the breast. The term should not be regarded as synonymous with 'breast infection' because although inflammation may be the result of infection, in over 50% of cases of mastitis it is not. Mastitis can be the result of milk leaking into the breast tissue because of a blocked duct or engorgement. The body's defence mechanism reacts in the same way as it would for infection by increasing the blood supply, which in turn is responsible for the redness and inflammation. Therefore antibiotics may not be required if self-help measures are initiated promptly.

Signs
- A red, swollen, usually painful area on the breast, often the outer, upper area.
- A lumpy breast that feels hot to touch.
- The whole breast may ache and become red.
- Flu-like symptoms which arise very quickly and rapidly get worse.

Predisposing factors
There are a number of factors that may make non-infective mastitis more likely; these include:
- Incorrect positioning and attachment, which may lead to inadequate draining of the breast
- Restriction of the breast as a result of tight clothing or by pressing the fingers too firmly into the breast when feeding
- Engorgement
- Blocked duct/s
- Stress and tiredness
- Sudden changes in the baby's feeding pattern.

Prevention of non-infective mastitis
The condition is often a consequence of engorgement and the following simple measures can help to avoid or reduce the risk of mastitis:
- Ensure correct positioning and attachment
- Avoid suddenly going longer between feeds—reduce gradually if possible
- Avoid pressure on the breasts by either clothing or the fingers
- Commence self-help measures as soon as symptoms occur.

Self-help measures

These measures will help to relieve engorgement and blocked ducts as well as mastitis:

- Breastfeeding must be continued if possible, it is the most effective way to reduce the symptoms
- Reassure the mother that her milk will not harm the baby
- Ensure correct positioning and attachment
- Increase the frequency of feeds and if the breasts are uncomfortably full express between feeds
- Ensure adequate drainage of the breasts and express gently following feeds until resolved
- Feed from the affected breast first
- Try using different positions for feeding
- Prior to feeding, apply warmth to the breast and gently express to soften the breast enabling the baby to attach more effectively
- If necessary, express breast milk by hand or pump until breastfeeding can be resumed
- Gently massage the breast towards the nipple to help the milk flow while feeding
- Check positioning of the fingers when feeding and check to see if clothing is restrictive
- Rest
- Plenty of fluids
- An anti-inflammatory agent may help, e.g. ibuprofen. Aspirin should not be taken by breastfeeding mothers. It can result in rashes, platelet abnormalities, bleeding and the potentially fatal Reye's Syndrome is nursing infants. 4–8% of maternal dose can be transferred.

If no improvement has occurred 12–24h after onset of symptoms, or infective mastitis is suspected refer to the doctor.

Infective mastitis

Bacterial infections result from organisms breaching the preventative barrier of the skin and multiplying in spite of the body's defence system. The epithelium of the breast and nipple may be damaged by:

- Incorrect positioning and attachment
- Sensitivity to creams, lotions, and sprays.

Treatment of infective mastitis

- The self-help measures above should be initiated.
- Systemic antibiotics compatible with breastfeeding should be commenced. This may be needed for 10–14 days.
- Beneficial bacteria killed by the antibiotics can be restored by taking live yogurt or *Acidophilus*.

Abrupt discontinuation of feeding increases the chances of a breast abscess, as will unresolved mastitis.

Breast abscess

This is a rare but serious medical condition. The mother will be pyrexial, have severe flu-like symptoms, and the affected area will be very painful and swollen. It presents as a localized breast infection with the presence of pus. The pus is not considered harmful to the baby but if blood is also present, the baby may vomit. It may occur without prior symptoms but often results from unresolved mastitis.

Actions
- Refer immediately to a doctor, who will prescribe antibiotics.
- Aspiration of the abscess or surgical drainage may be required.
- The mother should continue to feed on the unaffected breast.
- It is preferable for the mother to continue breastfeeding on the affected breast but she may prefer to express and discard the milk especially if the baby is vulnerable e.g. on SCBU.
- The mother may need to boost the milk supply on the affected side once the infection has cleared.

Insufficient milk supply

This is one of the most commonly quoted reasons for women discontinuing breastfeeding. The mother may express concern that she has an insufficient milk supply because the baby is not settling after a feed, is waking frequently for feeds, or the baby is not gaining weight.

Action
- Reassure the mother that this can usually be dealt with because actual insufficient milk is extremely rare.
- A breast feed should be observed and the positioning and attachment improved as necessary.
- There should be no time limit on the frequency or duration of feeding.
- The baby should drain one breast before being offered the second.
- Different feeding positions may be suggested, as this will assist drainage of all areas of the breast.
- Women should be encouraged and supported to continue breastfeeding. Supplementary feeds should not be suggested.
- If after the above action has been taken, the baby fails to gain weight refer to a breastfeeding adviser or breastfeeding clinic.

Breast refusal

There are two types of breast refusal: the baby who has never had a successful breastfeed and the baby who has breastfed well but then starts to refuse to go to the breast. Forty per cent of mothers who discontinue breastfeeding within the first week postnatally do so because the baby would not suck or rejected the breast,[2] therefore it is important for midwives to have the knowledge to help mothers overcome this problem.

Causes when breastfeeding not established
Breast refusal in the initial stages of establishing breastfeeding may be caused a number of factors including:
- Pain relief the mother received in labour
- Breast engorgement as the milk 'comes in'
- Baby being forced on to the breast
- Incorrect positioning and attachment
- Powerful let-down
- Let-down inhibited
- Baby prefers bottles.

Action
- Reassure the mother and try to establish a relaxed environment.
- Observe a feed and check positioning and attachment.
- If the breasts are overfull, express a small amount to soften the area around the areola to enable the baby to attach easier.
- Stimulate the let-down reflex by massaging the breast prior to attaching the baby.
- Express some breast milk onto the nipple or drip EBM in the baby's mouth to attempt him or her to suckle.
- Attempt to put the baby to the breast before they are fully awake.
- Try skin-to-skin stimulation and do not offer the breast, let the baby find it.
- Co-bathing—where the mother and baby bathe together, this is thought to re-create the birth experience for the baby and has been shown to help. The baby needs to be kept warm by a helper pouring warm water over the baby as it lies on the mother's chest.
- If supplements of EBM are given to the baby this should be given by either cup or spoon.

Breast refusal once feeding is established
The following are various factors that may cause a baby to refuse the breast but a cause may not be found:
- Baby ill
- Hormonal changes in the mother, e.g. menstruation, ovulation, contraceptive pill, pregnancy
- Mother using different toiletries or mother eating spicy or garlicky food
- If the mother has undertaken prolonged, vigorous exercise, lactic acid may alter the taste of the milk—but this is usually short lived
- If the mother has had mastitis the milk may taste saltier for a short time afterwards.

Action
- Check the baby's health. If he or she appears ill refer to the doctor.
- If thrush is present, 📖 see Candida (thrush) infection for action.
- If the baby is teething, offer a cool toy to chew on.
- Continue to offer the breast.
- Change the setting in which the baby is fed.
- Try feeding when the baby is sleepy.
- Check whether the mother wishes to continue feeding or if she had thought of discontinuing.
- If the baby is ill and refusing the breast offer EBM. The baby may take it better by spoon or cup.

Candida (thrush) infection

This is an occasional cause of sore nipples although the incidence appears to be increasing. It is caused by a microorganism *Candida*, which is a yeast. It commonly occurs after the mother has received antibiotic treatment. It often occurs after a period of trouble-free feeding and is commonly bilateral.

Signs
- Hypersensitive or itchy nipples even when wearing loose clothing.
- Pink and shiny nipples and areola.

- Shooting pains deep in the breast after feeding which may continue for up to an hour.
- Cracked nipples that will not heal.
- Loss of colour in the nipple or areola.
- Pain in both breasts.

The baby may also exhibit signs of a thrush infection, such as:

- Creamy white spots in the mouth which do not rub off
- Baby keeps pulling away from the breast, which may be a result of a sore mouth
- A windy unsettled baby
- Nappy rash.

Action

- Ensure correct positioning and attachment.
- Continue breastfeeding.
- Refer to the GP for treatment. Effective treatment enables the mother to continue pain-free breastfeeding. When left untreated, many mothers find the severity of pain difficult to deal with and will discontinue feeding earlier than they wish.
- Both the mother and baby need to be treated simultaneously to prevent reinfection even if only one shows signs of infection.
- Surface infection on the nipple is treated by application of an antifungal cream (usually miconazole) is prescribed.
- Oral treatment is required for infected milk ducts (usually nystatin or fluconazole is prescribed). Poor absorption of nystatin in the gut can delay resolution of symptoms. Fluconazole is not licensed for lactating mothers although the WHO recognizes it as compatible with breastfeeding.[3]
- Babies are usually prescribed nystatin drops, or miconazole oral gel. However, due to change in the manufacture's licence, use of miconazole oral gel is no longer considered suitable for use in babies <4 months old due to being a potential choking risk. Responsibility for use in a baby <4 months remains the responsibility of the person who prescribes or recommends its use.
- Any teats, dummies, or nipple shields used should be sterilized.
- Strict hygiene should be observed—washing of hands and use of separate towels for each member of the family.
- Any EBM collected during the infected period is best discarded to prevent reinfection.
- Acidophilus capsules may help restore the normal, healthy bacterial flora which helps prevent thrush infections.
- Painkillers may help the mother to cope with the pain.

1 UNICEF UK Baby Friendly Initiative (2008). *Breastfeeding Assessment Form*. Available at: ℘ www.babyfriendly.org.uk/page.asp?page=60 (accessed 12.4.10).

2 Bolling K, Grant C, Hamlyn B, Thornton A (2007). *Infant Feeding Survey 2005*. London: The Information Centre.

3 World Health Organization (2002). *Breastfeeding and Maternal Medication*. Geneva: WHO. Available at: ℘ http://whqlibdoc.who.int/hq/2002/55732.pdf (accessed 12.4.10).

Breastfeeding in special situations

Twins and higher multiples

The production of breast milk is based on a demand and supply system; therefore, provided the infants are suckling effectively, nature will supply the milk. In the early days postnatally, the mother will require a lot of reassurance and assistance to get breastfeeding established.

There are no rights and wrongs for whether the babies should be fed separately or together. The RCM[1] advocates that in the early days the babies should be fed separately, so that common early problems can be resolved, whereas the Twins and Multiple Births Association[2] believes that feeding the babies together in the early days will help to stimulate the milk supply, and feeding them together at night will ensure that the mother gets more sleep. Ultimately, the decision is up to the mother and the babies, as the infants' feeding patterns may not synchronize. One option is to mix and match so that at some feeds the babies are fed together and at others separately. The mother may decide that each baby has its own breast, or she may wish to swap breasts at each feed.

Positions for breastfeeding twins

When breastfeeding both babies at the same time, positioning of the babies at the breast may take some time and practice to get it right. The mother should:

- Ensure she has adequate cushions to provide support for both herself and the babies
- Use a footstool under her feet if necessary, to create a lap
- Find a position in which she feels comfortable to feed the babies. This may be the 'double football position', where the babies are tucked under the mother's arms and their heads are opposite each other at the front. This enables the mother to support each baby's head. Alternatively, one baby could be held conventionally in the cradle hold and the other held in the football position, so that the babies are parallel to each other. Another position is the criss-cross, where both babies could be held conventionally, one lying across the other.

A mother who is breastfeeding twins must remember her own needs, she should eat well, and try to obtain some rest each day to prevent exhaustion.

Cleft lip and palate

Cleft lip and palate are congenital malformations that result in the incomplete fusion of the upper lip and jaw.

Cleft lip should not present any problems for breastfeeding. Following surgery, some surgeons encourage breastfeeding soon afterwards, while others prefer an initial period of spoon-feeding.

A cleft palate, however, may present major difficulties. The baby is unable to form an effective seal between mouth and the breast, so that the breast and nipple cannot be formed into a teat. There are feeding plates/ palate seals (palatal obturator), which can assist in 'closing' the defect. A baby with a cleft palate will not usually stimulate the breast effectively, which will result in a diminished milk supply. A mother with large, elastic breasts and a ready milk ejection reflex may succeed in breastfeeding, but normally mothers will need to supplement with a nursing supplementer (📖 see Alternative methods of giving EBM/formula, p. 701). Alternatively, mothers may wish to express breast milk and feed it to the baby with a special bottle, teat, or spoon. Breastfeeding is both possible and beneficial following surgical repair, but the mother will need practical and accurate support from appropriately skilled professionals.

Breastfeeding and HIV

Mother-to-child transmission of HIV can occur through breastfeeding. WHO[3] advises that HIV-infected, pregnant mothers should consider their infant feeding options. It stipulates that 'when replacement feeding (formula milk) is acceptable, feasible, affordable, sustainable, and safe, HIV infected mothers should avoid breastfeeding completely'. This view is endorsed by the DH,[4] which recommends that HIV-infected women should avoid breastfeeding. Advice and counselling should be given to mothers during the antenatal period. If a mother decides to breastfeed once she has received advice, there may be a child protection issue, especially if she has a high viral load, which will place the baby at severe risk.

Breastfeeding and diabetes

Diabetes is not a contraindication to breastfeeding. It can be advantageous to the mother's and baby's health.
- For the mother it can: facilitate better management of diabetes and improve the mother's long-term health; this is because breastfeeding is a natural response to childbirth and the hormones responsible for lactation allow the physiological changes that follow childbirth to occur more gradually.
- For the baby it may: reduce the risk of developing diabetes.[5]

Considerations for diabetic mothers when breastfeeding
- Mothers may require extra carbohydrate to facilitate breastfeeding. An extra 50g of carbohydrate per day has been suggested.[6] These extra carbohydrates are best spread equally over the day, remembering especially to increase the supper snack to cover the night-time feeds.
- Warnings should be given to all diabetic mothers about the possibility of hypoglycaemia especially when breastfeeding. They should be advised to eat before breastfeeding the baby or have a snack handy while feeding.
- Mothers who are breastfeeding are at an increased risk of mastitis and candida (thrush), especially if their blood sugar levels are poorly controlled. Therefore they should be informed of the symptoms of mastitis and thrush, how they can help themselves and where help is available e.g. midwife, health visitor, breastfeeding peer supporter, National Childbirth Trust, etc.
- Diabetic mothers may find a delay in their milk production (lactogenesis II) and the milk may not 'come in' until the fourth or fifth postnatal day. Expressing (if mother and baby are separated) or breastfeeding every 2–3h during the first few days following delivery can help reduce the delay.

Care of the new born infant of a diabetic mother

- Babies of diabetic mothers are more prone to hypoglycaemia this is because in intrauterine life the hypertrophic islets of Langerhans produce more insulin in response to the maternal blood sugar levels. After birth the pancreas initially continues to produce excess insulin thus causing hypoglycaemia.
- Preparation for prevention of neonatal hypoglycaemia can commence in pregnancy with the expressing and storage of colostrum for use in the immediate postnatal period. Expression and storage of colostrum should be discussed with the hospital during the antenatal period.
- The baby should be given its first feed as soon as possible (within 30min of birth) and then 2–3h until pre-feeding blood glucose levels are maintained at 2 mmol/L or more.[7]
- The baby's blood glucose levels should be monitored until stabilized. The frequency and timing of testing neonatal blood glucose levels may vary according to hospital policies but NICE[7] recommends routine testing 2–4h after birth and prior to feeds until the blood sugar levels are stabilized.
- The mother and baby should not be transferred to community care until the baby's blood sugar levels have stabilized and feeding is established.
- The mother should be given the opportunity for peer support with breastfeeding.[8]

Separation

There are many reasons why a baby may be separated from its mother. The usual cause of separation of mother and baby immediately following delivery is that the baby requires specialist care in a special care baby unit, neonatal surgical unit, or paediatric ward. Alternatively, the mother may be seriously ill, requiring care in either an intensive care or high-dependency unit. Whenever possible, mothers and babies should be cared for together.

If the mother intends to breastfeed, expression of breast milk should commence as soon as her condition allows (if the mother is ill) or as soon as possible following delivery (if the baby is on a special care baby unit). The mother should be encouraged to express breast milk and will need extra reassurance and support in these circumstances, especially if the baby is in a unit where there are no midwives to assist and support her. For detailed guidance on expression and storage of breast milk 📖 see Expression of breast milk, p. 680.

Breast surgery

- Advice should be sought from the surgeon prior to surgery if the woman is of an age where she may wish to breastfeed.
- There are two types of breast reduction, pedicle and free-nipple. With the former, the mother may be able to breastfeed but with the latter, it is not possible.
- Augmentation is not a contraindication to breastfeeding but if a peri-areolar surgical technique has been used then the mother may find she has an insufficient milk supply.
- Women can breastfeed successfully following unilateral mastectomy.

Alternative methods of giving EBM/formula

Breastfeeding is the natural way to feed infants, but occasionally some infants may not be able to breastfeed immediately or the mother may require assistance to help improve her milk supply. The method of choice will depend upon the individual situations, and the aim of any alternative method of feeding should be to attain full breastfeeding as soon as possible. The alternative methods of feeding include cup, syringe, dropper, spoon, pipette, Lact-Aid®, and nasogastric feeding. The means used will depend upon the age of the baby and the reason for not breastfeeding. The main methods discussed in this text are nasogastric feeding, cup feeding, and supplementing with a Lact-Aid® device.

Nasogastric feeding
- Sometimes, if a baby is so premature, ill, or weak that oral feeding is not possible, the option is to tube feed the baby.
- A baby requiring nasogastric feeds would usually be cared for in a special care baby unit.
- Staff require training in the technique.
- Encourage the mother to express breast milk so that the baby can receive it via the nasogastric tube.
- A baby that has been fed via a nasogastric tube may present with sensory defensiveness and aversive behaviour once oral feeding commences, thought to be a result of a sore throat or irritated nasal passages.[5]

Cup feeding
- Cup feeding prevents exposure of the baby to artificial teats.
- In some countries, where teats are difficult to obtain and to clean, cup feeding is widely practised.
- Once the skill of cup feeding is mastered, then it is no more stressful than bottle feeding.
- Cup feeding is very useful to promote the early acquisition of oral skills.
- Cup feeding also accelerates the transition from nasogastric feeding to established functional breastfeeding by providing a positive way to learn suck/swallow/breathing coordination.
- Caution needs to be taken with premature or compromised babies if their cough reflex is immature. This could lead to an increased risk of aspiration.
- There is also a higher level of spillage when cup feeding, and this needs to be taken into account if trying to calculate the amount taken.
- It is important that mothers be taught the correct technique.

Technique for cup feeding
- Stabilize the baby's head and body.
- Place the baby in an upright position on your lap.
- Have the cup at least half full (if possible).
- Place the rim of the cup at the corners of the baby's mouth. Rest the side of the cup lightly on the lower lip. Do not apply pressure to the lower lip.
- Tilt the cup so that the milk just touches the upper lip.
- The baby can then control the intake, pausing as necessary.

- In effect, the baby laps from the cup, rather than milk being poured into the baby's mouth.
- It is important that the milk is offered but never poured.

The Lact-Aid ®

- This is a feeding tube device that allows the infant to be supplemented at the breast with either EBM or formula.[9]
- The aim of these devices is to deliver a faster flow of milk to the baby while he or she is still suckling at the breast.
- Feeding tube devices are helpful for mothers who have a very poor milk supply, are trying to re-establish lactation, or if attempting to induce lactation for an adopted baby.
- Mothers need supervision when first using these devices.
- They are more effective if the baby is able to latch onto the breast, although an augmented flow may assist a baby to suck better because he or she is being rewarded for their efforts.

Technique

- The tube is usually positioned on the nipple so that it enters the baby's mouth centred along the palate. However, the positioning of the tube may need to be adapted to enable the baby to obtain the flow of milk more effectively.
- The flow of milk from the receptacle is determined by a combination of the baby's suck and its position/height.
- Adjustments will be required to establish the correct flow for the baby.

1 Royal College of Midwives (2002). *Successful Breastfeeding*. Edinburgh: Churchill Livingstone.

2 Twins and Multiple Births Association (2004). *Breastfeeding Twins, Triplets or More*. Guildford: TAMBA.

3 World Health Organization (2004). *HIV Transmission Through Breastfeeding: A Review of Available Evidence*. Geneva: WHO.

4 Department of Health (2004). *HIV and infant feeding: Guidance from the UK Chief Medical Officers' Expert Advisory Group on AIDS*. London: Department of Health Publications.

5 Jackson W (2004). Breastfeeding and Type 1 diabetes mellitus. *British Journal of Midwifery* **12**(3), 158–65.

6 De Swiet M (1995). Medical disorders in pregnancy. In: Chamberlain G (ed.) *Turnbull's Obstetrics*, 2nd edn. Edinburgh: Churchill Livingstone.

7 National Institute for Health and Clinical Excellence (2008). *Diabetes in Pregnancy: Management of Diabetes and its Complications from Pre-conception to the Postnatal Period*. London: NICE.

8 National Institute for Health and Clinical Excellence (2008). Improving the nutrition of pregnant and breastfeeding mothers and children in low income households. NICE public health programme guidance 11. London: NICE.

9 Wilson-Clay B, Hoover KL (2002). *The Breastfeeding Atlas*, 2nd edn. Austin, Texas: LactNews Press.

Lactation and nutrition

All new mothers need to eat a healthy diet for their own well-being and to help them to replenish stores of certain nutrients that become depleted during pregnancy. They also need a healthy diet to assist them to cope with the demands of a new baby and possibly older siblings. Even if eating a suboptimal diet, either in calories or content, they will still produce high-quality milk which will satisfy their infant's nutrition requirements.

A healthy diet should be based on the five food groups and a breastfeeding mother should include:

- Group 1—Carbohydrates—a portion of bread, rice, potatoes, pasta or other starchy food should be eaten with each meal. Wholegrain should be eaten whenever possible.
- Group 2—Fruit and vegetables should be included in each meal aiming for five portions a day.
- Group 3—Dairy products—two to three portions of milk, cheese and yogurt should be eaten a day and they can be of low-fat varieties if desired.
- Group 4—Protein—meat, fish, nuts, and pulses should be included in two meals per day. Non-meat eaters should ensure they include eggs, nuts, and pulses in their diet on a regular basis.
- Groups 5—High fat and sugar foods and drinks—these should be kept to a minimum and the diet basically based on the other four food groups.

Fluids and breastfeeding

Breastfeeding mothers do not need to drink excessive amounts of fluid but should drink to their thirst. A minimum of eight drinks a day is recommended and can include a range of sources including water, fruit juice, milk, tea, coffee, and soups. Milk is not necessary to produce breast milk. In hot weather more fluid may be required to quench the mother's thirst.

Food to avoid whilst breastfeeding

Generally women who are breastfeeding do not need to avoid certain foods, however, there are several recommendations;

- Oily fish—can be included in the diet but no more than two servings a week.
- Large fish—shark, swordfish, and marlin should be avoided all together as they contain large amounts of mercury.
- Alcohol—passes into the blood stream and levels peak at 30–90min after consumption. The recommendation is that daily consumption should not exceed 1 unit per day.
- Peanuts—mothers are advised to avoid eating peanuts if they, the infant's father or siblings suffer from allergic conditions such as hay-fever, asthma, or eczema.
- Caffeine—in tea, coffee, cola, energy drinks, and chocolate should be limited as it can make some babies restless and may cause breast pain in some women.

Mothers who are overweight or obese should not embark on very low-calorie diets while breastfeeding but should eat a balanced diet and limit high fat and high sugar foods. Once breastfeeding is established some regular physical activity of at least 30min on all or most days of the week will help weight loss and women can still breastfeed successfully and lose about 450g (1lb) in weight each week.

Even with a healthy diet it is difficult to get an adequate intake of vitamin D in the UK. Breastfeeding mothers are therefore advised to take 10micrograms of vitamin D each day to prevent vitamin D deficiency in both them and their baby. Vitamin D is needed for bone health and the immune system. Babies of mothers who did not take vitamin D supplements during pregnancy may be born with low levels of vitamin D. There is a very small chance that these babies may have fits due to low levels of calcium. Older babies and toddlers with very low levels of vitamin D can develop rickets.

The NHS Healthy Start vitamins for women contain 10micrograms vitamin D along with 400micrograms folic acid and some vitamin C and are ideal for breastfeeding mothers. The vitamins are free for mothers included within the Healthy Start Scheme (see ℘ www.healthystart.nhs. uk). Vegan mothers may need a supplement containing vitamin B_{12} and calcium in addition to vitamin D.

Chapter 25

Artificial feeding

Introduction

Although breastfeeding is best for mother and infant there will always be some mothers who choose to artificially feed their infants. This is usually for social, psychological, or cultural reasons, but there will be some cases where breastfeeding is contraindicated for medical reasons (📖 see Contraindications to breastfeeding, p. 661). There will also be mothers who commence breastfeeding but, for a variety of reasons, discontinue earlier than they intended.

All pregnant women should be told of the benefits of breastfeeding but ultimately it is the mother's choice which feeding method she adopts. If the mother decides to bottle feed, give her guidance to ensure that she does so safely, but do not give her the impression that formula milk is equivalent to breastfeeding, or that it is without risk.[1]

1 Royal College of Midwives (2002). *Successful Breastfeeding*. Edinburgh: Churchill Livingstone.

Suppression of lactation

If a mother does not wish to breastfeed her infant, has a late miscarriage or a stillbirth, lactation will still occur and she may experience discomfort for several days.

Aetiology
- The classical theory is that milk secretion is controlled principally by the maternal hormones prolactin and oxytocin.
- However, removal of milk from the breasts has also been found to be a crucial element in milk secretion.
- If milk is not removed from the breast, a chemical (autocrine inhibitor) in the whey protein fraction prevents further production by exerting a negative feedback control. This is known as the feedback inhibitor of lactation.
- A build-up of this autocrine inhibitor then accelerates the breakdown of milk components already produced.

Management
- If unstimulated, the breasts will naturally stop producing milk.
- The breasts should be well supported, but binding has not been shown to contribute towards suppression of lactation.
- If there is severe discomfort with engorgement, encourage the mother to express very small amounts of milk once or twice. This can help relieve the discomfort without interfering with the regression of lactation.
- Give mild analgesics to assist in relieving the pain and discomfort felt.
- Do not restrict fluids.
- Pharmacological suppression using dopamine receptor agonists is effective, but is not advised for routine use.[1]

International code of marketing of breast milk substitutes

In May 1981, the World Health Assembly approved an International Code of Marketing of Breast Milk Substitutes.[2] The purpose of this code was to protect the practice of breastfeeding and to help control the marketing of products for the artificial feeding of infants. Nowhere does it seek to enforce breastfeeding, and the code does not prevent mothers from bottle feeding if that is what they choose to do. At present the code is voluntary in the UK, but some countries have chosen to enshrine it in law. Employees in Baby Friendly Hospitals and community healthcare facilities are required to ensure that their practice is in line with the International Code and not just with the UK law.[3] The code has major implications for the work of the midwife. The major recommendations are included in Box 25.1.

Box 25.1 Recommendations of the international code of marketing of breast milk substitutes

- No advertising or promotion of these products in hospital, shops, or to the general public.
- No free samples of breast milk substitutes to be given to mothers or members of their families.
- No free gifts relating to the products within the scope of the code to be given to the mothers.
- No promotion of products in healthcare facilities.
- No gifts or personal samples to be given to health workers, nor any free or subsidized supplies to hospitals or maternity wards.
- No words or pictures idealizing bottle feeding, including pictures of infants on product labels.
- All information on infant feeding, including product labels, should explain the benefits of breastfeeding and the costs and hazards associated with bottle feeding.
- Information provided by manufacturers to health care workers should include only scientific and factual material, and should not create or imply that bottle feeding is equivalent or superior to breastfeeding.
- Unsuitable products (i.e. sweetened condensed milk) should not be promoted for babies.
- All products should be of a high quality and should take into account the climate and storage conditions of the country where they are to be used.
- Healthcare workers should encourage and protect the practice of breastfeeding.

1 Inch S (2009). Infant Feeding. In: Fraser DM, Cooper MA (eds). *Myles: Textbook for Midwives.* Chapter 41. Edinburgh: Churchill Livingstone.

2 World Health Organization (1981). *International Code of Marketing Breast Milk Substitutes.* Geneva: WHO

3 UNICEF UK Baby Friendly Initiative (2008). *Three-day Course in Breastfeeding Management: Participant's Handbook.* London: UNICEF.

Selecting an appropriate substitute

All artificial milks are highly processed, factory-produced products. Under UK law it is an offence to sell any infant formula as being suitable from birth unless it conforms to the compositional and other criteria set out in the Infant Formula and Follow-on Formula Regulations 1995.

- Health professionals must not recommend one brand of formula over another.
- There is no scientific basis for recommending one brand over another.
- There is no reason for a mother to remain with one brand.
- All common baby milks suitable for home use are supplied in dried powder form so they can be stored and transported without risk of deterioration.
- Many manufacturers also supply individual feed sachets and ready-to-feed cartons. These are handy to use but tend to be more expensive.
- The DH recommends that soya formula should only be used for babies who are intolerant of cow's milk or lactose, and only with medical guidance.
- For babies and infants who are intolerant of standard formulas, alternative formulas, such as hydrolysate and amino-acid-based formulas, are medically prescribed.

Types of formula milks

Whey and casein are proteins found in milk. Formulas are modified to vary the ratio of these proteins. There are two main types, whey-dominant and casein-dominant formulas.

Whey-dominant formulas

- Whey is the dominant protein in human milk.
- Whey-based formulas have been modified so that the whey:casein ratio (60:40) is closer to that of human milk.
- These formulas are more easily digested, which affects gastric emptying times and leads to feeding patterns similar to those of breastfed babies.
- These formulas are suitable for use from birth to 1 year.

Casein-dominant formulas

- Casein is the dominant protein in cow's milk.
- Casein-dominant formulas have been modified so that the whey:casein ratio is 20:80 and is nearer to the type found in cow's milk.
- These formulas are not comparable to breast milk.
- Such feeds form large, relatively indigestible curds in the stomach, which are intended to make the infant feel full for longer. However, there is little evidence to support this.[1]
- They are advertised for the hungrier bottle-fed baby and can be used from birth to 1 year.
- There may be an even greater metabolic demand on the infant when these formulas are given.[2]
- Babies who are settled and gaining weight on whey-dominant formulas will not need casein-dominant formulas.

Additional ingredients

Whey- and casein-dominant formulas may also have additional ingredients, for example long-chain fatty acids (LCPs), nucleotides, β-carotene, and selenium. The ingredients and their sources vary from one brand to another.

LCPs

- Occur naturally in breast milk.
- Aid brain, eye, and, CNS development.
- Are added to formulas in the form of fish oils or egg yolk.
  Research into both the long- and short-term effects of adding LCPs to formulas is continuing.

β-carotene

- Occurs naturally in breast milk.
- Can be metabolized by the baby to produce vitamin A.

Nucleotides

- Nucleotides are present in breast milk.
- Assist with development of the baby's immune system.
- Aid adsorption of other nutrients from breast milk.

Selenium

- An antioxidant found in breast milk.

Specially modified formula
Several formula manufactures have recently introduced specially modified formulas which they claim aids digestion and helps reduce some of the common problems associated with formula feeding, e.g. constipation, colic. These products are available over the counter but their efficacy needs further research.

Follow-on milks
These milks are made from slightly modified cow's milk and they have added vitamin D and iron.
• They are *not* to be given to infants <6 months old.[3,4]
• The large amounts of iron may make some babies constipated.
• Full-fat cow's milk has low levels of iron and vitamin D and should *not* be used as a main drink for an infant under 1 year of age. However, it can be used for preparing baby weaning foods from 4–6 months of age.
• If an infant tolerates a well-balanced and varied diet, full-fat cow's milk can be used from the age of 1 year.

Good night milks
• 'Good night milks' have added starch and rice flakes, and are represented as helping to settle babies at bedtime and are promoted for use as a bedtime liquid feed from a bottle or feeding cup.
• The Scientific Advisory Committee on Nutrition[5] has identified no scientific evidence that demonstrates 'good night' milk products offer any advantage over the use of currently available infant formulas.
• Concern expressed that their promotion will encourage parents to believe that it is desirable for a baby to sleep longer at an age when healthy infants show considerable variation in normal sleeping patterns.
• There is a potential risk that mothers may consider the product suitable for 'settling' their infant more than once a day and use these products on occasions additional to bedtime.
• An even greater concern is that they may be used to 'settle' infants <6 months. Such unintended use would be contrary to advice that gluten-containing products should not be given to infants <6 months of age.[5]

Thickened formulas
• Pre-thickened formulas are advertised for infants with reflux or possetting.
• They are casein-based infant formulas with added pre-gelatinized starch. They thicken when in contact with the acid in the stomach and this increases the feed thickness while still flowing easily through the teat.
• Infants taking these formulas should not be prescribed thickeners or anti reflux medication such as Gaviscon®.
• Can be purchased over the counter or they may be prescribed.
• Most infants do not need this sort of preparation once solids have been established as part of their diet. However, they are suitable for use up to the age of 1 year.
• Extra care is needed when making up some of these feeds as they require cooled boiled water. Water at 70° will cause the feed to thicken in the bottle.

1 White A, Freeth S, O'Brien M (1992). *Infant Feeding 2000*. London: HMSO.

2 Inch S (2009). Feeding. In: Fraser DM, Cooper MA (eds) *Myles Textbook for Midwives*. Chapter 41. Edinburgh: Churchill Livingstone, 1990.

3 Department of Health (1994). *Weaning and the Weaning Diet*. Report on Health and Social Subjects No. 45. London: HMSO.

4 Statutory Instruments No. 77 (1995). *Food. The Infant Formula and Follow on Formula Regulations*. London: HMSO.

5 Scientific Advisory Committee on Nutrition (2008). *Consideration of the Place of Good Night Milks Products in the Diet of Infants Aged 6 Months and Above*. London: SACN. Available at: ℘ www.sacn.gov.uk/reports_position_statements/position_statements/index.html (accessed November 2009).

Alternatives to modified cow's milk formulas

Specialized formula milks are available for parents who wish their baby to have vegetarian feeds. These should only be given under the direction of a dietitian.

Soya formula

- It is recommended by the DH that these milks should only be used if a baby/infant is intolerant to cow's milk or lactose; and, generally, only under medical guidance.
- There are concerns about the possible effects of oestrogen-like compounds produced by soyabeans (phyto-oestrogens), and unacceptable levels of manganese and aluminium, in such formulas.[1]
- They may contain genetically modified ingredients.

Specialist formulas for babies intolerant to standard formulas

Predicting allergies is an inexact science. The likelihood has been estimated[2] to be:

- 30–35% if one parent is affected
- 40–60% if both parents are affected
- 50–70% if both parents suffer the same allergy.

Lactose-free formulas

- Appropriate for infants who are intolerant to lactose but can tolerate the milk protein.
- Cow's milk protein based with lactose replaced by glucose.
- Prescribable or may be purchased in pharmacies.
- Glucose in these formulas may be dangerous to teeth.

Hydrolysate formulas

- Used if breastfeeding is not possible.
- Prescription only.
- Some are designed to treat an existing allergy; some are designed to prevent an allergy.
- Prescribing guidelines: some hydrolysate formulas need proven intolerance, whereas others do not.

Amino-acid-based formulas

- Have a completely synthetic protein base.
- Are very expensive.

1 Minchin M (1998). *Breastfeeding Matters*, 4th edn. Australia: Alma Publications.

2 Brostoff J, Gamlin L (1998). *The Complete Guide to Allergy and Food Intolerance*. London: Bloomsbury Publishing.

Nutritional requirements of formula-fed babies

Three areas need to be taken into consideration:
- Energy requirements
- Fluid requirements
- Balance of ingredients.

Energy requirements
- The average healthy baby will thrive on 440kJ/kg of bodyweight per day.
- Breast milk and formula milk contain approximately 90kJ/30mL.
- A 3.5kg baby would therefore require 1540kJ in 24h = approximately 525mL of milk.

This is only a guide, and individual babies will take as much as they require at each feed to satisfy their needs. This amount may vary from feed to feed and the overall picture should be considered, e.g. the general health and weight gain of the baby.

Fluid requirements
- An average healthy baby requires 150–165mL of fluid per kg of bodyweight per day to remain hydrated.
- A 3.5kg baby would therefore require approximately 525–575mL per day.

Balance of ingredients
Formula feeds are developed from cow's milk, which is balanced to meet the needs of calves and therefore requires modification for human infants. 'Modified milks' are those that have had the balance of ingredients adjusted to resemble human milk as closely as possible.

Modifications include:
- Most of the casein is removed and replaced by whey protein
- Some of the milk fat is removed and replaced by vegetable fat
- Lactose is added to increase the energy value
- Vitamins are added to resemble levels in human milk
- Minerals are adjusted to resemble levels in human milk
- Higher levels of iron are required as it is less bio-absorbable from formulas than from breast milk.

Management of artificial feeding

Sterilization of infant feeding equipment

All infant feeding equipment must be completely clean and sterilized prior to use. This includes any equipment used for breastfed babies or for storing EBM, e.g. bottles, teats, breast pumps, and nipple shields. This is to protect babies against any potential sources of infection. Due to their immature immune system, babies are at risk of infection, particularly gastroenteritis (potentially life-threatening for newborn babies) and fungal infections (which can be difficult to treat).

Demonstrations of sterilization of equipment are best given on a one-to-one basis in the mother's home environment.

Types of sterilization
- Boiling
- Chemical sterilization
- Steam sterilization
- Microwave sterilization using a microwave sterilization unit. This is not suitable for metal items or certain types of plastic.

For all types of sterilization
Before sterilization
- Wash all bottles and other equipment thoroughly in hot, soapy water, using a bottle brush. Scrub both inside and outside to remove fatty deposits. Pay special attention to the rim.
- Clean the teat by either:
  - Using a small teat brush
  - Turning inside out and washing in hot, soapy water.
- Rinse all the washed equipment thoroughly with non-soapy water before sterilizing.

After sterilization
Always wash your hands before removing equipment from the sterilizer.

To sterilize by boiling
- Put the equipment in a large pan filled with water, ensuring that there is no air trapped in the bottles or teats. Cover the pan with a lid and bring to the boil.
- *Boil for 10min*, ensuring that the pan does not boil dry.
- Allow the water to cool and store the equipment in the covered pan until required. Use the equipment within 12h (if longer, repeat the process).
- Remove equipment from the saucepan carefully, to avoid desterilization.
- Check bottles and teats regularly for any signs of deterioration. If this is detected, discard them. Prolonged boiling of teats may destroy them.

To sterilize using chemicals (cold water sterilization)
- Use the liquid or tablets to make up the solution following the manufacturer's instructions.
- Either use a sterilizing tank or a large container with a well-fitting lid.

- Submerge the equipment, ensuring that no air bubbles are trapped in the bottles or teats.
- Keep all the equipment under the water, using the plunger provided or a plate.
- Leave in the solution for a minimum of 30min.
- Discard the solution and make up fresh every 24h.
- Use cooled, boiled water if you wish to rinse the equipment prior to use.

Sterilization using a steam or microwave sterilizer
- Follow the manufacturer's instructions.
- Sterilizing in a microwave without a microwave sterilizer is not advisable.

Preparing a formula feed

The correct preparation of infant formula feeds is important to prevent such conditions as dehydration, constipation, and gastroenteritis. The Food Standards Agency and the DH[1] have produced new guidelines on the safe preparation of infant formulas to reduce the risk of gastroenteritis. Powdered infant formula is not a sterile product and may contain bacterial contaminants. *Enterobacter sakazakii* and *Salmonella* are those of greatest concern. Both NICE and UNICEF UK recommend that all mothers who are artificially feeding their infants should be shown the correct method of preparing a formula feed prior to discharge from hospital.[2,3]

Methods of making up formula feeds
- Scoop method
- Individual feed sachets
- Ready-to-feed cartons.

Scoop method
- A fresh bottle should be made up for each feed. This is because bacteria multiply quickly at room temperature and may survive and multiply slowly in some fridges, therefore storing formula milk can increase the risk of gastroenteritis.
- The feed should be made up with water of around 70°C as this will destroy most bacterial contaminants. This means boiling the kettle and leaving it to cool for no longer than 30min. Do *not* use bottled or artificially softened water.
- Read the tin or pack to find out how much water and formula you require.
- Clean a surface on which to prepare the feed. Wash your hands thoroughly with soap and water, and dry on a clean towel.
- All equipment used for making up the feed must have been freshly sterilized.
- If using a sterilizer, remove the lid, turn upside down and place the teat(s) and cap(s) in it. If using a chemical (cold water) sterilizer rinse with cool, boiled water (not tap water) if wished.
- Remove the bottle rinse with cooled, boiled water (if wished) and stand on a clean, flat surface. Pour cool boiled water which should

still be hot into the bottle, up to the required mark. This is better if undertaken at eye-level.
- Measure the exact amount of formula using the scoop provided. Level the formula in the scoop using the knife or spatula provided.
- Do *not* compress or compact the formula in the scoop.
- Add the formula to the water in the bottle *never* the other way round. In the UK all baby formulas use one scoop to 1oz (30mL) of water.
- Do *not* add anything else to the feed unless medically prescribed.
- Apply the top or teat and cover. Shake the bottle well until all the formula is dissolved.
- Cool the feed down to required temperature by holding the bottle with the cap in place, under cold running water.
- Check the temperature of the formula prior to feeding the baby, by dripping a little on to the inside of your wrist; it should be lukewarm but not hot.
- Discard any formula that has not been used within 2h, clean and re-sterilize the bottle.

When it is not practical to make up feeds just before feeding
It is best to make up feeds individually as required but this may not always be practical. Ready to use formula is the safest option but this is more expensive.

Feeding the baby away from home
It is safest to carry a measured amount of formula powder in a small, clean, dry container, a flask of hot water that has been boiled and an empty sterilized feeding bottle. The feed is then made up fresh as required. The water should still be hot when used and therefore the bottle will need to be cooled before giving to the baby.

Making-up and transporting feeds for later use
If the above advice is difficult to follow, e.g. if preparing and transporting feeds either to a nursery or child minder the following steps should be adopted.
- Prepare feeds individually, not in one large container.
- Make the feeds up the day they are required not the night before. This reduces storage time therefore reduces the risk.
- Once prepared store at the back of a fridge at below 5°C.
- Ensure the feed has been in the fridge for at least 1h before transporting.
- Store for the minimum of time.
- Remove from the fridge just before leaving home and transport in a cool bag with ice packs.
- Use within 4h. If arriving at the destination in <4h, remove from the cool bag and store in the back of a fridge below 5°C.
- Never store reconstituted feeds for more than 24h.
- Re-warm before use.

Re-warming stored feeds
- Only remove the feed from the fridge just before it is needed.
- Re-warm using a bottle-warmer, or placing in a container of warm water.

- *Never* use a microwave to re-warm a feed.
- *Never* warm for more than 15min.
- Shake the bottle to ensure even heating of the feed.
- Check the temperature before feeding the baby.

Principles of artificial feeding

- Feed the baby when he or she is hungry.
- Let him or her take as little or as much as desired.
- Ideally, the minimum of caregivers should feed the baby and he or she should not be passed from person to person for feeding.
- *Never* feed babies by 'bottle propping' and *never* leave them unattended when feeding from a bottle.
- Make up feeds individually as required.
- Test the temperature of the feed on the inside of your wrist before offering it to the baby.
- Feeding times should be enjoyable and relaxed.
- Hold the baby securely, and close to your body, in a similar position to that used in breastfeeding.
- Maintain eye contact.
- Ensure that the teat covers the baby's tongue, and tip the bottle up sufficiently so that air is excluded from the teat.
- The baby will suck and pause while retaining the teat in their mouth.
- During the feed, when necessary, sit the baby in an upright position so he or she can bring up wind; this may be once or twice.
- It is normal for babies to regurgitate small amounts (posseting).
- If the baby is sucking but the feed does not appear to be reducing, check the teat for blockages.
- The baby will stop feeding when he or she has had enough.
- If the baby is draining the full amount offered, the amount should be increased.
- Any feed left at the end of the feed should be discarded and should *never* be reheated.

1 Food Standards Agency/Department of Health (2007). *Guidance for Health Professionals on Safe Preparation, Storage and Handling of Powered Infant Formula.* London; FSA.

2 National Institute for Health and Clinical Excellence (2008). *Improving the Nutrition of Pregnant and Breastfeeding Mothers in Low-income Households.* London: NICE.

3 UNICEF (1998). *Implementing the Ten Steps to Successful Breastfeeding.* London: UNICEF.

Problems associated with formula feeding

Constipation

It is the consistency, not the frequency, of bowel movements that should be considered when discussing constipation. Babies may go several days without a bowel movement, but if the stools are soft and yellow, then no treatment is required. Constipation results from reabsorption of water from the stools and stools present as hard, round pellets.

Management

- Check that the condition is constipation and not just infrequent stools.
- Ensure that the feeds are being prepared correctly, i.e. the water is being placed in the bottle prior to the formula, the powder in the scoop is not being compressed, and extra scoopfuls are not being added.
- Offer the baby cooled, boiled water between feeds. There should be *no* additives to the water, e.g. brown sugar or orange juice.
- Try an alternative make of formula; not all formulas suit all babies.
- If the above strategies do not work, seek a medical opinion.

Posseting

It is normal for a baby to regurgitate a small amount of milk following a feed. Reassure the mother that it is normal and take no action unless it becomes persistent or projectile vomiting, in which case medical aid should be sought immediately.

Disadvantages associated with formula feeding

The following disadvantages for the formula-fed infant have been identified.[1]
Formula milk is deficient in:
- Some nutrient compounds (e.g. epidermal growth factors)
- Cells (e.g. leucocytes, macrophages) which are important in protecting the infant from a wide variety of pathogens
- Antibodies, antibacterial, and antiviral factors (e.g. IgA, IgG, IgM, lactoferrin)
- Hormones (e.g. prolactin, thyroid hormones)
- Enzymes (e.g. mammary amylase, milk lipase, lysozyme)
- Prostaglandins.

These deficiencies are important to the infant's immunological and hormonal responses, as well as neonatal development and cell maturation.

The formula-fed infant may be further compromised by:
- The presence of cow's milk or soya proteins
- Possibility of errors during manufacture, including incorrect manufacture, bacterial contamination, foreign bodies, etc.[2]
- Addition of new ingredients on an uncertain scientific basis
- Frequent errors in the preparation of feeds, which alter their concentration[3]
- Variability of the mineral and trace element content in the water used to reconstitute feeds.

Formulas may be contaminated with bacteria and/or pathogens:
- During manufacture
- While preparing feeds at home with unclean utensils and/or contaminated water.

Examples of specific types of formulas

This is not a comprehensive list of all Infant formulas. There may be other specific types of formulas that have not been included as brand names change frequently due to constant research and re-branding by formula companies.

Examples of whey- and casein-dominant formulas (Table 25.1)

Table 25.1 Examples of whey- and casein-dominant formulas

Whey-dominant formula	Casein-dominant formula
(60% whey, 40% casein)	(80% casein, 20% whey)
Aptamil First®	Aptamil Extra Hungry®
Cow and Gate First Milk®	Cow and Gate for Hungrier Babies®
Heinz Nurture Newborn®	Heinz Nurture Hungry baby®
SMA First Infant Milk: Stage 1®	SMA Extra Hungry®
HIPP Organic First Infant Milk®	HIPP Organic Second Infant Milk®

Examples of soya infant formulas
- Heinz Nurture Soya®
- Infasoy (Cow & Gate)®
- Isomil (Abbott)®
- Prosobee (Mead Johnson)®
- Wysoy (SMA)®

Examples of specially modified formulas
- Aptamil Easy Digest®
- Cow and Gate Comfort First®
- Heinz Nurture Gentle®

Examples of follow-on milks
- Aptimil Follow-on®
- Cow & Gate Complete Care Follow-on®
- Cow & Gate Comfort Follow-on®
- Heinz Nurture Growing Baby Follow On®
- Heinz Nurture Gentle Follow-on®
- HIPP Organic Follow-on Milk®
- SMA Follow-on Milk: Stage 2®

Examples of pre-thickened formulas
- Enfamil AR (Mead Johnson)®
- SMA Stay Down®

Examples of 'good night milks'
- Cow & Gate Good Night Milk®
- HIPP Organic Good Night Milk®

1 Henschel D, Inch S (1996). *Breastfeeding: A Guide For Midwives*. Cheshire: Books for Midwives Press, p. 20.

2 Minchin M (1998). *Breastfeeding Matters*, 4th edn. Australia: Alma Publications.

3 Lucas A, Lockton S, Davies PS (1992). Randomized trial of ready-to-feed compared with powered formula. *Archives of Diseases in Childhood* **67**, 935–9.

Health risks associated with formula feeding

The RCM[1] stated that, taking breastfeeding as the 'gold standard', bottle-feeding has been shown to be associated with certain health risks.

For the infant:
- Increased risk of gastrointestinal infections
- Increased risk of respiratory infections
- Increased incidence of otitis media
- Increased risk of urinary infections
- Increased risk of atopic disease in families where there is a history of this disease
- Increased risk of sudden infant death
- Increased risk of insulin-dependent diabetes mellitus
- Reduced cognitive development
- Decreased visual acuity
- Reduced intelligence quotient (IQ) in preterm infants
- Increased risk of NEC.
  Some risks that manifest in later life have been demonstrated, including:
- Cardiovascular disease
- Obesity
- Some childhood cancers.

For the mother:
- Increased risk of ovarian and premenopausal breast cancer. The exact mechanisms whereby breastfeeding affords protection against these cancers are not fully understood. However, in the case of breast cancer it is thought to be linked with increased circulating hormones, which result in systemic metabolic effects as well as structural changes in the breast; whereas in the case of ovarian cancer it is believed that breastfeeding may afford a protective effect as a result of inhibition of ovulation.[2]
- Increased risk of hip fractures and reduced bone density. Prolactin, which is released during breastfeeding, increases the rate at which vitamin D is converted to its active form, and this enhances calcium utilization.[3]

  For full reference sources and details of further associated risks see Appendix 5 in RCM (2002)[1] and the UNICEF UK Baby Friendly website (🔗 www.babyfriendly.org.uk).

1 Royal College of Midwives (2002). *Successful Breastfeeding*. Edinburgh: Churchill Livingstone.

2 Heinig MJ, Dewey KG (1997). Health effects of breastfeeding for mothers: a critical review. *Nutrition Research Reviews* **10**, 35–56.

3 Palmer G (1988). *The Politics of Breastfeeding*. London: Pandora Press.

Index